CLINICAL CHEMISTRY

(Organ Function Tests, Laboratory Investigations and Inborn Metabolic Diseases)

CLINICAL CHEMISTRY

(Organ Function Tests, Laboratory Investigations and Inborn Metabolic Diseases)

Dr (Brig) MN Chatterjea
BSc MBBS DCP MD (Biochemistry)
Ex-Professor and Head of the Department of Biochemistry
Armed Forces Medical College, Pune

(Specialist in Pathology and Ex-Reader in Pathology)
Ex-Professor and Head, Department of Biochemistry
Christian Medical College, Ludhiana

Ex-Professor and Head of the Department of Biochemistry
MGM's Medical College, Aurangabad, Maharashtra, India

Dr Rajinder Chawla
MSc DMRIT PhD
Professor of Biochemistry, Faculty of Medicine
Addis-Ababa University, Ethiopia

Ex-Professor of Biochemistry
Christian Medical College, Ludhiana, Punjab, India

®

JAYPEE

JAYPEE BROTHERS MEDICAL PUBLISHERS
The Health Sciences Publisher
New Delhi | London

Jaypee Brothers Medical Publishers (P) Ltd

Headquarters
EMCA House, 23/23-B
Ansari Road, Daryaganj
New Delhi 110 002, India
Landline: +91-11-23272143,
+91-11-23272703
+91-11-23282021, +91-11-23245672
e-mail: jaypee@jaypeebrothers.com

Corporate Office
4838/24, Ansari Road, Daryaganj
New Delhi 110 002, India
Phone: +91-11-43574357
Fax: +91-11-43574314
e-mail: jaypee@jaypeebrothers.com

Overseas Office
JP Medical Ltd.
83, Victoria Street, London
SW1H 0HW (UK)
Phone: +44-20 3170 8910
e-mail: info@jpmedpub.com

EU GPSR Authorised Representative
Logos Europe, 9 rue Nicolas Poussin
17000, La Rochelle, France
Phone: +33 (0) 6 67 93 73 78
e-mail: contact@logoseurope.eu

Website: www.jaypeebrothers.com
Website: www.jaypeedigital.com

Inquiries for bulk sales may be solicited at: jaypee@jaypeebrothers.com

CLINICAL CHEMISTRY (Organ Function Tests, Laboratory Investigations and Inborn Metabolic Diseases)

First Edition: **1999**
Second Edition: **2010**

Reprint: **2026**

ISBN 978-81-8448-795-4

Printed in India at Purewall Ventures Pvt Ltd

Preface to the Second Edition

I take this opportunity to present the next revised edition of the book to my beloved students and teachers. The book has been found to be useful to undergraduates and extremely useful specially to postgraduate students of various disciplines viz. Pathology, Biochemistry, Medicine, Pediatrics, etc.

There has been a demand from some professors to include a chapter, rather a part on Inborn Metabolic Diseases (Inborn Errors of Metabolism). On my request, the task was taken by Professor Rajinder Chawla, Professor of Biochemistry (Faculty of Medicine), Addis Ababa University of Ethiopia. He has been kind enough to contribute the chapter on "Inborn Metabolic Diseases". He has taken considerable time and energy for compilation and preparation of the chapter and he has incorporated latest up-to-date information/materials. It is emphasized that there is a paucity of materials/information on Inborn Metabolic Diseases. I hope this chapter (part) will be of great help to the undergraduates as well as postgraduate students of various disciplines. I am extremely grateful to him for this job.

I have also included one more chapter on "Pancreatic Function Tests" in the part of "Organ Function Tests". This chapter has also been contributed by Professor Rajinder Chawla.

Considerable time and energy have been spent in revising the new edition of the book. I hope that the book will be appreciated by students and teachers. I shall look forward for valuable comments and fruitful suggestions from all quarters of medical fraternity, both teachers and students for further improvement of the book.

I am grateful to Shri Jitendar P Vij (Chairman and Managing Director), Mr Tarun Duneja (Director-Publishing), Mr PG Bandhu (Director-Sales), and other staff members for their sincere and untiring efforts to bring out the new edition of the book.

Dr (Brig) MN Chatterjea

Preface to the First Edition

Clinical chemistry is an important branch of biochemistry. It primarily deals with the various methods used for estimation of different biomolecules in blood and body fluids, establishing the normal values in health and study the alterations found in disease states with their interpretations.

The role of laboratory in diagnosis and treatment continues to gain importance as newer tests and analytical methods become available. The exponential growth of technology in the last decade has provided the clinicians with a plethora of tests which not only gives an astonishing insight into the metabolic and pathological changes but allows diagnosis to be made precisely which were not possible before.

Laboratory tests and investigations have become the mainstay for clinical practice. Clinicians found the laboratory tests as confidence building tools. Now many diagnosis can only be established or etiologies confirmed and appropriate therapy selected by laboratory investigations. The emphasis seems to be shifting from the study of patients to the study of laboratory investigative data.

Quite a number of books by foreign authors are available which deal with the various methods of estimation of different biomolecules in blood and body fluids and their interpretations in health and diseases. These books are voluminous, bulky and difficult to handle.

As a student and teacher of pathology and biochemistry, I felt the need for a handy, concise and comprehensive book which deals with the various organ function tests and laboratory investigations of various biochemical/pathological parameters *viz.* Laboratory investigation of hypoglycaemia, hypercalcaemia, polyuria, haemolytic anaemia, etc. under one roof. There is a paucity of such a book by Indian authors.

The book in the present form is divided mainly into two parts. First part deals with the various organ function tests which have been written to give a lucid and brief account with classification, basic principles of the tests and discussing their application to the clinical context. The second part of the book deals with the laboratory investigations of various biochemical and pathological parameters which are frequently encountered by the clinicians. The causes and steps of investigation have been discussed. An attempt has been made to give a flow chart at the end of each chapter of Laboratory investigation. ***The details of methodology have been omitted intentionally so as not to perplex the reader with unnecessary laboratory jargon.***

Considerable time and energy have been spent in preparation of the book. The book in the present form is an attempt to fill the existing vacuum and to quench the thirst of necessity of this type of book. I hope the efforts put in preparation of the book will not go waste and the book will be appreciated and get a welcome from the students and teachers.

Inspite of careful scrutiny, it is likely that a few mistakes might have crept in inadvertently. I welcome constructive criticisms and fruitful suggestions from the readers which would help me to bring further improvement in future.

I am grateful to Mr Jitendar P Vij (Chairman and Managing Director), Mr RK Yadav, Editorial Consultant and the staff members of M/s Jaypee Brothers Medical Publishers (P) Ltd., for their sincere and untiring efforts to bring out the book.

Dr (Brig) MN Chatterjea

Contents

Part 1: Organ Function Tests 1-82

Part 2: Laboratory Investigations 83-262

Part 3: Miscellaneous *263-290*

Part 4: Inborn Metabolic Diseases (Inborn Errors of Metabolism) *291-376*

Part One

Organ Function Tests

Chapter 1

Renal Function Tests

INTRODUCTION

The body has a considerable factor of safety in renal as well as hepatic tissues. One healthy normal kidney can do the work of two, and if all other organs are functioning properly, less than a whole kidney can suffice.

On the other hand, there are ***certain extra-renal factors which can interfere with kidney*** function, specially circulatory disturbances. Hence, methods that appraise the functional capacity of the kidneys are very important. Such tests have been devised and are available, but it is stressed that ***no single test can measure all the kidney functions.*** Consequently, more than one test is indicated to assess the kidney function.

PRELIMINARY INVESTIGATIONS

Assessment of renal function begins with the appreciation of:

- ***Patient's history:*** A proper history taking is important, particularly in respect of oliguria, polyuria, nocturia, ratio of frequency of urination in day time and night time. Appearance of oedema is important.
- ***Physical examination:*** This is followed by side room analysis of the urine specially for presence/or absence of albumin, and microscopic examination of urinary deposits specially for pus cells, RB cells and casts.
- ***Biochemical parameters:*** Certain biochemical parameters also help in assessing kidney function.

A ***stepwise increase in three nitrogenous constituents of blood is believed to reflect a deteriorating kidney function.*** Some authorities claim that serum uric acid normally rises first, followed by urea and finally increase in creatinine. ***By determining all the above three parameters a rough estimate of kidney function can be made.*** However, other causes of uric acid rise should be kept in mind.

Other biochemical parameters which may help are determination of total plasma proteins, and albumin and globulins and total cholesterol. In nephrosis there is marked fall in albumin and rise in serum cholesterol level.

PHYSIOLOGICAL ASPECT

Main functions of the kidney are:

- To get rid the body of waste products of metabolism,
- To get rid of foreign and non-endogenous substances,
- To maintain salt and water balance, and
- To maintain acid-base balance of the body.

A. Glomerular Function

The glomeruli act as *"filters"*, and the fluid which passes from the blood in the glomerular capillaries into Bowman's capsule is of the same composition of protein-free plasma.

The ***effective filtration pressure*** which forces fluid through the filters is the result of:

i. the blood pressure in the glomerular capillaries and

ii. the opposing osmotic pressure of plasma proteins, renal interstitial pressure and intratubular pressure. Thus,

- Capillary pressure = 75 mmHg
- Osmotic pressure of plasma proteins = 30 mmHg
- Renal interstitial pressure = 10 mmHg
- Renal intratubular pressure = 10 mmHg

Hence, net effective filtration pressure
= 75 – (30 + 10 + 10)
= 25 mmHg

Rate of filtration is influenced by:

- Variations in BP in glomerular capillary,
- Concentration of plasma proteins,
- Factors altering intratubular pressure, viz.,
  a. rise with ureteral obstruction;
  b. during osmotic diuresis.
- State of blood vessels.

If the efferent glomerular arteriole is constricted, the pressure in the glomerulus rises and the effective filtration pressure is increased. On the other hand, if the afferent glomerular arteriole is constricted, the filtration pressure is reduced.

The volume of glomerular filtrate formed depends on:

- the number of glomeruli functioning at a time;
- the volume of blood passing through the glomeruli per minute; and
- the effective glomerular filtration pressure.

Under normal circumstances, about 700 ml of plasma (contained in 1300 ml of blood or approximately 25% of entire cardiac output at rest) flow through the kidneys per minute and 120 ml of fluid are filtered into Bowman's capsule. The volume of the filtrate is reduced in extrarenal conditions, such as dehydration, oligaemic shock and cardiac failure which diminish the volume of blood passing through the glomeruli, or lower the glomerular filtration pressure, and when there is constriction of the afferent glomerular arterioles or, changes in the glomeruli such as occur in glomerulonephritis. If the volume of glomerular filtrate is lowered below a certain point, the kidneys are unable to eliminate waste products which accumulate in blood.

B. Tubular Function

Whereas the glomerular cells act only as a passive semipermeable membrane, the tubular epithelial cells are a highly specialised tissue able to reabsorb selectively some substances and secrete others. About 170 litres of water are filtered through the glomeruli in 24 hours, and only 1.5 litres is excreted in the urine. Thus, ***nearly 99% of the glomerular filtrate is reabsorbed in the tubules.***

Glucose is present in the glomerular filtrate in the same concentration as in the blood but practically none is excreted normally in health in detectable amount in urine and the tubules reabsorb about 170 gm/day. At an arterial plasma level of 100 mg/100 ml and a GFR of 120 ml/minute, approximately 120 mg of glucose are delivered in the glomerular filtrate in each minute. ***Maximum rate at which glucose can be reabsorbed is about 350 mg/minute (Tm G), which is an 'active' process.*** About 50 grams of urea are filtered through the glomeruli in 24 hours, but only 30 grams are excreted in the urine, this is a passive diffusion.

Certain substances foreign to the body, e.g. diodrast, para-aminohippuric acid (PAH) and phenol red are:

i. filtered through the glomeruli, and in addition are
ii. secreted by the tubules. Thus, the amount of these substances excreted per minute in the urine is greater than that filtered through the glomeruli per minute. At low blood levels, the tubular capacity for excreting these compounds is so great that plasma passing through the kidneys is almost completely cleared of them.

Another group of substances, e.g. inulin, thiosulphate, and mannitol are eliminated exclusively by the glomeruli and are neither reabsorbed nor secreted by the tubules. Hence, amount of these substances excreted per minute in the urine is the same as the amount filtered through the glomeruli per minute, thus they give the glomerular filtration rate (GFR).

CLASSIFICATION

Based on the above functions, the renal function tests can be classified as follows:

A. Tests Based on Glomerular Filtration

a. Urea clearance test.
b. Endogenous creatinine clearance test.
c. Inulin clearance test.
d. Radio-isotopes in measurement of GFR.
   1. ^{51}Cr—EDTA clearance.
   2. ^{99m}Tc—DTPA clearance.

B. Tests to Measure Renal Plasma Flow (RPF)

a. Para-amino hippurate (PAH) test.
b. Measurement of ERPF by radioisotope-^{131}I-labelled hippuran.
c. Filtration fraction (FF).

C. Tests Based on Tubular Function

a. Concentration and dilution tests.
b. 15 minute—PSP excretion test.
c. Measurement of tubular secretory mass.

D. Certain Miscellaneous Tests

These tests can determine size, shape, asymmetry, obstruction, tumour, infarct, etc.

A. GLOMERULAR FILTRATION TESTS

These are used to examine for impairment of glomerular filtration. Recently, ^{51}Cr-EDTA and ^{99m}Tc-DTPA clearance tests have been described.

What is meant by clearance test?

As a means of expressing quantitatively the rate of excretion of a given substance by the kidney, its "clearance" is frequently measured. This is defined as, "a volume of blood or plasma which contains the amount of the substance which is excreted in the urine in one minute", ***or alternatively,*** "the clearance of a substance may be defined as that volume of blood or plasma cleared of the amount of the substance found in one minute's excretion of urine".

I. Urea Clearance Test

Ambard was the first to study the concentration of urea in blood and relate it to the rate of excretion in the urine, and ***"Ambard's coefficient"*** was, for a while, the subject of much clinical study. At present, the blood/plasma urea clearance test of **Van Slyke is widely used.**

Blood urea clearance is an expression of the number of ml of blood/plasma which are compeletely cleared of urea by the kidney per minute. As a matter of fact, the plasma is not completely cleared of urea. Only about 10% of the urea is removed. Consequently, 750 ml of plasma pass through the kidney per minute and 10% of the urea is removed, this is equivalent to completely clearing 75 ml of plasma per minute.

A. Maximum Clearance

If the urine volume exceeds 2 ml/minute, the rate of urea elimination is at a maximum and is ***directly proportional*** to the concentration of urea in the blood. Thus, provided the blood urea remains unchanged, urea is excreted at the same rate whether the urinary output is 4 ml or 8 ml/minute.

Volume of blood cleared of urea per minute can be calculated from the formula,

$$\boxed{\frac{U \times V}{B}}$$

where

U = Concentration of urea in urine (in mg/100 ml)
V = Volume of urine in ml/minute
B = The concentration of urea in blood (in mg/100 ml)

Substituting average values, the number of ml of blood cleared of urea per minute =

$$\boxed{\frac{1000 \times 2.1}{28} = 75}$$

A urea clearance of 75 does not mean that 75 ml of blood have passed through the kidneys in one minute and were completely cleared of urea. ***It means that the amount of urea excreted in the urine in one minute is equal to the amount found in 75 ml of blood.*** The clearance which occurs when the urinary volume exceeds 2 ml/ minute is termed as ***Maximum urea clearance (C_m)*** and average normal value is 75.

C_m = 75 ml (normal range = 75 ± 10)

B. Standard Clearance

When the urinary volume is less than 2 ml/ minute, the rate of urea elimination is reduced, because relatively more urea is reabsorbed in the tubules, and is proportional to the square root of the urinary volume. Such clearance is termed as ***standard clearance of urea (C_s)*** and ***average normal value is 54.***

$$C_s = \frac{U\sqrt{V}}{B} = 54 \text{ ml (Normal range} = 54 \pm 10)$$

Note

Provided no prerenal factors are temporarily reducing the clearance of urea, the volume of blood cleared of urea per minute is an index of renal function.

- If a larger volume than normal is cleared/ minute renal function is satisfactory.
- If a smaller volume is cleared, renal function is impaired.

Expression As %

Sometimes the result of a urea clearance test is expressed as a % of the normal maximum or of the normal standard urea clearance depending on whether the urinary output is greater or lesser than 2 ml/minute.

Expressed as % of normal

$$C_m = \frac{UV}{B} \frac{100}{75} \% = 1.33$$

$$C_s = \frac{U\sqrt{V}}{B} \times \frac{100}{54} \% = 1.85$$

Relation with Body Surface

The urea clearance is proportional to the surface area of the body and if the result is to be expressed as a % of normal, a correction must be made in the case of children and those of abnormal stature. The C_m is directly proportional to the body surface and if any correction is required the result should be multiplied by 1.73/*BS*, where BS = the patient's body surface derived from the height and weight. In the case of C_s, the correction factor is $\frac{\sqrt{1.73}}{BS}$.

Procedure

The test should be performed between breakfast and lunch, as excretion is more uniform during this time.

- The patient, who is kept at rest throughout the test, is given a light breakfast and 2 to 3 glasses of water.
- The bladder is emptied and the urine is discarded, the exact time of urination is noted.
- One hour later, urine is collected and a specimen of blood is withdrawn for determining urea content.
- A second specimen of urine is obtained at the end of another hour.

The volume of each specimen of urine is measured accurately and the concentration of urea in the specimen of blood and urine is determined. The average value of the two specimens of urine is used for assessing the quantity and urea content of urine.

Interpretation

Urea clearance of 70% or more of average normal function indicates that the kidneys are excreting satisfactorily. Values between 40 and 70% indicates mild impairment, between 20 and 40% moderate impairment and below 20% indicates severe impairment of renal function.

- ***In acute renal failure,*** the urea clearance C_m or C_s, is lowered, usually less than half the normal and increases again with clinical improvement.

- ***In chronic nephritis*** the urea clearance falls progressively and reaches a value half or less of the normal before the blood urea concentration begins to rise. With values below 20% of normal, prognosis is bad, the survival time rarely exceeds two years and death occurs within a year in more than 50% cases.
- ***Terminal uraemia*** is invariably found when the urea clearance falls to about 5% of the normal values.
- ***In nephrotic syndrome*** the urea clearance is usually normal until the onset of renal insufficiency sets in and produces the same changes as in chronic nephritis.
- ***In benign hypertension*** a normal urea clearance is usually maintained indefinitely except in few cases which assume a terminal malignant phase when it falls rapidly.

Note

A very low protein diet can lead to low clearance value even in normal persons and in patients with mild renal disease.

II. Endogenous Creatinine Clearance Test

At normal levels of creatinine, this metabolite is filtered at the glomerulus but neither secreted nor reabsorbed by the tubules. Hence, its clearance gives the GFR. This is a convenient method for estimation of GFR since

i. it is a normal metabolite in the body;
ii. it does not require the intravenous administration of any test material; and
iii. estimation of creatinine is simple. Measurement of 24 hour excretion of endogenous creatinine is convenient. This longer collection period minimizes the timing error.

Procedure

- An accurate 24-hour urine specimen is collected ending at 7 a.m. and its total volume is measured.
- Collect a blood sample for serum creatinine determination.
- Estimate the serum and urinary creatinine concentration.

Result

$$C_{cr} = \frac{U \times V}{P}$$

where,

U = Urine creatinine concentration in mg/dl
P = Serum creatinine in mg/dl
V = Volume of urine in ml/minute

Normal values for creatinine clearance varies from 95 to 105 ml/minute.

III. Inulin Clearance Test

Inulin, a homopolysaccharide, polymer of fructose is an ideal substance as;

i. it is not metabolized in the body;
ii. following IV administration, it is excreted entirely through glomerular filtration, being neither excreted nor reabsorbed by renal tubules. Hence, the number of ml of plasma which is cleared of Inulin in one minute is equivalent to the volume of glomerular filtrate formed in one minute.

Procedure

- Preferably performed in the morning. Patient should be hospitalized overnight and kept reclining during the test.
- A light breakfast is given consisting of half glass milk, one slice toast can be given at 7.30 a.m.
- At 8 a.m. 10 gm of inulin dissolved in 100 ml of saline, at body temperature, is injected IV at a rate of 10 ml per minute.
- One hour after (9 a.m.) the injection, the bladder is emptied and this urine is discarded.
- Note the time and collect urine one and two hours after. Volume of urine is measured and analyzed for inulin content.
- At the midpoint of each collection of urine, 30 and 90 minutes after the initial emptying of bladder, 10 to 15 ml of blood is withdrawn (in oxalated bottle), plasma is separated and analyzed for inulin concentration.

Calculation and Result

Values obtained from two samples of blood are averaged.

$$C_{In} = \frac{U \times V}{P}$$

where,

U = mg of inulin/100 ml of urine
V = ml of urine/minute
P = mg of inulin/dl of plasma (average of two samples)

Normal average: Inulin clearance in an adult (1.73 sqm) = 125 ml of plasma cleared of inulin/ minute. Range = 100 to 150 ml.

Note

- To promote a free flow of urine, one glass of water is given at 06.30 a.m. and repeated every half an hour until the test is completed. This step may be eliminated if administration of fluid is contraindicated.
- Inulin clearance test is definitely superior for determination of GFR but requires tedious and intricate chemical procedure for determination.

IV. Radioisotopes in Measurement of GFR

Clinical advances in management techniques that halt or retard the progression of renal impairment requires an accurate and practical method for monitoring a patient's renal function.

Endogenous creatinine clearance test described above tends to ***overestimate*** GFR as renal failure evolves; whereas inulin clearance measurements although accurate are too cumbersome to use routinely.

The above limitations have stimulated the discovery and use of several radioisotopes with renal clearance characteristics that make them useful in assessing GFR and RPF on patients with renal insufficiency.

Methods

Measurement of GFR, either on the basis of urinary clearance or plasma clearance of the isotope can be reliably undertaken using the following methods:

1. ^{51}Cr-Ethylene diamine tetra-acetic acid (^{51}Cr-EDTA clearance)
2. ^{99m}Tc diethylene triamine Penta acetic acid (DTPA)- for split renal function

To ensure accuracy in the measurement of GFR by urinary clearance of radionucleotide, it is essential that:

i. renal tubular secretion or reabsorption does not contribute to the elimination of the compound;
ii. plasma protein binding of the isotope is negligible; and
iii. patients completely empty their urinary bladder.

Plasma clearance of a radionucleotide measures GFR reliably only if non-renal clearance routes are negligible.

1. ^{51}Cr-EDTA Clearance

Currently simplified single injection method for determination of ^{51}Cr-EDTA plasma clearance is widely used, for routine assessment of glomerular filtration rate (GFR) in adults as well as in children.

It is particularly convenient in children where it is not easy to collect 24 hour urine sample. It has been used for children younger than one year.

A dose of 4.5 μci (0.17 MBq)/kg body weight of ^{51}Cr-EDTA is injected IV. Capillary blood samples are drawn at 5, 15, 60, 90 and 120 minutes after the injection and simultaneously the haematocrit (hct) is determined. The radioactivity is calculated as measured activity in 0.2 ml capillary blood/1-hct. The ^{51}Cr-EDTA plasma clearance is determined as the ratio between the injected amount of the 'tracer' (Q_o) and the total area under the plasma activity curve c (t) which is resoluted into two mono-exponential functions (Fig. 1.1).

The plasma clearance (cl) is then calculated as,

$$cl = \frac{Q_o}{c_1/b_1 + c_2/b_2}$$

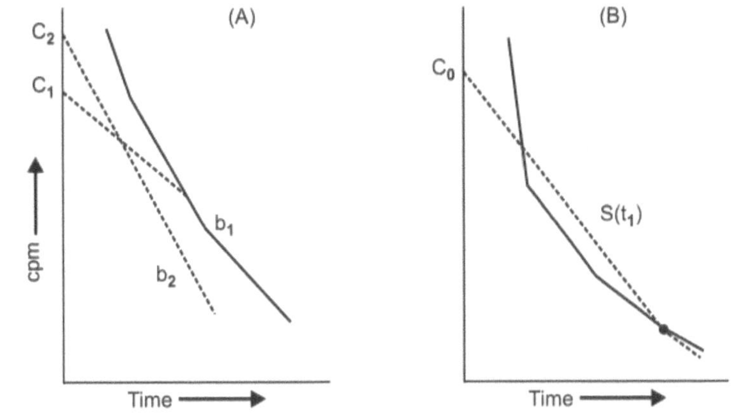

Figs 1.1A and B: ^{51}Cr-EDTA activity C(t) in capillary plasma samples. Disappearance of ^{51}Cr-EDTA. In curve (A) C_1 and C_2 are intercepts (monoexponential functions) and b_1 and b_2 rate constants. In (B) the disappearance curve is indicated by the solid line while the broken line shows the monoexponential curve that is used in estimating ^{51}Cr-EDTA clearance from a single sample drawn

To determine plasma clearance from a single sample the mean transit time and extracellular fluid volume are estimated, and then cl = Ecv/t gives the clearance value.

2. ^{99m}Tc-DTPA Clearance

This technique measures the split renal function. Separate estimation of GFR within the right and left kidneys is referred to as the split renal function technique

Gate's technique

Basis: This test is based on the fact that the fractional renal uptake of intravenously administered ^{99m}Tc-DTPA, within 2 to 3 minutes after radio-tracer arrival within the kidneys, is proportional to the GFR.

Thus, with this technique it is possible to determine both split renal function and total GFR.

The actual test is less time consuming and does not take more than 5 to 10 minutes.

B. TESTS FOR RENAL BLOOD FLOW

1. Measurement of Renal Plasma Flow (RPF)

Para-aminohippurate (PAH) is filtered at the glomeruli and secreted by the tubules. At low blood concentrations (2 mg or less/100 ml) of plasma, PAH is removed completely during a single circulation of the blood through the kidneys. Tubular capacity for excreting PAH of low blood levels is great. Thus, the amount of PAH in the urine becomes a measure for the value of plasma cleared of PAH in a unit time, i.e. PAH clearance at low blood levels measures renal plasma flow (RPF).

RPF (for a surface area of 1.73 sqm) = 574 ml/minute.

2. Mesurement of Effective Renal Plasma Flow (ERPF) by Radioisotope

Though PAH method is satisfactory but not very accurate. ERPF is a measurement of tubular secretory function combined with GFR. Selection of a suitable test substance requires that

i. the compound be minimally protein-bound to provide for glomerular filtration; and
ii. the non-filtered residual drug exiting the glomerulus in the efferent arteriole be completely secreted into the lumen of the tubule such that renal venous blood is fully cleared of the test substance.

It is to be noted that a small fraction of renal blood flow (approximately 8%) does not pass through fully active nephrons, and as a result, the renal blood extraction rate of the best test substance PAH is 90% +. Accordingly, estimating total renal blood flow with radiopharmaceutical counterpart, ^{131}I labelled hippuran it is possible to designate only ERPF.

This estimation of ERPF can be performed easily in patients. It typically requires measuring differential or split renal appearance of the radionuclide, 1 to 2 minutes after injection of the isotope and collecting peripheral blood 44 minutes after isotope injection to assess glomerular renal function.

3. Filtration Fraction (FF)

The filtration fraction (FF) is the fraction of plasma passing through the kidney which is filtered at the glomerulus is obtained by dividing the inulin clearance by the PAH clearance.

$$FF = \frac{C_{In}}{C_{PAH}} = \frac{GFR}{RPF}$$

If we take, GFR = 125 and RPF = 594, then

$$FF = \frac{125}{574} = 0.217\ (21.7\%)$$

Normal range = 0.16 to 0.21 in an adult.

Interpretations

- The FF tends to be normal in ***early essential hypertension,*** but as the disease progresses, the decrease in RPF is greater than the decrease in the GFR. This produces an increase in FF.
- In the ***malignant phase of hypertension,*** these changes are much greater, consequently the FF rises considerably.
- In ***glomerulonephritis,*** the reverse situation prevails. In all stages of this disease, a progressive decrease in the FF is characteristic because of much greater decline in the glomerular filtration rate (GFR), than the renal plasma flow (RPF).
- A rise in FF is also observed early in ***congestive cardiac failure.***

C. TESTS OF TUBULAR FUNCTION

Pathophysiological aspect: Alterations in renal tubular function may be brought about by:

i. ischaemia with reduction in blood flow through the peritubular capillaries;
ii. by direct action of toxic substances on the renal tubular cells; and
iii. by biochemical defects, e.g. impairing transfer of substances across the tubular cells.

Adequate renal tubular function requires adequate renal blood flow, a significant reduction in the latter is reflected in impaired tubular function. Hence, arteriolar nephrosclerosis and other diseases diminishing blood flow, causes inability to concentrate or dilute the urine with resulting ***"isosthenuria" ("fixation" of sp gr at 1.010).***

I. Concentration Tests

These tests are based on the ability of the kidneys to concentrate urine, and on measureing sp gr of urine.

They are ***simple bedside procedures,*** easy to carry out and extremely important. The tests are conducted either

i. under conditions of restricted fluid intake, or
ii. by inhibiting diuresis by injection of ADH.

1. Fishberg Concentration Test

This test imposes less strenuous curtailment of fluid intake and may be completed in a shorter period of time. Most commonly used simple bedside concentration test.

Procedure

- Patient is allowed no fluids from 8 p.m. until 10 a.m. next morning.
- The evening meal is given at 7 p.m. It should be high protein meal and must have a fluid content of less than 200 ml.
- Urine passed in the night is discarded
- Nothing orally next morning.
- Collect urine specimens next morning at 8 a.m., 9 a.m. and 10 a.m. and determine the specific gravity of each specimen.

Result and Interpretation

- If tubular function is normal, the sp gr of at least one of the specimens should be greater than 1.025, after appropriate correction made for temperature, albumin, and glucose.
- Impaired tubular function is shown by a sp gr of 1.020 or less and may be fixed at 1.010 in cases of severe renal damage.

Note

A false result may be obtained, if the patient has:

i. congestive cardiac failure because elimination of oedema fluid in night will simulate inability to concentrate;
ii. inability to concentrate is also characteristic of diabetes insipidus.

2. Lashmet and Newburg Concentration Test

This test imposes: (i) severe fluid intake restriction over a period of 38 hours; and (ii) involves the use of a special dry diet for one day.

3. Concentration Test with Posterior Pituitary Extract

The subcutaneous injection of 10 pressor units of posterior pituitary extract (0.5 ml of vasopressin injection) in a normal person will inhibit the diuresis produced by the ingestion of 1600 ml of water in 15 minutes.

The test has the advantage of short performance time, and minimising the necessity of preparation of the patient.

Posterior pituitary extract will also inhibit the diuresis seen in ***congestive heart failure*** under active treatment as well as that of ***diabetes insipidus,*** allowing sufficient concentration to determine degree of tubular function in these conditions.

Interpretation

Under the conditions of the test, individual with normal kidney function, excrete urine with sp gr 1.020 or higher. Failure to concentrate to this degree indicates renal damage.

II. Water Dilution/Elimination Test

Principle: The ability of the kidneys to eliminate water is tested by measuring the urinary output after ingesting a large volume of water.

Note

Water excretion is not only a renal function but also depends on extrarenal factors and prerenal deviation will reduce the ability of the kidneys to excrete urine.

Procedure

- The patient remains in bed throughout the test because elimination of water is maximal in the horizontal position.
- On the day before the test, the patient has an evening meal but takes nothing by mouth after 8 p.m.
- On the morning of the test, he empties his bladder at 8 a.m. which is discarded, and then drinks 1200 ml of water within half an hour.
- The bladder is emptied at 9 a.m., 10 a.m., 11 a.m. and 12 noon and the volume and the sp gr. of the four specimens are measured.

Interpretations

- If renal function is normal more than 80% (1000 ml) of water is voided in 4 hours, the larger part being excreted in the first 2 hours. The sp gr of at least one specimen should be 1.003 or less.
- If renal function is impaired, less than 80% (1000 ml) of water is excreted in 4 hours, and the sp gr does not fall to 1.003 and remains fixed at 1.010 in cases of severe renal damage.

III. Tests of Tubular Excretion and Reabsorption

Principle: The reserve function of secretion of foreign non-endogenous materials by the tubular epithelium is most conveniently tested for by the use of certain dyes and measuring their rate of excretion.

1. Phenol Sulphthalein (PSP) Excretion Test

Use of PSP (Phenol red) to measure renal function was first introduced by **Rowntree** and **Geraghty** in 1912. Later on, **Smith** has shown that with the amount of dye employed, 94% is excreted by tubular action and only 6% by glomerular filtration. Thus, the test measures primarily tubular activity as well as being a measure of renal blood flow.

15-minute PSP Test

It has been shown the test is reliable and sensitive if the amount of dye excreted in the first 15 minutes is taken as the criterion of renal function.

Test and Interpretation

When 1.0 ml of PSP (6 mg) is injected IV, normal kidneys will excrete 30 to 50% of the dye during the first 15 minutes. Excretion of less than 23% of the dye during this period regardless of the amount excreted in 2 hours indicates impaired renal function.

It is also used to determine the function of each kidney separately. Here, ***the appearance time as well as the rate of excretion of the dye is of importance.*** After IV injection, the normal appearance time of the dye at the tip of the catheters is 2 minutes or less and rate of excretion from each kidney is greater than 1 to 1.5% of the injected dye per ml. Increase in appearance time and decrease in excretion rate indicate impaired function.

2. Tests to Measure Tubular Secretory Mass

Principle: If diodone/or PAH concentration in the plasma is gradually raised above the level at which it is wholly excreted whilst traversing the kidney on a single occasion, the amount of diodone/PAH actually excreted per minute increases, but the removal of the presented diodone is no longer complete. Eventually a plasma concentration will be reached at which the tubules are excreting the "maximum" amount possible, they are said to be "saturated" and since they are working at their utmost capacity, further elevation of plasma diodone level produces no increase in the tubular excretion. Hence, the total excretion/minute under these conditions is the

i. amount excreted by glomerular filtration +
ii. the amount excreted by the tubules.

$$\text{Total excretion/minute} = U_D \times V$$

The glomerular contribution is the glomerular volume/minute (C_{In}) and diodone concentration in the glomerular filtrate (P_D), since filtrate and plasma contain the same concentration.

Maximum contribution by tubules

$$= U_D \times V - C_{In} \times P_D$$

The above represents the ***"tubular excretory capacity or mass"*** for diodone expressed in mg/minute and represented by the symbol "T_{mD}".

Normally, T_{mD} lies in the range 36 to 72 in adults.

D. OTHER MISCELLANEOUS TESTS TO ASSESS RENAL FUNCTION

1. Test of Renal Ability to Excrete Acid

A number of workers have studied the excretion of acid by the kidneys following stimulation by giving NH_4Cl.

Procedure

Method followed here is that of **Davies** and **Wrong** (1957).

- Give NH_4Cl, 0.1 gm/kg in grams or half gram gelatin coated capsules over a period of an hour, e.g., from 10 a.m. to 11 a.m.
- Empty the bladder an hour later and discard the specimen.
- Collect all urine specimens passed during the next 6 hours and empty the bladder at the end of that period.

Note:
Make sure that the urine is collected in specially cleaned vessels preferably under oil. A crystal of thymol can be placed in the vessel. Measure the pH of the urine specimens and determine the NH_3 content of the combined urine specimens.

Interpretation

- Normal persons pass urine during the 6-hour period with pH—5.3, and have an ammonia excretion between 30 and 90 micro-equivalents/minute.
- In most forms of renal failure, the pH falls in the same way, but the ammonia excretion is low.
- In renal tubular acidosis, pH remains between 5.7 and 7.0 and ammonia excretion is also low.

2. Intravenous Pyelography

When injected IV, certain radiopaque organic compounds of iodine are excreted by the kidneys in sufficient concentrations to cast a shadow of the renal calyces, renal pelvis, ureters and the bladder on an X-ray film and gives lot of informations regarding size, shape and functioning of the kidneys.

The most commonly used substances are:

- **Iodoxyl**—available as "Pyelectan" (Glaxo), Uropac (M & B), Uroselectan B, etc.
- **Diodone** 30%, which is recently introduced, and gives better results. Available as Perabrodil (Bayer), Pyelosil (Glaxo), etc.

Indications
IV pyelography is widely used in the investigation of diseases of urinary tract and should be a routine procedure for investigation with patients of:

- renal calculi,
- repeated urinary infections,
- renal pain; haematuria,
- prostatic enlargement,
- suspected tumours; and
- congenital abnormalities.

By pyelography the relationship of the renal tract to calcified abdominal shadows and masses can be demonstrated. The excretion and concentration of diodone may be used as a rough indication of renal function. If the calyces and pelvis of one kidney are outlined, while the other remains invisible, it can be assumed that the function of the invisible side is impaired.

Contraindications
IV pyelography should not be done in patients with:

- acute nephritis,
- congestive cardiac failure,
- severely impaired liver function,
- in frank uraemia
- in hypersensitive patients and sensitivity to organic iodine compounds. Sensitivity test should be done before injecting the drug.

3. Radioactive Renogram

^{131}I-labelled Hippuran is given IV and simultaneously the radioactivity from each kidney is recorded graphically in a stripchart recorder by electronic device. Hippuran-^{131}I is actively secreted by the kidney tubules and it is not concentrated in the liver.

A single dose 15 to 60 μci of Hippuran ^{131}I given IV slowly.

Interpretation

With the limitations and complexities of the interpretation of the results, the investigation is of great practical clinical use. The following information is obtained.

- Whether any major asymmetry in function between the two kidneys is present.
- A reasonable assessment of overall renal function—Given by the ratio of bladder activity/heart activity in 10 minutes time.
- The presence of obstruction to urine flow in renal pelvis or ureters.

No other means exist for obtaining so much information in a short time about the differential function of the kidneys.

4. Radioactive Scanning

A recent development is the renal scintiscan. This has the theoretical advantage over the renogram of being able ***to detect segmental lesions.***

In this technique, ^{203}Hg-labelled chlormerodrin or ^{197}Hg-labelled chlormerodrin is injected intravenously and a renal scan can be obtained by a scintillation counter over the lumbar region.

Renal scanning is helpful for detection of abnormalities in size, shape and position of the kidneys.

Renal tumours and renal infarcts are shown in scintiscan which may be missed in Pyelography.

Chapter 2

Liver Function Tests

INTRODUCTION

Numerous laboratory investigations have been proposed in the assessment of liver diseases. From among these host of tests, the following battery of blood tests; total bilirubin and VD Bergh test, total and differential proteins and A:G ratio and certain enzyme assay as aminotransferases; alkaline phosphatase and γ-GGT have become widely known as ***"Standard Liver Function Tests" (LFTs).***

Urine tests for bilirubin and its metabolites and the prothrombin time (PT) and index (PI) are also often included under these headings but ***tests such as turbidity/flocculation test, icteric index, etc. are now becoming outdated. "Second generation" LFTs*** attempt to improve on this battery of tests and to gain a genuine measurement of liver function, i.e. quantitative assessment of functional hepatic mass. These include the capacity of the liver to eliminate exogenous compounds such as aminopyrine or caffeine or endogenous compounds such as bile acids which have gained much importance recently. However, such investigations are not yet routinely or widely used due to lack of facilities and are useful for research purpose only.

Hence in our discussion we will confine to "Standard LFTs" which are routinely done and possible in any standard laboratory. ***It is stressed that with the advent of more sophisticated techniques for the diagnosis of liver diseases, particularly ultrasound*** and ***CT scanning together*** with ***percutaneous*** and ***endoscopic cholangiography*** and ***liver biopsy,*** routine use of standard LFTs being questioned now.

FUNCTIONS OF THE LIVER

Liver is a versatile organ which is involved in metabolism and independently involved in many other biochemical functions. **Regenerating power of liver cells in tremendous.**

The reader may consult the textbook of medical biochemistry by the author for detailed account of various functions performed by the liver which have been discussed under their respective places, a summary of these functions is given below in brief, so that students can easily group the tests of liver associating with its functions.

- *Metabolic functions:* Liver is the key organ and the principal site where the metabolism of carbohydrates, lipids, and proteins take place.
  - **a.** Liver is the organ where ammonia is converted to urea.
  - **b.** It is the principal organ where cholesterol is synthesized, and catabolized to form bile acids and bile salts.
  - **c.** Esterfication of cholesterol takes place solely in liver.
  - **d.** In this organ, absorbed monosaccharides other than glucose are converted to glucose, viz, galactose is converted to glucose, fructose converted to glucose.

e. Liver besides other organs can bring about catabolism and anabolism of nucleic acids.

f. Liver is also involved in metabolism of vitamins and minerals to certain extent.

- *Secretory Functions:* Liver is responsible for the formation and secretion of bile in the intestine. Bile pigment bilirubin, formed from heme catabolism is conjugated in liver cells and secreted in the bile.
- *Excretory Function:* Certain exogenous dyes like **BSP (bromsulphthalein)** and **Rose Bengal dye** are exclusively excreted through liver cells.
- *Synthesis of Certain Blood Coagulation Factors:* Liver cells are responsible for conversion of preprothrombin (inactive) to active prothrombin in the presence of vitamin K. It also produces other clotting factors like factor V, VII and X. Fibrinogen involved in blood coagulation is also synthesized in liver.
- *Synthesis of Other Proteins*: Albumin is solely synthesized in liver and also to some extent α and β globulins.
- *Detoxication Function and Protective Function*: Kupffer cells of liver remove foreign bodies from blood by phagocytosis. Liver cells can detoxicate drugs, hormones and convert them into less toxic substances for excretion.
- *Storage Function:* Liver stores glucose in the form of glycogen. It also stores vitamin B_{12} and A, etc.
- *Miscellaneous Function:* Liver is involved in blood formation in embryo and in some abnormal states, it also forms blood in adult.

CLASSIFICATION

Tests used in the study of patients with liver and biliary tract diseases can be classified according to the specific functions of the liver involved.

I. ***Tests based on abnormalities of pigment metabolism:***
   a. Serum bilirubin and VD Bergh reaction
   b. Icteric index
   c. Urine bilirubin
   d. Urine and faecal urobilinogen
   e. Serum and urinary bile acids.

II. ***Tests based on liver's part in carbohydrate metabolism:***
   a. Galactose tolerance test
   b. Fructose tolerance test.

III. ***Tests based on changes in plasma proteins:***
   a. Estimation of total plasma proteins, albumin and globulin and determination of A:G ratio
   b. Determination of plasma fibrinogen
   c. Various flocculation tests.
   d. Amino acids in urine.

IV. ***Tests based on abnormalities of lipids:***
   a. Determination of serum cholesterol and ester cholesterol and their ratio
   b. Determination of faecal fats.

V. ***Tests based on detoxicating function of liver:***
   a. Hippuric acid synthesis test
   b. The amino anti-pyrime breath test.

VI. ***Excretion of injected substances by the liver (excretory function):***
   a. Bromsulphalein test (BSP-retention test)
   b. ^{131}I Rose Bengal test.

VII. ***Formation of prothrombin by liver:***
   a. Determination of prothrombin time.

VIII. ***Tests based on amino acid catabolism:***
   a. Determination of blood NH_3
   b. Determination of glutamine in CS fluid (Indirect Liver Function Test).

IX. ***Determination of serum enzyme activities.***

I. TESTS BASED ON ABNORMALITIES OF BILE PIGMENT METABOLISM

(a) VD Bergh Reaction and Serum Bilirubin

Principle: Methods for detecting and estimating bilirubin in serum are ***based on the formation of a purple compound "azo-bilirubin"*** where bilirubin in serum is allowed to react with a freshly prepared solution of VD Bergh's diazo reagent.

VD Bergh reaction consists of two parts—direct and indirect reactions. The latter serves as the basis for a quantitative estimation of serum bilirubin.

Ehrlich's diazo reagent: This is freshly prepared before use. It consists of two solutions:

- **Solution A:** Contains sulphanilic acid in conc. HCl.
- **Solution B:** Sodium nitrite in water. **Fresh solution is prepared by taking 10 ml of solution A + 0.8 ml of solution B.**

Procedure

Take 0.3 ml of serum into each of two small tubes. Add 0.3 ml of distilled water to one which serves as **"Control"** and 0.3 ml of freshly prepared diazo reagent into second **('test').** Mix both tubes and observe any colour change.

Basis of the reaction: Coupling of diazotized sulphanilic acid and bilirubin if present produces a "redish-purple" azo-compound.

Responses: Three different responses may be observed.

- ***Immediate direct reaction:*** Immediate development of colour proceeding rapidly to a maximum.
- ***Delayed direct reaction:*** Colour only begins to appear after 5 to 30 minutes and develops slowly to a maximum.
- ***No direct reaction is obtained:*** Colour develops after addition of methanol **(indirect reaction).**

• Determination of Serum Bilirubin

Indirect reaction is essentially a method for the quantitative estimation of serum bilirubin.

Principle: Serum is diluted with D.W. and methanol added in an amount insufficient to precipitate the proteins, yet sufficient to permit all the bilirubin to react with the diazo reagent. (**NB:** Absolute methanol gives a clear solution than 95% ethanol).

Colour developed is compared with a standard solution of bilirubin similarly treated.

Note

Bilirubin is a costly chemical hence an artificial standard may be used.

It is methyl red solution in glacial acetic acid of pH 4.6 to 4.7, which closely resembles the colour of azo-bilirubin.

Note

Before interpretation, students should know about Jaundice and its causes.

JAUNDICE

In jaundice there is yellow coloration of conjunctivae, mucous membrane and skin due to increased bilirubin level.

Jaundice is visible when serum bilirubin exceeds 2.4 mg/dl.

Classification of Jaundice

1. **Rolleston and McNee's (1929),** classification as modified by Maclagan (1964):

• *Haemolytic or Prehepatic Jaundice*

In this there is increased breakdown of Hb, so that liver cells are unable to conjugate all the increased bilirubin formed.

Causes: Principally there are two categories:

a. ***Intrinsic***: Abnormalities within the red blood cells by various haemoglobinopathies, hereditary spherocytosis, G6PD deficiency in red cells and favism.
b. ***Extrinsic:*** Factor external to red blood cells, e.g. incompatible blood transfusion, haemolytic disease of the newborn (HDN), autoimmune haemolytic anaemias, in malaria, etc.

• *Hepatocellular or Hepatic Jaundice*

In this there is disease of the parenchymal cells of liver. This may be divided into 3 groups, although there may be overlappings.

a. ***Conditions in which there is defective conjugation:*** There may be a reduction in the number of functioning liver cells, e.g., in chronic hepatitis. In this all liver functions are impaired or there may be a specific defect in the conjugation process e.g. in Gilbert' disease, Crigler-Najjar syndrome, etc. In these the liver function is otherwise normal.

b. ***Conditions such as viral hepatitis and toxic jaundice:*** There is extensive damage to liver cells, associated with considerable degree of intrahepatic obstruction resulting in appreciable absorption of conjugated bilirubin.

c. ***"Cholestatic" jaundice:*** This occurs due to drugs, (drug-induced) such as chlorpromazine and some steroids in which there is mainly intrahepatic obstruction, liver function being essentially normal.

- ***Obstructive or Posthepatic Jaundice***

In this there is obstruction to the flow of bile in the extrahepatic ducts, e.g. due to gallstones, carcinoma of head of pancreas, enlarged lymph glands pressing on bile duct, etc.

2. • **Rich's classification of jaundice:** According to this classification jaundice is divided into two main groups.

- ***Retention Jaundice***

In this there is impaired removal of bilirubin from the blood, or excessive amount of bilirubin is produced and not cleared fully by liver cells. This group includes haemolytic jaundice and those conditions characterized by impaired conjugation of bilirubin.

- ***Regurgitation Jaundice***

In this there is excess of conjugating bilirubin and it includes obstructive jaundice and those liver conditions in which there is considerable degree of intrahepatic obstruciton (cholestasis).

Interpretations

VD Bergh reaction: Correlation of different types of VD Bergh reaction is based on the fact how bilirubin reacts differently with the diazo reagent according to whether or not, it has been conjugated. Bilirubin formed from Hb and not passed through liver cells is called ***unconjugated bilirubin and it gives an indirect reaction.*** On the other hand, bilirubin which has passed through liver cells and undergoes conjugation is called ***conjugated bilirubin and gives direct reaction.***

- *In haemolytic jaundice:* there is an increase in unconjugated bilirubin, hence indirect reaction is obtained, occasionlly it may be a delayed direct reaction.
- *In obstructive jaundice:* conjugated bilirubin is increased, hence an immediate direct reaction is obtained.
- *In hepatocellular jaundice:* either or both may be present. In viral hepatitis, direct reaction is the rule because it is associated with intrahepatic obstruction.

An immediate direct reaction is also observed in "cholestatic jaundice". In low-grade jaundice present in some cases of cirrhosis liver, results are variable, but an indirect reaction is usually seen.

An immediate direct reaction is obtained whether the obstruction is intrahepatic or extrahepatic. This does not, therefore differentiate between an infectious hepatitis or toxic jaundice on one hand and posthepatic (obstructive jaundice) on the other. ***Hence a direct VD Bergh reaction is only of limited value.***

Serum bilirubin: It gives a measure of the intensity of jaundice. Higher values are found in obstructive jaundice than in haemolytic jaundice.

Usefulness of quantitative estimation of serum bilirubin:

- *In subclinical jaundice:* where the demonstration of small increases in serum bilirubin 1.0 to 3.0 mg/dl is of diagnostic value.
- *In clinical jaundice:* useful to follow the development and course of the jaundice.

(b) Icteric Index

It measures the degree of jaundice by measuring the intensity of the yellow colour of the serum.

Principle: Serum or plasma is diluted with physiological saline until it matches in colour a 1 in 10,000 solution of potassium dichromate (standard solution). ***The dilution factor is termed the icteric index.***

Precautions

- Turbidity may appear sometimes on diluting the serum with physiological saline. This is prevented by using phosphate buffer of pH 7.0 as dilution fluid.
- Lipaemia may also interfere with the comparison.
- Haemolysis may interfere which should be avoided.

Interpretations

- Normal range is from 4 to 6.
- In latent jaundice, the index is from 7 to 15.
- With an index over 15, clinically obvious jaundice should be present. *It has no advantages over serum bilirubin, and it is not done now and become obsolete.*

(c) Bile Pigments in Urine (Bilirubinuria)

Principle: Most of the tests used for detection of bile pigments depend on the oxidation of bilirubin to differently coloured compounds such as biliverdin (green) and bilicyanin (blue).

Interpretations

- Bilirubin is found in the urine in obstructive jaundice due to various causes and in "cholestasis". Conjugated bilirubin can pass through the glomerular filter.
- Bilirubin is not present in urine in most cases of haemolytic jaundice, as unconjugated bilirubin is carried in plasma attached to albumin, hence it cannot pass through the glomerular filter.
- ***Bilirubinuria is always accompanied with direct VD Bergh reaction.***

Note

Bilirubin in the urine may be detected even before clinical jaundice is noted

- **Bile Pigments in Faeces**

  Bilirubin is not normally present in faeces since bacteria in the intestine reduce it to urobilinogen.
- Some amount may be found if there is very rapid passage of materials along the intestine.
- Sometimes it is found in faeces of very young infants, if bacterial flora in the gut is not developed.
- It is regularly found in faeces of patients who are being treated with gut sterlizing antibiotics such as neomycin.
- Biliverdin is found in meconium, the material excreted during the first day or two of life.

(d) *Urinary and Faecal Urobilinogen*

1. *Faecal Urobilinogen*

Normal quantity of urobilinogen excreted in the faeces per day is from 50 to 250 mg. Since urobilinogen is formed in the intestine by the reduction of bilirubin, the amount of faecal urobilinogen depends primarily on the amount of bilirubin entering the intestine.

- Faecal urobilinogen is increased in haemolytic jaundice, in which dark-coloured faeces is passed.
- Faecal urobilinogen is decreased or absent if there is obstruction to the flow of bile in obstructive jaundice, in which clay-coloured faeces is passed. Complete degree of obstruction is found in tumours, whereas obstruction due to gall stones in intermittent.

  A complete absence of faecal urobilinogen is strongly suggestive of malignant obstruction. Thus, it may be useful in differentiating a non-malignant from a malignant obstruction.
- A decrease may also occur in extreme cases of disease affecting hepatic parenchyma.

2. *Urine Urobilinogen*

Normally there are mere traces of urobilinogen in the urine. Average is 0.64 mg, maximum normal 4 mg/24 hours.

- ***In obstructive jaundice:*** In case of complete obstruction, no urobilinogen is found in the urine. Since bilirubin is unable to get into the intestine to form it.

  The presence of bilirubin in the urine, without urobilinogen is strongly suggestive of obstructive jaundice either intrahepatic or posthepatic.
- ***In haemolytic jaundice:*** increased production of bilirubin leads to increased production of urobilinogen which appears in urine in large amounts. Thus, ***increased urobilinogen in urine and absence of bilirubin in urine are strongly suggestive of haemolytic jaundice.***
- Increased urinary urobilinogen may be seen in damage to the hepatic parenchyma, because of inability of the liver to re-excrete into the stool by way of the bile and urobilinogen absorbed from the intestine "entero-hepatic circulation" suffers.

(e) Serum and Urinary Bile Acids

Two primary bile acids are **cholic acid** and **chenodeoxy cholic acid.** They are formed in hepatocytes from cholesterol.

Bile acids are newly synthesized and also derived from plasma lipids. Such bile acids production is subject to negative "feed-back" by the quantity of bile acids returning to the liver in the entero-hepatic circulation.

Two primary bile acids, cholic and chenodeoxycholic, are conjugated with glycine and taurine via the COOH gr at C_{24} to form the corresponding bile salts glycocholate and taurocholate.

1. Serum Bile Acids

- Fasting serum contains conjugates of primary and secondary bileacids as well as some unconjugated bile acids
- Serum concentrations increase after meals. The peak value is obtained after 90 minute of the meal.
- Clinical importance of serum bile acid measurement lies mainly in the effect of liver disease on the organic anion transport process and the consequent ability to clear bileacids from blood.
- Other factors that affect the concentration and pattern are:
  - deficient reabsorption in diseases;
  - absence of distal ileum;
  - changes in proportion of conjugated and unconjugated forms caused by bacterial overgrowth and consequent increase in ileal deconjugation.

Methods

Methods available for determination of serum bile acids are given below:

a. ***Radioimmunoassay (RIA):*** It is very sensitive test and does not require any prior extraction. The test usually measures only conjugated forms of bile acids.

b. ***Gas liquid chromatography (GLC):*** This method measures several species simultaneously and requires serum extraction and deconjugation of the bile acids.

   The preparative procedures make possible to measure the bileacids and conjugates separately.

c. ***Enzymatic methods:*** Depends on the oxidation of 3 α OH group to 3-oxo groups by a "3 *α-hydroxysteroid dehydrogenase*" enzyme.

   NADH produced as a result of enzymatic reaction is measured fluorimetrically. Enzymatic methods measure total bile acids.

Interpretation

Normal values:
Different values have been given for different methods used:

- By GLC—0.6 to 4.7 μmol/L
- By RIA:
  - conjugated cholic acid 0.3 to 1.5 μmol/L
  - conjugated chenodeoxycholic acid: 0.4 to 2.5 μmol/L

- By enzymatic method
  - For males: 0 to 4.7 μmol/L
  - For females: 1.0 to 8.2 μmol/L
- Value of serum bile acid assay is still a matter of debate but its main usefulness lies in the discrimination of mild liver disease and in the assessment of the progress of chronic liver disease.
- An increased concentration of bile acids in non-fasting serum collected at 1200 to 1400 hours was found ***to be a highly sensitive indicator of hepatobiliary disease*** but fails to indicate the etiology.
- Serum bile acid assay has been claimed to be more specific in diagnosis of occult liver disease as a cause for a case of pruritus.
- Estimation of serum bile acids has been found to detect decompensation of cirrhosis liver earlier and becomes positive 1 to 4 months before the onset of ascites.
- Ratio of bile acid concentrations has been found to be useful. The ratio of trihydroxy to dihydroxy acids, i.e., cholic/chenodeoxycholic acid ratio, is affected by greater depression of chol synthesis in hepatocellular disease. Ratio is less than 1 in 80% cases of hepatocellular disease including cirrhosis liver. On the other hand, the ratio exceeds and is greater than 1 in cholestatic lesions. But ***it cannot differentiate between intrahepatic and extrahepatic cholestasis.***
- Thus, it has been claimed to be the best discriminatory factor in diagnosing parenchymal liver disease and obstructive liver diseases including malignancy.
- Serum Bile acid measurements are normal in Gilbert's syndrome and unhelpful in the diagnosis of the Dubin-Johnson syndrome.

2. Bile Acids in Urine

The detection and measurement of bile acid in urine is unstatisfactory and of less importance now.

II. TESTS BASED ON LIVER'S PART IN CARBOHYDRATE METABOLISM

Basis: The tests are based on tolerance to various sugars since liver is involved in removal of these sugars by glycogenesis or in conversion of other monosaccharides to glucose.

- **Glucose Tolerance Test**
  - Not of much value in liver diseases
  - Although glucose tolerance is sometimes diminished, it is often difficult to separate the part played by the liver from other factors influencing glucose metabolism.

(a) *Galactose Tolerance Test*

Basis: The normal liver is able to convert galactose into glucose, but this function is impaired in intrahepatic diseases and the amount of blood galactose and galactose in urine is excessive.

Advantages of this test:

- It is ***used primarily to detect liver cell injury.***
- It can be performed in presence of jaundice.
- As it measures an intrinsic hepatic function, it may be used to distinguish obstructive and non-obstructive jaundice.

Note

In prolonged obstruction, if untreated, secondary involvement of liver leads to abnormality in the gatactose tolerance.

Methods

This can be of two types:

a. Oral galactose tolerance test (Maclagan) and
b. IV galactose tolerance test.

1. Oral Galactose Tolerance Test (Maclagan)

- The test is performed in the morning after an overnight fast.
- A fasting blood sample is collected which serves as **"control"**.
- 40 gm of galactose dissolved in a cup-full of water is given orally.
- Further, four blood samples are collected at ½ hourly intervals for two hours (similar to GTT).

Interpretations

- Normally or in obstructive jaundice 3 gm or less of galactose are excreted in the urine within 3 to 5 hours and the blood galactose returns to normal within one hour.

- In intrahepatic (parenchymatous) jaundice, the excretion amounts to 4 to 5 gm or more during the first five hours.

Galactose Index (Maclagan): It is obtained by adding the four blood galactose levels.

Interpretations

- Upper normal limit of normal was taken as 160.
- ***In healthy medical students*** range varied from 0 to 110 and in hospital patients not suffering from liver disease the value ranged from 0 to 160.
- ***In liver diseases,*** very high values are obtained.
- In ***infective and toxic hepatitis*** values up to about 500 are seen, decreasing slowly as the clinical condition improves. In cirrhosis liver, increased values may be obtained up to 500, depending on the severity of the disease.

2. *Intravenous Galactose Tolerance Test (King)*

- The test is performed in the morning after a night's fast.
- A fasting blood sample is collected which serves as **"control"**.
- An IV injection of galactose, equivalent to 0.5 gm/kg body weight is given as a sterile 50% solution.
- Blood samples are collected after five minutes, ½, 1, 1½, 2 and 2½ hours after IV injection and blood galactose level is estimated.

Interpretations

- A ***normal response*** should have a curve beginning on the average at about 200 mg galactose/100 dl, falling steeply during the one hour and reaching a figure between 0 and 10 mg% by end of 2 hours.
- In most cases of ***obstructive jaundice,*** similar results are obtained, unless there is parenchymal damage.
- In ***parenchymatous diseases*** with liver cell damage, the fall in blood galactose takes place more slowly.

Normally, no galactose is detected in 2½ hours sample, but in parenchymatous disease, value is greater than 20 mg/dl.

(b) *Fructose Tolerance Test*

Method

- Fasting blood sugar is estimated.
- 50 gm of fructose is given to the fasting patient.
- Samples are taken at ½ hourly intervals for 2½ hours after giving the oral fructose. Blood sugar is estimated in all the samples. The usual methods for estimation of blood sugar measures both the glucose and fructose present.

Interpretations

- ***Normal response*** shows little or no rise in the blood sugar level. The highest blood sugar value reached during the test should not exceed the fasting level by more than 30 mg%.
- Similar result is obtained in most cases of ***obstructive jaundice*** cases (provided no parenchymal damage).
- ***In infectious hepatitis*** and ***parenchymatous livercells damage,*** rise in blood sugar is greater than above, but the increases obtained are never very great.

• *Epinephrine Tolerance Test (Storage Function)*

Principle: The response to epinephrine as evidenced by elevation of blood sugar is a manifestation of glycogenolysis and is directly influenced by glycogen stores of liver.

Method

- The patient is kept on a high carbohydrate diet for three days before the test.
- After an overnight fast, the fasting blood sugar is determined.

- 0.01 ml of a 1 in 1000 solution of epinephrine per kg body weight is injected.
- The blood sugar is then determined in samples collected at 15 minutes intervals up to one hour.

Interpretations

- *Normally,* in the course of an hour, the rise in blood sugar over the fasting level exceeds by 40 mg% or more.
- *In parenchymal hepatic disease,* the rise is less.
- It is of much use for ***diagnosis of glycogen storge diseases,*** specially in von Gierke disease, in which blood glucose rise is not seen due to lack of glucose-6-phosphatase.

III. TESTS BASED ON CHANGES ON PLASMA PROTEINS

(a) *Determination of Total Plasma Proteins, Albumin, globulin and A:G Ratio*

This yields most useful information in chronic liver diseases.

Liver is the site of albumin synthesis and also possibly of some of α and β-globulins.

Interpretations

- *In infectious hepatitis:* quantitative estimations of albumin and globulin may give normal results in the early stages. Qualitative changes may be present, in early stage rise in β globulins and in later stage γ-globulins show rise.
- *In obstructive jaundice:* normal values are the rule, as long as it is not associated with accompanying liver cells damage.
- *In advanced parenchymal liver disease, and in cirrhosis liver:* the albumin is grossly decreased and the globulins are often increased, so that A:G ratio is reversed, such a pattern is characteristically seen in cirrhosis liver.

The albumin may fall below 2.5 gm% and may be a contributory factor in causing oedema in such cases.

Fractionation of globulins reveals that the increase is usually in the γ-globulin fraction, but in some cases there is a smaller increase in β-globulins.

Note

- The severity of hypoalbuminaemia in chronic liver diseases is of diagnostic importance and may serve as a criterion of the degree of damage.
- A low serum albumin which fails to increase during treatment is usually a poor prognostic sign.

(b) *Estimation of Plasma Fibrinogen*

Fibrinogen is formed in the liver and likely to be affected if considerable liver damage is present.

Normal value is 200 to 400 mg%.

Values below 100 mg% have been reported in severe parenchymal liver damage. Such a situation is found in severe acute insufficiency such as may occur in

(i) acute hepatic necrosis,
(ii) poisoning from carbon tetrachloride, and
(iii) in advanced stages of liver cirrhosis

(c) *Flocculation Tests*

Principle: Flocculation tests depend on an alteration in the type of proteins present in the plasma. The alteration may be either quantitative or qualitative and most frequently involves one or more of the globulin fractions.

1. Thymol Turbidity Tests

Thymol turbidity: The degree of turbidity produced when serum is mixed with a buffered solutin of thymol is measured. Turbidity produced is compared with a set of protein standards, or turbidity is read in a colorimeter agaisnt a $BaSO_4$ standard.

Maclagan unit: Maclagan expressd the results in units, so that a turbidity equivalent to that of 10 mg/100 ml protein standard is one unit.

Basis of the reaction: The thymol turbidity test requires lipids (phospholipids). The turbidity/and flocculation in this test is a complex of **"lipothymoprotein."** The thymol seems to decrease the dispersion and solubility of the lipids, and the proteins involved is mainly β-globulin, though some γ-globulin is also precipitated.

Interpretations

- ***Normal range*** is 0 to 4 units.
- It measures only an acute process in the liver, but the degree of turbidity is not proportional to the severity of the disease.
- *In infectious hepatitis:* it is highest soon after the onset of the jaundice, but frequently remains raised for several weeks.
- Sera with high β and γ-globulin fractions, due to other causes may give a positive test.
- ***A negative thymol test in the presence of jaundice is very useful for distinguishing between hepatic and extrahepatic jaundice.***

Thymol Flocculation Test

After the turbidity has been measured, the tubes are kept in the dark for overnight and read the degree of flocculation if any. Flocculation is graded as –ve no flocculation, +ve flocculation as +, ++, +++, and ++++.

2. *Zinc Sulphate Turbidity Test*

When a serum having an abnormally high content of γ-globulin is diluted with a solution containing buffered $ZnSO_4$ solution, a turbidity develops. The amount of turbidity is proportional to concentration of γ-globulin. Turbidity is measured as discussed in thymol turbidity test.

Interpretations

- ***Normal range*** varies from 2 to 8 units.
- All cases of ***cirrhosis liver*** give +ve results.
- ***In infectious hepatitis***-γ-globulin is increased in later stage. $ZnSO_4$ turbidity becomes +ve later as compared to thymol turbidity which becomes +ve early.
- It may be +ve in other cases where there is increase in γ-globulin.

3. *Jirgl's Flocculation Test*

A flocculation test was described by **Jirgl**, in which he observed flocculation ++ to +++ in all obstructive jaundice cases. He suggested a negative thymol turbidity, and a +ve (++ to +++) Jirgl's flocculation test in a clinical jaundice with serum ALP more than 50 KA units % will be almost diagnostic for obstructive jaundice.

4. *Formol-Gel Test*

This test also ***detects increase in globulins.*** Add one drop of formalin to one ml of serum in a narrow test tube, shake and keep for sometime. When +ve serum solidifies within a few minutes, sometimes becoming opaque.

Interpretations

- A +ve test is mainly found in conditions in which there is increased serum globulins.
- It is found ***+ve in chronic liver diseases,*** but it is ***not specific.*** Positive test has been reported in conditions such as multiple myeloma, sarcoidosis, severe malarial infections, trypansomiasis, and in many other chronic infections.
- The test has been mainly used for diagnosis of kala-azar.

Other turbidity/and flocculation tests viz, cephalin-cholesterol flocculation test, Takata-Ara test, etc., have become outmoded.

(d) *Amino Acids in Urine (Amino Aciduria)*

The daily excretion of amino acid nitrogen in normal health varies from 80 to 300 mg. Amino-aciduria found in severe liver diseases is of "overflow" type, with accompanying increase in plasma amino acids level.

Clinical Importance

In severe liver diseases like acute yellow atrophy and sometimes in advanced cirrhosis of liver crystals of certain amino acids may be found in urinary deposits microscopically.

a. ***Tyrosine crystals:*** Tyrosine crystallizes in sheaves or tufts of fine needles.

b. ***Leucine crystals:*** Leucine has spherical shaped crystals, yellowish in colour, with radial and circular striations.

Both are insoluble in acetone and ether but soluble in acids/and alkalies. Tyrosine is only slightly soluble in acetic acid and insoluble in ethanol, whereas leucine is soluble in the former and slightly soluble in the latter.

IV. TESTS BASED ON ABNORMALITIES OF LIPIDS

- ***Cholesterol-Cholesteryl Ester Ratio***

The liver plays an active and important role in the metabolism of cholesterol including its synthesis, esterification, oxidation and excretion.

Interpretations

- ***Normal total blood cholesterol:*** ranges from 150 to 250 mg/dl and approximately 60 to 70% of this is in esterified form.
- ***In obstructive jaundice:*** an increase in total blood cholesterol is common, but the ester fraction is also raised, so that % esterified does not change. It has been observed that the ratio of free and ester cholesterol is usually not changed unless accompanied by parenchymal damage.
- ***In parenchymatous liver diseases:*** there is either no rise or even decrease in total cholesterol and the **ester fraction is always definitely reduced.** The degree of reduction roughly parallels the degree of liver damage.
- ***In severe acute hepatic necrosis:*** the total serum cholesterol is usually low and may fall below 100 mg/dl, whilst there is marked reduction in the percentage present as esters.

V. TESTS BASED ON THE DETOXICATING FUNCTION OF THE LIVER

(a) *Hippuric Acid Test of Quick*

- Best known test for the detoxicating function of liver.
- Liver removes benzoic acid, administered as sodium benzoate, either orally or IV and combines with the amino acid glycine, to form hippuric acid. The amount of hippuric acid excreted in urine in a fixed time is determined.
- The test thus **depends on two factors:**
  a. The ability of liver cells to produce and provide sufficient glycine and
  b. The capacity of liver cells to conjugate it with the benzoic acid.
- ***For reliable result-renal function must be normal.*** If there is any reason to suspect renal impairment, a urea clearance test should be done simultaneously.

Method

Both oral and IV forms of the hippuric acid test are in use

1. Oral Hippuric Acid Test

- Dissolve 6.0 gm of sodium benzoate in approximately 200 ml of water.
- The test may be started 3 hours after a light breakfast of toast and tea. Food should not be given until late in the test.
- The patient empties the bladder, the urine being discarded.
- The patient is allowed to drink the sodium benzoate solution and time is noted.
- The bladder is again emptied 4 hours later. Any urine passed during this 4 hours is kept and added to that passed at the end of 4 hours.
- The amount of hippuric acid excreted in this 4 hours period is estimated.

Interpretations

- Normally, at least 3.0 gm of hippuric acid, expressed as benzoic acid or 3.5 gm of sodium benzoate should be excreted in health.
- Smaller amounts are found when there is either acute or chronic liver damage. Amounts lower than 1.0 gm may be excreted by patients with infectious hepatitis.

2. *Intravenous Hippuric Acid Test*

Indications: Normally oral test is preferred. **An IV test is indicated:**

- When there is impairment of absorption due to absorption defects.
- If there is accompanying nausea/vomiting.

Procedure

- A sterile solution of sodium benozate 1.77 gm dissolved in 20 ml of DW is given intravenously.
- Shortly before the injection, the patient empties the bladder, which is discarded.
- The bladder is emptied after one hour and two hours after the injection.

Interpretations

- *In normal health,* hippuric acid equivalent to at least 0.85 gm of sodium benzoate, or to 0.7 gm of benzoic acid should be excreted in one hour, or equivalent to 1.15 gm of benzoic acid in the first two hours.
- Excretion of smaller amounts than above indicate the presence of liver damage.

(b) The Amino Antipyrine Breath Test

The test is based on detoxicating function of liver.

Principle: Aminopyrine is metabolized by the liver by N-demethylation to give CO_2.

Using (^{14}C) methyl-labelled aminopyrine, the appearance of $^{14}CO_2$ corresponds to the microsomal mixed function oxidase of liver cells.

Method

- After an overnight fast, 2 μc: of amino (^{14}C) Pyrine and 2 mg of unlabelled aminopyrine is administered orally.
- Breath, dried over calcium sulphate, is bubbled through a solution of 2 ml ethanol and 1 ml of hyamine hydroxide (1 mol/L containing 2 drops of phenolphthalein as indicator).
- When the indicator colour changes indicating the absorption of 1 mmol of CO_2, the activity of $^{14}CO_2$ is measured in a scintillation counter.

Interpretation

- $^{14}CO_2$ excretion is reduced in parenchymal liver diseases, such as cirrhosis of liver, acute and chronic hepatitis and in malignancy of liver.
- Overlapping of values in these conditions limits the disgnostic use of this test, but it is claimed that the test is more reliable than other conventional LFTs, to predict short term survival, clinical improvement and histological severity more reliably.

VI. TESTS BASED ON EXCRETORY FUNCTION OF LIVER

1. BSP-Retention Test (Bromsulphalein Test)

Principle:

- The ability of the liver to excrete certain dyes, e.g., BSP is utilized in this test.
- In normal healthy individual, a constant proportion (10–15% of the dye) is removed per minute. In hepatic damage and insufficiency, BSP removal is impaired by cellular failure, as damaged liver cells fail to conjugate the dye or due to decrease blood flow.
- Removal of BSP by the liver involves conjugation of the dye as a mercaptide with the cysteine component of glutathione. The reaction of conjugation of BSP with glutathione is ***rate-limiting,*** and thus it exerts a controlling influence on the rate of removal of the dye.

Procedure

- With the patient fasting, inject IV slowly, an amount of 5% BSP solution, which contains 5 mg of BSP/kg, body weight.
- Withdraw 5 to 10 ml of blood, 25 and 45 minutes after the injection and allow the specimens to clot. Separate the sera and estimate amount of the dye in each sample.

Interpretations

- ***In normal healthy*** individual not more than 5% of the dye should remain in the blood at the end of 45 minutes. The bulk of the dye is removed in 25 minutes and less than 15% is left at the end of 25 minutes.

- *In parenchymatous liver diseases,* removal proceeds more slowly. In advanced cirrhosis removal is very slow and 40 to 50% of the dye is retained in 45 minutes sample.

Contraindication: Since the dye is removed in bile after conjugation, this test can only be used in cases in which there is no obstruction to the flow of bile. **Hence the test is of no value if obstruction of biliary tree exists (obstructive jaundice).**

Clinical Significance

- BSP-excretion test is a useful index of liver damage, particularly when the damage is diffuse and extensive.
- The **test is most useful in:**
  - **(i)** Liver cell damage without jaundice;
  - **(ii)** Cirrhosis liver; and
  - **(iii)** Chronic hepatitis.

2. Rose Bengal Dye Test

Rose Bengal is another dye which can be used to assess excretory function. Ten ml of a 1% solution of the dye is injected IV slowly.

Interpretation

Normally 50% or more of the dye disappears within 8 minutes.

^{131}I-labelled Rose Bengal

Recently, ^{131}I-Rose Bengal has been used where isotope laboratory is present. ^{131}I-labelled Rose Bengal is administered IV. Then count is taken over the neck and abdomen. Initially, count is more in neck, practically nil over abdomen. **As the dye is excreted through liver, neck count goes down and count over abdomen increases.**

In parenchymal liver diseases, high count in the neck persists and there is hardly rise in count over abdomen, as the dye is retained.

3. Bilirubin Tolerance Test

One mg/kg body weight of bilirubin is injected IV. If more than 5% of the injected bilirubin is retained after 4 hours, the excretory and conjugating function of the liver is considered abnormal.

The bilirubin excretion test has been recommended by some authorities as a better test of excretory function of the liver as compared to dye tests as bilirubin is a normal physiologic substance and the dyes are foreign to the body. But the test is not used routinely and extensively due to its high cost.

Note

The three substances listed above, with the exception of BSP, are excreted almost entirely by the liver. No significant amounts are taken up by RE cells.

VII. FORMATION OF PROTHROMBIN BY LIVER

Prothrombin is formed in the liver from inactive *"pre-prothrombin"* in presence of vitamin K. Prothrombin activity is measured as prothrombin time (PT). The term prothrombin time was given to time required for clotting to take place in citrated plasma to which optimum amounts of **"thromboplastin"** and Ca^{2+} have been added.

The "one-stage" technique introduced by Quick, the prothrombin time is related inversely to the concentration not only to prothrombin, but also of factors V, VII and X and it can be more sensitive to a lack of VII and X than to prothrombin alone. In spite of above restriction, as it is simple and quick in performance, it is still much used.

Interpretations

- *Normal levels* of prothrombin in *control* give prothrombin time of approx 14 seconds. (Range 10–16 sec.) Results are always expressed as patient's prothrombin time in seconds to normal control value.
- *In parenchymatous liver diseases:* depending on the degree of liver cells damage

plasma prothrombin time may be increased from 22 to as much as 150 secs.

- *In obstructive jaundice:* due to absence of bile salts, there may be defective absorption of vitamin K, hence PT is increased, as prothrombin formation suffers.
- From above, it is observed that PT is increased both in obstructive jaundice and in diseases of liver cells damage. **Hence, PT cannot be used to differentiate between them.** However, if adequate vitamin K is administered parenterally, the PT returns rapidly to normal in uncomplicated obstructive jaundice, whereas in liver damage the response is less marked.

Other Clinical Uses

- PT is used mostly in controlling anticoagulant therapy.
- Determination of PT is also used to decide whether there is danger of bleeding at operation in biliary tract diseases.

Prothrombin index: Prothrombin activity is also sometimes expressed as *"prothrombin index"* in %, which is the ratio of prothrombin time of the normal control to the patient's prothrombin time multiplied by 100. Thus,

$$\text{Prothrombin index} = \frac{\text{PT of normal control}}{\text{PT of patient}} \quad 100$$

- *Normally,* index is 70 to 100%. The **"critical level"** below which bleeding may occur is not fixed one, but there is always a possibility of this occurring if prothrombin index is below 60%.

VIII. TESTS BASED ON AMINO ACID CATABOLISM

1. Determination of Blood Ammonia

Nitrogen part of amino acid is converted to NH_3 in the liver mainly by transamination and deamination (transdeamination) and it is converted to urea in liver only. Following are the **other sources of ammonia.**

- NH_3 is formed from nitrogenous material by bacterial action in the gut.
- In kidneys, by hydrolysis of glutamine by *glutaminase.*
- A small amount of NH_3 is formed from catabolism of pyrimidines.

Interpretations

- *The normal range* of blood ammonia varies from 40 to 75 μg ammonia nitrogen per 100 ml of blood.
- In parenchymal liver diseases, the ability to remove NH_3 coming to liver from intestine and other sources may be impaired.
- Increases in NH_3 can be found in more advanced cases of cirrhosis liver, particularly when there are associated neurological complications. In such cases blood levels may be over 200 μg/100 ml. Very high values may be obtained in hepatic coma.

2. Ammonia Tolerance Test

An ammonia tolerance test has been devised to test the ability of the liver to deal with NH_3 coming to it from the intestine.

Procedure

- The patient should come for the test after over night 12 hours fast, only small amounts of fluids can be taken during that time.
- Take fasting specimen of blood for NH_3 determination.
- After that, give orally 10 gm of ammonium citrate dissolved in water and flavoured with fruit juice/lemon.
- Take blood samples after 30, 60, 120 and 180 minutes and determine blood NH_3.

Note: In patients with increased initial levels, give smaller doses, e.g. only 5 grams.

Interpretations

- *In normal healthy persons:* little increase is found; blood NH_3 levels remaining within normal range.

- ***In advanced cirrhosis liver:*** marked rise to twice the initial level or more, exceeding 200 to 300 µg% are seen.
- Considerable increases are also seen when there is a collateral circulation and in patients who have a portocaval anastomosis.

3. Determination of Glutamine in Cerebrospinal Fluid (An Indirect Liver Function Test)

Glutamine, the amide of glutamic acid, is formed by *glutamine synthetase* by glutamic acid and NH_3.

Glutamine in cerebrospinal fluid can be estimated by the method of **Whittaker** (1955). The glutamine is hydrolyzed to glutamic acid and NH_3 by the action of dilute acid at 100°. A correction is made for a small amount of NH_3 produced from urea. No other substances present in CS fluid were found to form NH_3 under above conditions.

Interpretations

- ***The normal range:*** found to be 6.0 to 14.0 mg%.
- ***In infectious hepatitis:*** glutamine was found to range from 16 to 28 mg%, but usually less than 30 mg%.
- ***In cirrhosis liver:*** the increase is more; depending on the severity. It varied from 22 to 36 mg% or more.
- ***In hepatic coma:*** increase is very high, ranging from 30 to 60 mg% or more.
- ***In other types of coma:*** normal values are obtained.

Some authorities put ***40 mg% as a critical level.*** Prognosis of the case is fatal if CSF glutamine level is more than 40 mg%, in case of cirrhosis liver and hepatic coma.

IX. VALUE OF SERUM ENZYMES IN LIVER DISEASES

Quite a large number of enzyme estimations are available which are used to ascertain liver function. But most commonly and routinely employed in laboratories are two:

(i) serum transaminases (aminotransferases), and

(ii) serum alkaline phosphatase.

1. Serum Transaminases (Aminotransferases)

Interpretations

- ***Normal ranges:*** for these enzymes are as follows:
    - ***SGOT (aspartate transaminase):*** 4 to 17 IU/L (7–35 units/ml)
    - ***SGPT (alanine transaminase):*** 3 to 15 IU/L (6–32 units/ml)
- *Both these enzymes* are found in most tissues, but the relative amounts vary. Heart muscles are richer in SGOT, whereas liver contains both but more of SGPT.
- ***Increases in both transaminases:*** are found in liver diseases, with SGPT much higher than SGOT. Their determination is of limited value in differential diagnosis of jaundice because of considerable overlapping. But their determination is of extreme use in assessing the severity and prognosis of parenchymal liver diseases specially acute infectious hepatitis and serum hepatitis. In these two conditions, highest values in thousand units are seen.
- ***In outbreak of infectious hepatitis (viral hepatitis):*** it is the most sensitive diagnostic index. The increase can be seen in prodromal stage, when jaundice has not appeared clinically. Such cases can be isolated and segregated from others, so that spread of the disease can be checked.
- ***Very high values are also obtained in toxic hepatitis:*** due to carbontetrachloride poisoning. Increases are comparatively less in drug hepatitis (cholestatic) like chloropromazine.
- ***In obstructive jaundice (extrahepatic)*** also, increases occur but usually do not exceed 200 to 300 IU/L.

2. Serum Alkaline Phosphatase

Alkaline phosphatase enzyme is found in a number of organs, most plentiful in bones and liver, than in small intestine, kidney and placenta. **Placental isoenzyme of alkaline phosphatase is heat-stable.**

Interpretations

- *Normal range:* for serum ALP as per King-Armströng method is 3 to 13 KA U/100 ml (23–92 IU/L).
- It is ***used*** for ***many years in differential diagnosis of jaundice.*** It is increased in both infectious hepatitis (viral hepatitis) and posthepatic jaundice (extrahepatic obstruction) but the rise is usually much greater in cases of obstructive jaundice. **Dividing Line which has been suggested is 35 KA U/100 ml.** A value higher than 35 KA U/100 ml is strongly suggestive of diagnosis of obstructive jaundice, in which very high figures even up to 200 units or more may be found. There is certain amount of overlapping mostly in the range of 30 to 45 KA U/ 100 ml.
- Very high values are occasionally found in certain liver diseases, e.g. xantomatous biliary cirrhosis in which there is no extrahepatic obstruction.
- Higher values are also obtained in ***space-occupying lesions of liver,*** e.g., abscess, primary carcinoma (hepatoma), metastatic carcinoma, infiltrative lesions like lymphoma, granuloma and amyloidosis. **A diagnostic triad suggested is:**
  - ***High serum ALP,***
  - ***Impaired BSP-retention,*** and
  - ***Normal/or almost normal serum bilirubin.***
- Serum ALP is found to be normal in haemolytic jaundice.

Mechanism of increase in ALP in liver diseases: Increase in the activity of ALP in liver diseases is not due to hepatic cell disruption, nor to a failure of clearance, but rather **to increased synthesis of hepatic ALP.** The stimulus for this increased synthesis in patients with liver diseases has been ***attributed to bile duct obstruction*** either ***extrahepatically by stones, tumours, strictures or intrahepatically by infiltrative disorders*** or ***"space occupying lesions."***

Note: The relation of the aminotransferase to ALP level may provide better evidence than either test alone, as to whether or not the jaundice is cholestatic.

- ***High ALP with low aminotransferase activity is usual in cholestasis and the converse occurs in non-cholestatic jaundice.*** It is, however, stressed that there are several intrahepatic causes of cholestasis such as primary biliary cirrhosis, acute alcoholic hepatitis and sclerosing cholangitis in which laparotomy is in-appropriate. Hence, even after a confident diagnosis of cholestatic jaundice based on the LFTs, further investigation to define the site of obstruction is imperative.

OTHER ENZYMES

Other enzymes which have been found to be useful but not routinely done in the laboratory are discussed below briefly.

3. Serum 5'-Nucleotidase

This enzyme hydrolyzes nucleotides with a phosphate group on carbon atom 5′ of the ribose, e.g., adenosine 5′-P, hydrolytic products being adenosine and inorganic PO_4. These nucleotides are also hydrolyzed by nonspecific phosphatases such as alkaline phosphatase present in the serum. However, ***5′-nucleotidase is inactivated by nickel, hence if hydrolysis is carried out with and without added nickel, the difference gives the 5′-nucleotidase activity.***

Interpretations

- ***Normal range:*** is 2 to 17 IU/L
- ***Liver diseases:***
  - Serum 5′-nucleotidase is raised along with serum ALP in diseases of liver and biliary tract in a roughly parallel man-

ner. It is thus highest in posthepatic obstructive jaundice frequently over 100 units. ***It has added advantage over serum ALP in that enzyme is not affected in bone diseases.***

- Smaller increases are found in hepatic jaundice, e.g. in infectious hepatitis, in some cases of which normal results are obtained.

- In bone diseases such as Paget's disease, 5'-nucleotidase is normal in patients with increased serum ALP.

4. Serum Lactate Dehydrogenase (LDH)

LDH enzyme is widely distributed, found in all cells in man, but is specially plentiful in cardiac and skeletal muscle, liver, kidney and the red blood cells.

Interpretations

- ***Normal range:*** is 70 to 240 IU/L
- ***In liver diseases*** an increased activity is found, particularly in infectious hepatitis, but the increase is not so great as that of the transaminases and its behaviour is less predictable.
- ***The enzyme is less specific*** and as it is widespread, increase of the enzyme activity is also seen in many other diseases like leukaemias, pernicious anaemia, megaloblastic and haemolytic anaemias, in renal diseases and in generalized carcinomatosis.
- ***In cirrhosis liver and posthepatic jaundice (obstructive jaundice),*** normal results are often found.

Isoenzymes LDH

LDH has ***five isoenzymes*** which differ at the level of quarternary structure. Active LDH molecule has mol. wt. 130,000 daltons, it is a **tetramer,** ***four subunits of two types 'H' and 'M'*** each having a mol. wt. of 34,000 daltons. Only the tetrameric form possesses the catalytic activity.

Five Isoenzymes	*Subunits*	*mol. formula*
• LDH-1	HHHH	H_4
• LDH-2	HHHM	H_3M
• LDH-3	HHMM	H_2M_2
• LDH-4	HMMM	HM_3
• LDH-5	MMMM	M_4

In starch gel electrophoresis, LDH-1 moves farthest towards the anode and fast moving LDH-1 is found between albumin and α_1-globulins. LDH-2 moves in position of α_2, LDH-3 in β region, LDH-4 with fast γ and LDH-5 rather behind γ-globulins (slowest moving).

Interpretations

- ***Cardiac muscle:*** is richest in LDH-1 (H_4) with diminishing proportions of LDH-2 to LDH-5, in that order.
- ***In liver:*** *LDH-5* is preponderant isoenzyme, with diminishing proportions of LDH-4 to 1.
- ***Marked increase of LDH-5*** *iso-enzyme* occurs in liver diseases.

5. Serum Iso-citrate Dehydrogenase (ICD)

A specific enzyme found in liver.

- ***Normal range*** 0.9 to 4.0 IU/L
- ***In liver diseases:*** A marked increase in ICD activity seen whether it is inflammatory like infectious hepatitis, malignancy or from taking drugs. Large increases are seen in infectious hepatitis; serum activity almost returns to normal by the 3rd week after the onset of jaundice.
  - ***In obstructive jaundice:*** normal values are the rule.
  - In most cases of cirrhosis liver, serum enzyme activity is either normal or slightly raised.

6. Serum Cholinesterases

Cholinesterases are enzymes which hydrolyze esters of choline to give choline and acid. Two types have been distinguished:

(i) "True", and

(ii) "Pseudo".

- ***'True' cholinesterase:*** It is thought to be responsible for the destruction of acetylcholine at the neuromuscular junction and is found in nerve tissues and RBC.
- ***'Pseudo' cholinesterases:*** These are found in various tissues such as liver, heart muscle and intestine and it is this type which is present in plasma.

Interpretations

- ***Normal range:*** is 2.17 to 5.17 IU/ml. (130 to 310 units of de la Huerga)
- ***Liver diseases:***
  - The enzyme is formed in liver and serum activity is reduced in liver cells damage. Hence, determination has been **used for recognising liver damage. (Protein synthesis?)**
  - Low values are also obtained in advanced cases of cirrhosis liver.
- Normal serum activity seen in obstructive jaundice cases.
- Serial estimations has been found to be of value in prognosis of infectious hepatitis and cirrhosis liver.

7. *Serum Ornithine Carbamoyl Transferase (OCT)*

This enzyme catalyzes the following reaction:

$$\text{Ornithine} + \text{Carbamoyl-P} \underset{}{\overset{\text{OCT}}{\rightleftarrows}} \text{Citrulline} + PO_4.$$

It is involved in urea synthesis.

Note: Note that this enzyme is exclusively found in liver and virtually no activity in other tissues.

Interpretations

- Serum enzyme activity ***in normal healthy individuals*** usually very low and ranges from 8 to 20 m-IU.
- ***In liver diseases:***
  - The enzyme level is markedly elevated 10 to 200 fold in patients with acute viral hepatitis depending on the severity and also those with other forms of hepatic necrosis.
  - Relatively slight elevations occur in obstructive jaundice, cirrhosis liver, metastatic carcinoma, etc.
- **Serum OCT appears to be a specific and sensitive measure for hepatocellular injury.**

8. *Serum Leucine Amino Peptidase (LAP)*

It is a ***proteolytic enzyme*** which splits off N-terminal residues from certain L-peptides and amides having a free NH_2 group, especially when the N-terminal residue is leucine or related aminoacid.

Interpretations

- ***Normal range*** is 15 to 56 m-Iu.
- ***In viral hepatitis:*** there is mild to moderate increase and ranges from 30 to 130 m-Iu.
- Increases also seen **in cirrhosis liver** but rise is less. It has been observed by some workers and corroborated by PM studies that ***marked increase in cirrhosis liver is usually associated with superimposed hepatoma.***
- ***In obstructive jaundice:*** marked increase is seen like alkaline phosphatase. Increase is more in malignant obstruction than that of benign obstruction. In one series benign obstruction showed 75 to 184 m-Iu (average 101.25 m-Iu), whereas malignant obstruction showed 67 to 340 m-IU (average 105 m-Iu)
- ***Advantage over serum ALP is that LAP does not rise in osseous involvement.***
- Marked rise has been seen **in liver cell carcinoma (hepatoma).**

9. Serum Hydroxy Butyrate Dehydrogenase (SHBD)

An enzyme acting on α-hydroxy butyric acid has been identified in the serum and studied as a diagnostic aid in liver diseases.

Interpretations

- ***Normal SHBD:*** is 56 to 125 IU/L
- ***In liver diseases:*** elevated levels of this enzyme is observed in acute viral hepatitis. Also elevated level is seen in myocardial infarction.

Ratio of LDH/SHBD:

To Differentiate the two, ratio of $\frac{\text{LDH}}{\text{SHBD}}$ has been found more useful.

- **Normal ratio of** $\frac{\text{LDH}}{\text{SHBD}} = 1.18$ to 1.60
- Less than 1.18 is observed in most cases of myocardial infarction.
- Greater than >1.60 is observed in Liver diseases.
- In infectious hepatitis, the ratio is frequently > 2.0. In chronic hepatitis and obstructive jaundice the ratio ranges from 1.6 to 2.0.

10. Serum Aldolase and Phosphohexose Isomerase

These are both markedly increased in serum of patients with acute hepatitis. No increase is found in cirrhosis, latent hepatitis or biliary obstruction.

11. Serum Amylase

Liver is a major, if not the only source of amylase found in the serum under normal physiologic conditions. Studies have shown low serum amylase levels in liver diseases like acute infectious hepatitis.

12. Serum Sorbitol Dehydrogenase (SDH)

SDH catalyzes the following reaction:

$$\text{Sorbitol} + \text{NAD}^+ \underset{}{\overset{\text{SDH}}{\rightleftarrows}} \text{Fructose} + \text{NADH}$$

Interpretation

- ***Normal serum values:*** are found to be less than 0.2 m-IU.
- Striking elevation seen in acute viral hepatitis and carbontetrachloride poisoning up to 17 mIU. In viral hepatitis, values of SDH return to normal before transaminases.
- ***In chronic hepatitis and in obstructive jaundice,*** serum levels of SDH are normal or only slightly elevated.
- Myocardial and other extrahepatic diseases do not lead to elevated levels.

Advantages

- Like OCT, it is a ***hepato-specific enzyme.***
- The serial estimation is of immense value in diagnosis and follow-up for prognosis of Infectious hepatitis.
- Also of immense value in differential diagnosis of jaundice.
- Enzyme has been recently demonstrated in small amount in kidney and prostate but no increase in activity in the diseases of these organs noted.

- ***Serum γ-Glutamyl Transferase (γ-GT)***
- ***Normal range:*** is 10 to 47 IU/L

Table 2.1: Enzyme assays as per priorities useful in detecting alterations in liver diseases

	Alterations detected	*Principal enzyme assays*
a.	Hepatocellular damage/or increased permeability of liver cells.	• Transaminases (aminotransferases): SGOT and SGPT. • Ornithine carbamoyl transferase (OCT) • Sorbitol dehydrogenase (SDH)
b.	Extrahepatic or intrahepatic obstruction benign/malignant.	• Alkaline phosphatase • 5′-Nucleotidase • γ-GT • LAP
c.	Protein synthesis	• Pseudo cholinesterase
d.	Alcohol abuse	• γ-GT

Table 2.2: Differentiation of three types of jaundice

	Haemolytic or prehepatic jaundice	*Hepatic or parenchymatous jaundice*	*Obstructive or posthepatic jaundice*
I. *Causes*	Due to excessive haemolysis i. Intrinsic defects in RBC ii. Extrinsic causes external to RBC	Disease of parenchymal cells of Liver e.g. Viral hepatitis, toxic jaundice. Cirrhosis liver, fibrosis	Due to obstruction of biliary passage i. extrahepatic gall-stones, tumours, enlarged lymph nodes, etc. ii. Intrahepatic cholestasis.
II. *Clinical findings*			
• Degree of jaundice	Usually low +	Marked jaundice ++ to +++	Marked jaundice ++ to +++
• Faeces	Dark coloured	Variable, usually pale	Clay coloured
III. *Biochemical findings* Based on bile pigment metabolism			
• *VD Bergh reaction*	Indirect, may be delayed positive	Biphasic	Direct
• *Type of bile pigment in circulation*	Unconjugated bilirubin	Mixture of conjugated and unconjugated bilirubin	Conjugated bilirubin
• *Serum bilirubin*	Usually low, 3 to 5 mg%	High, up to 20 mg%	Very high, may be up to 50 mg%
• *Bile pigments in urine*			
a. Bilirubin	Not detected	Present	Present ++
b. Urobilinogen	Increased ++	May be increased + or normal	Decreased or Absent
• *Faecal stercobilinogen*	Increased ++	Decreased	Decreased or absent
IV. *Steatorrhoea*	Not present	Present	Present
V. *Other biochemical features*			
• **Prothrombin time (PT)**	Normal	Increased	Increased, After parental vit K becomes normal
• **Turbidity and flocculation tests**			
a. Thymol turbidity	Negative	++ to +++	Negative
b. Jirgl's flocculation test	Negative	± to +	++ to +++
• *Enzyme assays*			
a. *Aminotransferase activity* ALT (SGPT)	Usually normal	Marked increase +++ to ++++ (goes in thousand units). Usually 500 to 1500 IU/L or may be more	Increased to ++. Usually 100 to 300 IU/L Do not exceed 300 IU/L
b. *Alkaline phosphatase (ALP)*	Normal	Increased slightly (+), usually less than 30 KA U %	Marked increase, 30 to 100 KA U %, more than 35 KA U % suggests obstructive jaundice.
c. *5'-Nucleotidase*	Normal	Increased (+) Slight	Marked increase ++ to +++

- **Recently, the importance of this enzyme in alcohol abuse has been stressed.** The activity of this microsomal enzyme has been found to increase in most of hepatobiliary diseases but, largely because of the enzyme's wide tissue distribution, the specificity of a high value is very low. Unlike the aminotransferases, the elevated levels do not necessarily indicate liver cell disruption but may be due to enzyme induction by drugs such as, phenobarbitone, phenytoin, warfarin and alcohol.

These severe limitations have meant that this test has now only two, practical uses:

(*i*) an elevated γ-GT implies that an elevated ALP is of hepatic origin, and

(*ii*) it may be useful in screening for alcohol abuse. ***Sudden increase in γ-GT in chronic alcoholics suggests recent bout of drinking of alcohols.***

Chapter 3

Gastric Function Tests

INTRODUCTION

In diseases of the stomach and duodenum alterations of gastric secretion often occur. Chemical examination of gastric contents has a limited but specific value in the diagnosis and assessment of disorders of the upper gastrointestinal tract, e.g., peptic ulcer, cancer of the stomach, etc. In order to obtain complete data regarding gastric function, the contents of the stomach should be examined

(i) during the resting period;
(ii) during the period of digestion after giving a meal; and
(iii) after stimulation.

In 24 hours the normal healthy stomach secretes about 1000 ml of gastric juice when the subject is fasting. But the stomach of a person taking a normal diet secretes 2000-3000 ml of juice per 24 hours.

The chief constituents of gastric juice are:

- *HCl:* secreted by the parietal cells
- *Pepsinogen:* secreted by zymogen cells or "chief" cells
- *Rennin:* only found in infants/babies and not in adult gastric juice
- *Intrinsic factor:* required for absorption of vitamin B_{12}
- Other cells produce an alkaline mucus.

INDICATIONS OF GASTRIC FUNCTIONS TESTS

Gastric analysis may be of value in the following:

- Diagnosis of gastric ulcer.
- Exclusion of diagnosis of pernicious anaemia and of peptic ulcer in a patient with gastric ulceration.
- Diagnosis of pulmonary tuberculosis.
- Presumptive diagnosis of Zollinger-Ellison syndrome.
- Determination of the completeness of surgical vagotomy.

The above are the only situations in which gastric analysis has significant clinical value.

Cytologic examination of gastric juice fluid has not been included as part of gastric analysis.

CLASSIFICATION

Tests commonly employed for assessing gastric function are:

I. ***Examination of resting contents in resting juice (gastric residuum).***
II. ***Fractional gastric analysis using a test 'meal'.***
III. ***Examination of the contents after stimulation.***
   a. "Alcohol" stimulation.
   b. Caffeine stimulation.
   c. i. Histamine stimulation
      ii. Augmented histamine test
   d. Insulin stimulation
   e. Pentagastrin test
IV. *Tubless gastric analysis*

COLLECTION OF CONTENTS OF STOMACH

- The stomach contents are collected after introducing a stomach tube by nasogastric route into the stomach and removing the contents by aspiration. The resting gastric contents are completely removed for examination.

- Gastric contents are removed after a "test meal" to see the response of stomach. In this, small samples 5 to 6 ml of the gastric contents are removed after every 15 minutes and the samples are collected in small sterile clean Bottles.

Types of St omachT ubes

- The stomach tubes is made of rubber or plastic and has an external diameter of 4 mm.
- **Two types of tubes** are in use:
  - *Rehfuss tube:* This has an uncovered metal end with openings about the size of the bore of the tube
  - *Ryle's tube:* This is commonly used. It has a covered end containing a small weight of lead, the holes being in the tube a short distance from the end.
- *Markings on the tubes:* Both tubes have markings to indicate how far the tube has been swallowed by the patient. The markings are in the form of **black rings.**
  - When the single ring reaches the lips, sufficient tube has been swallowed so that tip reaches the cardiac end.
  - When the double ring reaches the lips, the tube should be in body of the stomach, sometimes almost to pylorus (about a distance of 50 cm).

Suhfdxwlrq

The tube should be boiled in water and before passing it should be lubricated with liquid paraffin or glycerol.

Note:

- Ryle's tube is easier to swallow and less likely to cause trauma.
- But disadvantage is that the Ryle's tube tends to block more easily.

Huuruv#lq#Froohfwlrq#ri#Vdpsohv

Common errors are as follows:

- Tube may be blocked with mucus or food residues, so that the stomach is wrongly assumed to be empty.
- Tube may not be placed properly in the stomach so that either no specimen is obtained or if saliva is being swallowed, a series of samples containing saliva may be sent for analysis and a wrong diagnosis of achlorhydria may be made.
- Too much tubing may be swallowed resulting to aspiration of heavily bile stained duodenal contents.

EXAMINATION OFRESTING CONTENTS

The **tube is passed after a night's fast** and the stomach contents are removed completely. Valuable informations can be obtained by the examination of resting stomach contents. The following physical and chemical characteristics are important from diagnostic point of view of diseases of stomach.

ˇ Yroxph

In most normal cases after a night's fast only 20 to 50 ml of resting contents is obtained. Volume > than 100 to 120 ml is considered abnormal. An increase in volume of resting contents may be due to:

- hypersecretion of gastric juice;
- retention of gastric contents due to delayed emptying of the stomach;
- due to regurgitation of the duodenal contents.

ˇ Frqvlvwhqf|

The normal resting gastric juice is fluid in consistency and does not contain food residues. It may contain small amounts of mucus. ***Food residues are present in carcinoma of the stomach.***

ˇ Frorxu

In more than 50% of normal individuals, the gastric residuum is clear or colourless, or it may be slightly yellow or greenish due to regurgitation of bile from duodenum. A bright red or dark red or brown colour in the residuum is due to presence of blood—fresh/or altered blood.

Eloh

Bile may be found occasionally but is not usually of any particular significance. A small amount may be regurgitated from the duodenum as stated above, as a result of nausea which some people may experience in swallowing the tube.

Increase quantities of bile is abnormal which may result from intestinal obstruction or ileal stasis.

- Normally blood should not be present.
- A small amount of fresh bright blood may be traumatic.

Eorrg

- *Pathologically*
  - i. Blood which has stayed for sometime in stomach is usually brown or reddish-brown in colour. In the presence of HCI, red blood cells are haemolyzed and dark brown acid haematin is formed. This can occur in gastric ulcer (bleeding) and occasionally in gastric carcinoma
  - ii. When bleeding is associated with delayed emptying of stomach, the blood is usually mixed with food residues giving dark brown colour—***called as coffee-grounds appearance. This is characteristically seen in gastric carcinoma.***
  - iii. Occasionally bleeding can occur from gastritis.
- Sudden bleeding from swallowing aspirin tablets is due to irritation of mucous membrane of stomach and erosion of small capillaries.

Note

Possibility of blood arising from a lesion of upper or lower respiratory tract which may be swallowed, appear as altered blood in gastric contents.

Pxfxv

Normally mucus is present in only small amounts.

Increase mucus is found in gastritis and in gastric carcinoma. Presence of mucus is inversely proportional to the amount of HCI present.

Note

Swallowed saliva may account for excess of mucus.

Iuhh#dqg#Wrwdo#Dflglw|

Determined by titrating a portion of the filtered specimen with a standard solution of NaOH. Two indicators are used in succession. The indicators most commonly used are:

- ***Methyl orange:*** 0.1% aqueous solution or ***Topfer's reagent*** (0.5% solution of dimethyl amino azobenzene in absolute ethanol). It measures pH 2.9 to 4.4 (change from red to yellow colour).
- ***Phenolphthalein:*** 1% solution in 50% ethanol. This indicator measures, pH 8.3 to 10.0, colour change yellow to red again.

Inferences: The following inferences should be drawn

- ***Free acidity***: The first titration to about pH 4.0 measures the amount of free HCI present, i.e., free acidity.
- ***Total acidity***: The complete titration is said to give the total acidity. Some protein hydrochloride and any organic acids present are titrated. Proteins present include mucin in the gastric secretion and protein in meal (this will be in juice obtained after test meal).
- ***Combined acid:*** The difference between the two titrations gives the combined acid.

Uhvxow

Result of titration is expressed as ml of 0.1 N HCI per 100 ml of gastric contents. This is same as mEq/L. To get this figure multiply the above titration by 10.

Normal values:

- ***Free acid:*** 0 to 30 mEq/L
- ***Total acid:*** 10 mEq/L higher (10-40 mEq/L)

Note

- ***Thymol blue*** can be used as indicator. It has the advantage of having two colour changes. First, red to yellow at pH 1.2 to 2.8, and the other, from yellow to blue at pH 9.0 to 9.5. Titration to the first colour change has been used for free acid and second titration colour change for total acid.
- Concentration of free acid above 50 mEq/L indicate hyperacidity.

- ***Rujdqlf#Dflgv***

Lactic acid and butyric acid may be present in large amounts in cases where there is achlorhydria and hypochlorhydria and residual foods must remain in stomach. In absence of HCI, the microorganisms can thrive well and ferment the food residues to produce the organic acids, lactic acid and butyric acid. ***Achlorhydria associated with retention of food materials is exclusively found in carcinoma stomach.***

FRACTIONAL GASTRIC ANALYSIS: USING TEST MEALS

- ***Iudfwlrqdo#Jdvwulf#Dqdo|vlv***

Fractional gastric analysis is also called fractional test meal (FTM) It consists of the following steps:

- Introduction of Ryle's tube in stomach of a fasting patient (overnight).
- Removal of residual gastric contents and its analysis.

These have already been discussed above.

- Ingestion of "test meal".
- Removal of 5 to 6 ml of gastric contents after meal by aspiration using a syringe and analysis of the samples.

Whvw#Phdov

Several types of test meals have been used:

- ***"Ewald" test meal:*** It consists of two pieces (35 gm) of toast and approximately 8 ounces (250 ml) of light tea.
- ***"Oatmeal" porridge:*** This is prepared by adding 2 tablespoonfuls of oat meal to one quart of boiling water and straining the porridge through fine thin muslin.
- ***"Riegel" meal:*** It consists of 200 ml of beef broth, 150 to 200 gm of broiled beef steep and 100 gm of smashed potatoes. This meal is not used normally in India.

Ewald meal has to be consumed by the patient before the introduction of Ryle's tube and the tube is introduced after one hour. This is a little disadvantageous. ***In the case of oat porridge, it can be taken by the patient with tube in situ after clipping the tube.***

Froohfwlrq#ri#Vdpsohv

At intervals of exactly 15 minutes, about 10 ml of gastric contents are removed by means of syringe attached to the tube. If the stomach is not empty at the end of 3 hours, the remaining stomach contents are removed and the volume noted.

Dqdo|vlv#ri#wkh#Vdpsohv

Each sample is strained through a fine mesh cheese cloth. The residue on the cloth is examined for mucus, bile, blood and starch. The strained samples are analyzed for free and total acidity.

Uhvxowv#dqg#Lqwhusuhwdwlrq#ri#wkh#Whvw

- ***Normal response:*** In normal health, after taking the meal, free acid is again found after 15 to 45 minutes (Fig. 3.1). The free acid then rises steadily to reach a maximum at about 15 to 30 minutes, after which the concentration of free acid begins to decrease. ***Free acid ranges from 15 to 45 mEq/L at the maximum with total acid at about 10 units higher.*** About 80% of normal people fall within these limits.

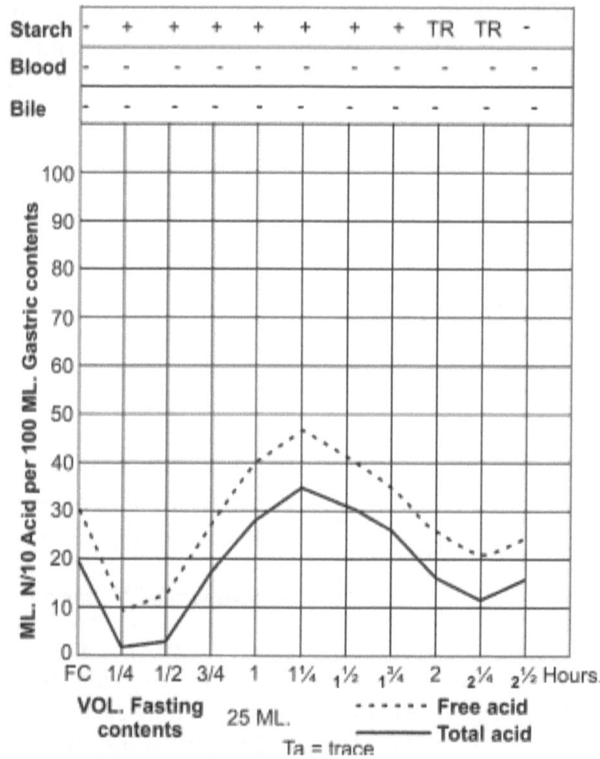

Fig.3.1: Fractional test meal: Normal result

Blood should not be present and there should not be any appreciable amount of bile.

- ***Abnormal responses:*** Three types of abnormal responses are seen.
  - ***Hyperacidity (hyperchlorhydria):*** in which free acid reaches a higher concentration than in normal persons.
  - ***Hypoacidity (hypochlorhydria):*** in which though free acid is present, its concentration is below the normal range.
  - ***Achlorhydria:*** in which there is no secretion of free acid at all.

- ***K|shufkoruk|guld***

This occurs when the maximum free acidity exceeds 45 mEq/L, some prefer to keep at 50 mEq/L, combined acid remains the same as in normal persons.

Causes Hyperacidity is found in the following conditions.

- ***In duodenal ulcer:*** a climbing type of curve is seen.
- ***In gastric ulcer:*** though hyperacidity is common, 50% cases may give normal results, whilst in some chronic cases, due to associated gastritis, hypoacidity may be found. Blood may be present in gastric contents. ***Blood together with hyperchlorhydria is suggestive of gastric ulcer.***
- ***In gastric carcinoma:*** a small percentage of cases show hyperacidity and blood.
- ***Jejunal and gastrojejunal ulcers occur as sequelae to gastroenterostomy:*** they are often found associated with hyperacidity after operation.

Other disorders where hyperacidity may be found are—gastric neurosis, hyperirritability and pylorospasm, pyloric stenosis, chronic cholecystitis, chronic appendicitis, etc.

- ***K | s rfkoruk|guld***

It is difficult to define this zone. Low acidities are found in carcinoma of stomach and in atonic dyspepsia. In pernicious anaemia, free HCI is absent in gastric secretion. Gastro-enterostomy-hypoacidity seen.

- ***Dfkoruk|guld***

This term is used when there is no secretion of HCI, but enzyme like pepsin is present. ***Achlorhydria can be differentiated from hypochlorhydria by stimulation test with histamine.*** In hypochlorhydria, histamine stimulation shows rise in free HCI. ***In achlorhydria, histamine stimulation does not show response.***

Causes

- Found in some normal people increasing with age about 60 to 75 years.
- High incidence in carcinoma of stomach.
- *In chronic gastritis:* tendency of gastric acidity to be reduced. As the disease progresses, increasing incidence of achlorhydria as seen.
- **Partial gastrectomy** leads to reduction of gastric acidity often and to achlorhydria in a considerable number of cases.
- **In pernicious anaemia.**
- **Other diseases** are microcytic hypochromic anaemia (in 80% cases), hyperthyroidism and myxoedema may be associated with achlorhydria.

- ***Dfk|old#Jdvwulfd***

The term is used when ***both enzymes and acids are absent*** indicating there is a complete absence of gastric secretion.

Causes

It is found in the following conditions:

- In advanced cases of cancer of stomach.
- Advanced cases of gastritis.
- Typically found in pernicious anaemia and of subacute combined degeneration of the spinal cord (100% cases).

STIMULA TION TESTS

4 Dofrkro#Vwlpxodwlrq

*7% **ethyl alcohol*** is used as a stimulant of gastric secretion.

Surfhgxuh

- After an overnight fast, the Ryle's tube is passed into the stomach and resting contents are removed for analysis.
- One hundred ml (100 ml) of 7% ethyl alcohol is administered.

  Note

  A little of methylene blue can be added in alcohol meal so that it gives an indication of emptying time of the stomach.
- Samples of gastric contents are removed every 15 minutes.

All the collected samples are analyzed for free and total acidity, peptic activity, presence of blood, bile and mucus.

Dgydqwdjhv

Advantages of alcohol test meal over "oatmeal" porridge are:

- More easily administered and prepared.
- It is consumed better than porridge.
- Specimens are clear and easily analyzed.
- The gastric response is more rapid and more intense.
- The stomach empties more quickly as compared to porridge meal.

Glvdgydqwdjhv

- Stimulus with alcohol is not so strictly physiological as with oat meal porridge.
- Stimulus is more vigorous as compared to oat meal.
- Rather higher levels of free acidity are obtained and the limits of normal are wider.

2 Fdiihlqh#Vwlpxodwlrq

Caffeine can be used as a stimulus instead of alcohol. Procedure remains the same as described above.

Surfhgxuh

- Ryle's tube is introduced after an overnight's fast and the resting gastric contents are removed and analyzed.
- Caffeine sodium benzoate, 500 mg, disolved in 200 ml of water, is given to the patient orally.
- Samples of stomach contents are removed every 15 minutes and analyzed for free and total acidity, peptic activity and blood, bile and mucus.

Advantages of caffeine stimulation is similar to alcohol stimulation.

3 Klvwdplqh#Vwlpxodwlrq#Whvw

Histamine is a powerful stimulant for the secretion of HCI in the normal stomach. It acts on receptors on the oxyntic cells, increasing the cyclic AMP level, which causes secretion of an increased volume of highly acidic gastric juice with low pepsin content.

Lqglfdwlrqv

- *To differentiate "true" achlorhydria from "false" achlorhydria due to various causes.*

"True" achlorhydria which is histamine-resistant is seen in achylia gastrica. Demonstration of such an achlorhydria is useful in the diagnosis of subacute combined degeneration of the cord and pernicious anaemia.

W|shv#ri#Klvwdplqh#Whvw

a. Standard histamine test
b. Augmented histamine test.

D1 Vwdqgdug#Klvwdplqh#Whvw

Surfhgxuh

- After an overnight fast, Ryle's tube is passed into the stomach and stomach contents are removed for analysis.
- Patient is given a subcutaneous injection of histamine, 0.01 mg/kg body weight.
- After the injection, 10 ml of stomach contents are removed every 10 minutes for one hour. The samples are analyzed for free and total acidity, peptic activity, and for presence of blood, bile and mucus.

Clinical Significance

- Absence of free HCI in the secretions after histamine indicate *"achylia gastrica' ("true" achlorhydria).*
- In duodenal ulcer, more juice may be secreted and a higher concentration of acid may be found in the specimen obtained after histamine administration than in normal cases.

Note
Standard histamine test may be combined with the FTM. If no free acid is found in the resting contents in FTM by the end of an hour after giving the gruel meal, histamine can be given and standard test can be carried out.

E1 Dxjphqwhg#Klvwdplqh#Whvw#+Ndl,

It is a more powerful stimulus than the original standard test used, and provides a more reliable proof of an inability to secrete acid.

Glvdgydqwdjh

Larger doses of histamine used in this test sometimes cause untoward severe reactions and hence an antihistaminic will have to be given side by side to prevent any such reactions.

Note
The antihistamine does not interfere in gastric stimulation action of histamine.

Lqglfdwlrqv

The test has been *used for two purposes:*

- To show an inability to secrete acid which is present with pernicious anaemia and subacute combined degeneration of the cord.
- To assess the maximum possible acid secretion as in the diagnosis and surgical treatment of duodenal ulcer.

Surfhgxuh

- After an overnight fast, pass a Ryle's tube and remove the residual gastric contents for analysis.
- Collect resting contents every 20 minutes for an hour.
- Halfway through this period, give 4 ml of Anthisan (100 mg of mepyramine maleate) intramuscularly (IM).
- At the end of the hour, give histamine (0.04 mg histamine acid phosphate per kg body weight) subcutaneously (SC) and remove gastric contents every 15 minutes for one hour (4 specimens) or three 20-minute interval specimens.

  Thus specimens obtained are:
- Resting contents,
- An hour prehistamine specimen, and
- Three 20-minute posthistamine specimens.

Folqlfdo#Vljqlilfdqfh

- *In pernicious anaemia:* no free HCl is secreted after augmented histamine stimulation (achylia gastria), but in other forms of achlorhydria (false achlorhydria), some amount of free HCl is secreted after histamine stimulation.
- *In normal persons:* up to 10 mEq/hour acid is present in the prehistamine specimen, with 10 to 25 mEq in the combined posthistamine ones.
- *In duodenal ulcers:* higher values are obtained sometimes reaching or even exceeding 100 mEq. The maximum acidity, reached in the second 20-minute specimen has been used by some workers for duodenal ulcers.

Note

Recently, a histamine analogue, called 'histalog' (3β β-amino ethyl pyrazole) has been used in place of histamine.

Dose: Recommended dose is 10 to 50 mg.

Dgydqwdjhv

- No side effects like histamine hence no antihistaminic is required to be administered along with.
- It is highly effective in stimulating gastric secretion.

4 Lqvxolq#Vwlpxodwlrq#Whvw#+Kroodqghu¶v#Whvw,

Hypoglycaemia produced by administration of insulin is a potent stimulus of gastric acid secretion. **Hollander** suggested that to be effective blood sugar must be brought below 50 mg%, whereas other workers have recommended a level below 45 mg% is a necessity for a reliable test.

Lqglfdwlrq

To ascertain the effectiveness of vagotomy (vagal resection) in patients with duodenal ulcer. Insulin test meal was suggested by Hollander to determine whether the section of vagus has been successfully performed.

Surfhgxuh

- After an overnight fast, pass a Ryle's tube and empty the stomach.
- Then give 15 units of soluble insulin intravenously (IV)
- After injecting the insulin, withdraw approximately 10 ml samples of gastric contents every 15 minutes for 2 ½ hours.
- Samples to be analyzed for free and total acidity, peptic activity and presence of blood, bile and starch. **No starch should be present.**

Note

- The test is not without hazard as blood sugar may go down to dangerously low level in some, which may require glucose treatment and should be readily available.
- Blood sugar may be determined at least once, half an hour after giving insulin in order to make sure a sufficiently low value 45 to 50 mg% has reached.

Folqlfdo#Vljqlilfdqfh

- In suffering from duodenal ulcer, before operation, there is a marked and prolonged

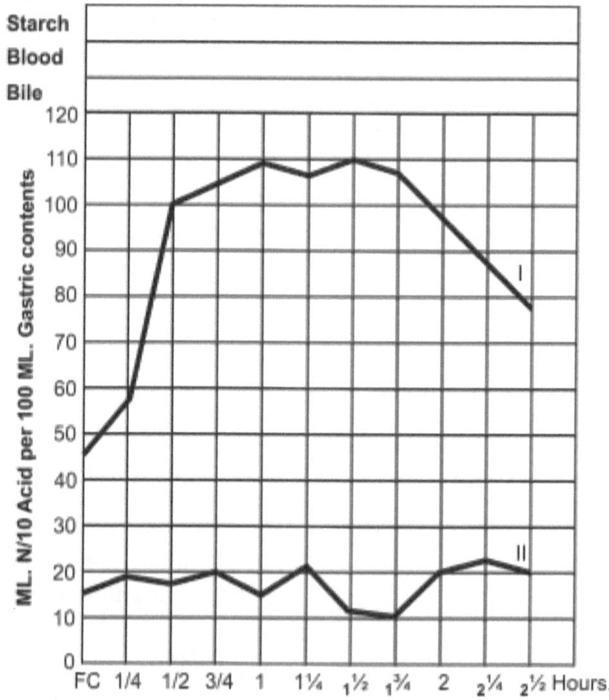

I Free acid curve before vagotomy
II Free acid curve after vagotomy

Fig. 3.2: Insulin 'test meal'

output of acid in response to insulin. The concentration of free acid may rise well over 100 mEq/L.

- After a successful vagotomy there is no response to insulin and the gastric acidity remains at a low level of 15 to 20 mEq/L, before and after insulin injection (Fig. 3.2).

Note

- Some surgeons prefer to have the test done preoperatively and then soon after the operation and once more several months later. Others have suggested that it is sufficient and quite satisfactory to do it once only at least six months after the operation.
- The degree of stimulation of acid secretion is related to the degree of hypoglycaemia obtained and hence indirectly to the dose of insulin given.

5 Shqwdjdvwulq#Whvw

Pentagastrin is a synthetic peptide in which N-terminal end is blocked by butyl-oxycarbonyl-β-alanine.

Trp-Met-Asp-phe ($CONH_2$). The four C-terminal amino acids form the "active" part of the molecule.

Pentagastrin is a potent stimulator, and involves the maximal stimulation of stomach after a period of assessment of the basal secretion rate. ***This is thus a measure of the total parietal mass.***

Lqglfdwlrqv

- Useful in investigation of patients with "active" duodenal ulcer, which may suggest appropriate surgical measures.
- In pernicious anaemia.

- Useful in suspected cases of Zollinger-Ellison syndrome.

Surfhgxuh

- After an overnight fast, stomach tube (Ryle's tube) is passed into the stomach and the resting contents completely removed.
- After emptying the stomach of resting contents, collect two 15 minute specimens to have the ***"basal secretion"***.
- Then injection of pentagastrin- 6 μg/kg body weight is given subcutaneously (SC) and four specimens are collected, accurately timed at 15 minutes intervals.
  All the specimens are analyzed.

Folqlfdo#Vljqlilfdqfh

- ***Normal basal secretion*** rate is 1 to 2.5 mEq/hour. After pentagastrin stimulus, maximal secretion in normal persons roughly varies from 20 to 40 mEq/hour.
- ***In duodenal ulcer:*** the range was 15 to 83 mEq/hour with a mean of 43. Values above > 40 mEq/hour has been kept which is suggestive of duodenal ulcer.
- ***Zollinger-Ellison syndrome:*** it is characterized by a high basal secretion usually above 10 mEq/hour; if as it may be, it is maximal then, there will be no further rise after giving pentagastrin, otherwise only a small to moderate increase is seen.
- ***In gastric ulcer:*** the test is of little value.
- ***In cancer of the stomach:*** "true" achlorhydria is found in about 50% of cases, and hypochlorhydria in about 25%.
- Output of acid is also reduced transiently in ***acute gastritis,*** and permanently in chronic gastritis.
- ***In pernicious anaemia:*** the basic pathology is gastric mucosal atrophy with lack of intrinsic factor and in great majority of cases "true" achlorhydria. Some occasional young persons with pernicious anaemia have been found to have acid secretion.

Note

- ***Zollinger-Ellison syndrome:*** Zollinger-Ellison syndrome is characterized by a peptic ulcer, intractable to medical treatment, gastric hyper secretion and diarrhoea in patient with "gastrin", secreting pancreatic islet cell (δ-cells) adenoma. It is sometimes accompanied by other endocrine adenomas or hyperplasias, especially parathyroid adenomas with hyperparathyroidism.
- ***Peptic activity:*** Pepsinogen determination has been used to investigate the gastric secretion of this enzyme. A convenient method using the digestion of dried serum has been used.

Folqlfdo#Vljqlilfdqfh

- Gastric secretion of pepsin occurs after stimulation with pentagastrin or insulin.
- After insulin, the secretion of pepsin parallels acid secretion and is dependant on the dose of stimulant.
- The relative merits of determining pepsin or HCI are yet to be established but the latter is technically easier and quicker to determine.
- Gastric pepsin is not homogenous and a particular fraction, "pepsin I" has been claimed to show a greater association with the tendency to develop a peptic ulcer.

Vljqlilfdqfh#ri#Ghwhuplqdwlrq ri#Vhuxp#Shsvlqrjhq

- ***Normal value:*** ranges from 30 to 160 units/ml.
- ***In pernicious anaemia:*** serum pepsinogen is absent or very low.
- ***In duodenal ulcer:*** an increase is often found up to and above twice the upper limit of normal. If the serum pepsinogen is less than < 80 units/ml, it is considered that an ulcer is not present.

TUBELESS GASTRIC ANALYSIS

Swallowing a stomach tube (Ryle's tube) is an unpleasant and cumbersome procedure and sometimes inadvisable, hence attempts have been made to devise tests which can be done without using a stomach tube.

Initially **Segal and co-workers** used a quininium resin indicator given orally, from which H^+ ions if present in stomach could liberate quinine ions (QH^+ cation) at a pH less than 3.0. The quinine, thus liberated, forms quinine HCI which is absorbed in small intestine and then excreted in the urine from which quinine is extracted and determined fluorimetrically. Thus, it gives indirect measure for acid secretion.

Prglilfdwlrq

Subsequently the test was simplified. They introduced ***"Diagnex Blue"*** prepared by reacting carbacrylic cation exchange resin with ***"Azure A"***, an indicator. The hydrogen ions of the resin exchanged with "Azure A" ions, the reaction is reversed in the stomach when acid, if present, in a concentration giving a pH less than 3.0. By the action of acid, the indicator "Azure A" is released, which is absorbed in the small intestine and excreted in the urine, the colour of which can then be matched with known standards.

Folqlfdo#Vljqlilfdqfh

The test is of value if it is used as a ***"screening test"*** only.

- **A positive result,** provided no other cations such as K^+, Ba^{++}, Fe^{++}, etc. are present, indicates that acid is being secreted by the stomach.
- **A negative result** is an unreliable indicator of "true" achlorhydria since 50% of these cases secrete acid in response to pentagastrin.
- The test is not reliable in patients suffering from renal diseases, urinary retention, malabsorption, pyloric obstruction and after gastrectomy and gastroenterostomy.

Note

Vitamin preparations should not be taken on the day preceding the test or medicaments which might contain substances decolourised by ascorbic acid.

Chapter 4

Thyroid Function Tests

INTRODUCTION

The **main objectives** for the laboratory procedures in evaluation of thyroid diseases are:

- To assess the functional status of the gland;
- To characterize the anatomical features of the thyroid gland; and
- To possibly evaluate the cause for the thyroid dysfunction.

With the advent of **"tracers"** especially ^{131}I,

(i) uptake studies reflecting substrate input in hormone synthesis; and

(ii) scanning, characterizing benign and malignant lesions, localizing "ectopic" thyroid tissue or functioning metastasis, have contributed a great deal in improving the thyroid diagnostic acumen.

This was followed by the development of radioimmuno assays (RIA) and the prospect of determining the actual minute circulating quantities of thyroid hormones, viz. T_4, T_3 and TSH, further augmented the precision in diagnosis of thyroid diseases. It must be emphasized that a single thyroid function test is not absolute in diagnostic accuracy and thus, a ***careful selection of tests, so that their combination can give comprehensive data, would enhance the diagnostic accuracy.***

CLASSIFICATION

Classification of various tests can be made on the basis of the functions of the gland.

I. ***Tests based on Primary function of thyroid, viz. substrate input and hormone synthesis:***
   - Radioiodine "uptake" studies and turnover (RAI or RIU) studies,
   - PB ^{131}I in serum
   - T_3-suppression test
   - TSH-stimulation test
   - TRH-stimulation test

II. ***Tests measuring blood levels of thyroid hormones:***
   - Serum PBI and BEI
   - Circulating T_4 and T_3 level
   - Circulating TSH level
   - *In vitro* resin uptake of T_3
   - Plasma tyrosine level

III. ***Tests based on metabolic effects of thyroid hormones:***
   - BMR
   - Serum cholesterol level
   - Serum creatine level
   - Serum uric acid
   - Serum CK enzyme

IV. ***"Scanning" of thyroid gland***

V. ***Immunological tests to detect autoimmune diseases of thyroid gland***
   - Agar gel diffusion test (precipitation test)
   - TRCH test—tanned red cells haemagglutination test.
   - Complement fixation test.

Newer tests:

- ***Determination of antithyroid peroxidase antibody (anti-TPo antibodies)***
- ***Determination of thyrotropin receptor antibodies (TR ab)***

I. TESTS BASED ON PRIMARY FUNCTION OF THYROID

1. *Radioactive "Uptake" Studies*

Iodine plays a key role in the metabolism of the thyroid gand. ^{131}I "tracer" is most commonly used for thyroid function studies because of low cost, easy availability, and convenient shelf life. Short lived isotopes of iodine like ^{132}I and ^{123}I are preferred for use in paediatric practice and in pregnant and lactating women. Recently, ^{99m}Tc has also been used as it behaves like iodine and has added advantage of lower radiation dose to the patient.

Dose of ^{131}I = 10 μci is given orally. Thyroid accumulation of radioiodine is measured externally over the gland. Radioiodine uptake of the gland reflects the iodine "trapping" ability. Thyroid uptake of ^{131}I is routinely measured 24 hours after the administration of oral dose, although 4 or 48 hours uptakes are also measured when rapid turnover or delayed uptake situation is expected.

"Turnover" is faster in "active" and hyperfunctioning gland and slower in underactive hypofunctioning gland.

- ***Normal range:*** is 20 to 40%.

In Indian subjects, a value of 15 to 35% has been found. The range varies from one population to another depending on dietary iodine intake.

Interpretations

- An abnormally high RAI uptake is usually consistent with hyperthyroid state.
- In endemic goitre and some cases of nontoxic sporadic goitre also may be high.
- Abnormally low thyroid uptake is characteristic of hypothyroidism, but not specific since subacute thyroiditis and administration of large doses of iodine and thyroid hormones may also lower the ^{131}I uptake of the gland.

2. *Urinary excretion of ^{131}I and "T-Index"*

Renal excretion of ^{131}I is an indirect evidence of thyroid function. Proportion of the administered dose excreted is ***inversely proportional*** to thyroid uptake.

If uptake is "more", less of ^{131}I will be excreted and vice versa.

Twenty-four hours urine is collected accuratley and radioactivity is measured.

- ***Normal range:*** is 30 to 60% of the administered dose.

"T"-index

Activity is measured in urine sample—0 to 8 hours after, 0 to 24 hours and 0 to 48 hours.

'T'-index is calculated as follows:

$$T = \frac{\text{0-8 hours excretion expressed as \% x 100}}{\text{(0-24 hours excretion expressed as \%)} \times \text{(0-48 hours excretion expressed as \%)}}$$

- ***Normal value of "T":*** 2.5 to 12

Interpretations

- A "T"-index greater than 17 indicates hyperfunctioning of the gland.
- A "T"-index less than 2.5 indicates hypothyroidism.

3. *Thyroid "Clearance" Rate*

The amount of ^{131}I that is accumulated in thyroid over a fixed interval, in relation to the mean plasma concentration of ^{131}I midway in that time period provides the index of rate at which the thyroid gland is handling ^{131}I. (Rationale is similar to the concept of renal clearance).

Hence,

$$\text{Thyroid clearance rate} = \frac{\text{Thyroid } ^{131}I \text{ accumulation rate}}{\text{Plasma } ^{131}I \text{ concentration.}}$$

(Midway between the time period)

The above gives a direct index of thyroid activity with regard to iodine accumulation.

- ***Normal value:*** 60 ml/minute.

Interpretations

- Clearance rate is high with thyroid hyperfunction, the value has been distinctly high with no overlap.

- The value is also high when "intrathyroidal iodine pool" is small.
- Lower values are indicative of hypothyroid status.

4. *Serum $PB^{131}I$*

Administered ^{131}I accumulates in the thyroid gland and appears as "labelled" hormone bound to proteins. Normally it is a ***slow process,*** but in hyperthyroidism level of protein-bound radioactivity increases in plasma, which can be measured accurately by a scintillation counter. The result is conveniently expressed as **"conversion ratio",** which indicates the proportion of the total plasma radioactivity at 24 hours.

- *Normal value:* is 35%.

Interpretations

- ***In hyperthyroidism*** it is usually greater than 50%.
- It is of no value in the assessment of patients who have been treated for hyperthyroidism, either surgically or with radioactive iodine, as high values may persist for a long time after such treatments.
- PB ^{131}I is found to be elevated in 50% of the patients with ***Hashimoto's thyroiditis, when the thyroid uptake is usually normal or low, a combination of findings which is very suggestive of this condition.***

The reason for these discrepancies is that PB ^{131}I is not a measure of plasma thyroxine concentration. The level of serum PB ^{131}I is dependant on several factors.

- The initial proportion of the "tracer" dose accumulated by the thyroid.
- The rate of secretion of the thyroid hormones.
- The size of the "intrathyroidal iodine pool".

In primary hyperthyroidism, the intrathyroidal iodine pool is similar to that of the normal thyroid gland so that in untreated hyperthyroidism, the elevated PB ^{131}I is largely a reflection of increased secretion rate. On the other hand, the "intrathyroidal iodine pool" is markedly reduced after treatment either surgically or with radioiodine, and ***also a striking feature in Hashimoto's thyroiditis,*** so that under these circumstances an elevated $PB^{131}I$ is mainly due to markedly reduced intrathyroidal iodine pool, the secretion rate of the thyroid hormones being normal or even reduced.

5. *T_3-Suppression Test*

- After 24 hours RIU studies and obtaining the basal value and serum T_4 values, 20 µg of T_3, four times daily is given for 7 to 10 days (or alternatively 25 µg three times a day for 7 days).
- RIU is repeated after T_3 administration and serum T_4 values are also determined.

Interpretations

- A suppression is indicated by the 24 hours RIU falling to less than 50% of the "initial" uptake (as exogenous T_3 suppresses TSH) and total T_4 to approximately 2 µg/100 ml or less.
- Non-suppression indicates autonomous thyroid function. In Graves' disease, no change seen as the action is due to LATS (long-acting thyroid stimulator) and is not under control of hypothalamopituitary axis.

Use: To differentiate borderline high normal from primary hyperthyroidism (Graves' disease).

6. *TSH-Stimulation Test*

- Following completion of 24 hours RIU studies, 3 injections of TSH, each 5 USP units are given at 24 hours intervals.
- 24-hour thyroidal RIU is measured 42 hours after the final TSH dose.

Interpretations

- ***In primary hypothyroidism,*** there is failure of stimulation of the gland.
- ***In secondary hypothyroidism,*** there is stimulation of the gland showing increase RIU.

Use: The test is useful in differentiating primary hypothyroidism from secondary hypothyroidism.

7. *TRH-Stimulation Test*

With the availability of synthetic TRH, which is a tripeptide, suitable for human use, it is now possible to assess the functional integrity of thyrotropic cells or the factors that influence the secretory response.

Procedure

TRH 200 to 400 μg is administered IV and blood samples at 0, 20, 40, and 60 minutes are analyzed for TSH content.

Interpretations

- Peak response ***in normal*** is about 4 times elevation of TSH levels at 20 and 40 minutes sample as compared to basal TSH level.
- ***In primary hypothyroidism:*** the response will be exaggerated and prologned.
- ***In secondary hypothyroidism:*** the response will be blunted.
- ***In tertiary hypothyroidism:*** i.e., hypothalamic in origin, the increase in TSH is delayed.

Use: Currently this test is used to locate the site of pathological lesion for hypothyroid states.

II. TESTS MEASURING BLOOD LEVELS OF THYROID HORMONES

1. *Serum PBI Levels*

Chemical estimation of protein-bound iodine (PBI) is in use for a long time as a test for thyroid function. It is an indirect measure of thyroid hormones and is useful where isotope techniques are not available. But it is technically time consuming lengthy procedure, and also measures non-hormonal iodine and iodotyrosines.

- ***Normal value:*** ranges from 4.0 to 8.0 μg%

Interpretations

- More than 95% of hyperthyroidism cases show greater than 8.0 μg%.
- About 87% of hypothyroidism cases show value below 3 μg%.
- Care should be taken to interpret values between 4.0 and 5.0 μg%.

Precautions and Limitations

- Easily affected by iodine contamination, both exogenous and endogenous.
  Exogenous: to eliminate exogenous contamination, all glass wares and syringes should be iodine free.
  Endogenous: iodides, iodine containing drugs and radiological contrast media can give false high results.
- The test is also affected by "trace" elements and chemicals that interfere iodine-reduction reaction.
- Values are also affected by alterations in serum TBG level. Increased serum TBG gives higher values, whereas decreased TBG gives lower values.

Serum TBG may be increased in:

- pregnancy;
- oestrogen therapy, and
- on oral contraceptive pills.

Serum TBG may be decreased in:

- hypoproteinaemic states;
- nephrotic syndrome;
- androgen therapy and anabolic drugs like danazol;
- dicoumarol therapy; and
- inherited TBG deficiency.
- Certain drugs may give misleading results by competing with T_4 for protein binding sites, e.g. phenytoin sodium, salicylates, etc.

2. *Serum BEI Levels*

Butanol-extractable iodine (BEI) involves extraction of serum with n-butanol and subsequent washing of the extracts with alkaline solution. This removes the inorganic iodine and iodotyrosines.

Interpretations

- *In normal:* value ranges from 3.5 to 7.0 μg%.
- *In hyperthyroidism:* values are more than 10 μg%.

3. Serum T_4 Levels

Most commonly used methods are listed below.
- Competitive protein binding assay (CPBA)
- Radioimmunoassay (RIA)
- ELISA technique

See the principles of these techniques at the end of this chapter.
- *Normal range of serum* T_4: is 4.0 to 11.0 μg%.
- *In hyperthyroidism:* the value is usually more than 12.0 μg% and
- *In hypothyroidism:* less than 2.5 μg%.

4. Effective Thyroxine Ratio (ETR)

This integrates into a single procedure the measurement of total serum thyroxine and also binding capacity of thyroid hormone proteins. At the present time, the ETR provides the most reliable single test of thyroid function available which can be readily carried out on a sample of serum and only requires radioisotope laboratory.

Advantage

It is not affected by oral contraceptives, pregnancy, excess iodine or any other drugs.

5. Serum T_3 Level

Radioimmunoassay is the method of choice for measurement of serum T_3 level. CPBA is not good and accurate as T_3 has very low affinity for TBG.
- *Normal range:* is 100 to 250 ng% (mμg%). Values in females tend to be slightly on higher side compared to males.
- *In hyperthyroidism:* it is usually more than 350 ng% and
- *In hypothyroidism:* less than 100 ng%.

It may be ***a useful test for hyperthyroidism, but it is less useful for diagnosis of hypothyroidism.***

6. Serum TSH Level

Measurement of serum TSH also provides a very sensitive index of thyroid function. It is of particular value in the diagnosis of primary hypothyroidism.
- By radioimmunoassay the ***normal range*** is 0 to 3 μ (U/ml) average being 1.6 μ U/ml.
- Recently an ***immunoradiometric assay (IRMA)*** for TSH has been developed which is specific and sensitive enough to detect the very low (and hitherto usually undetectable) plasma TSH levels found in hyperthyroidism. A number of investigators have indicated that this test would be a suitable screening test for hyperthyroidism and hypothyroidism.
- Also recently, ***"sensitive" TSH (sTSH) assay*** has been developed. Enzymatic, fluorimetric assays and chemiluminescence being assessed for their clinical utility.

Assay of very sensitive TSH (sTSH) has allowed low and suppressed basal TSH levels to be clearly demonstrated. Thus, in the absence of hypothalamic-pituitary disease, a very low, less than 0.1 mU/L of serum TSH is strongly supportive of a diagnosis of thyrotoxicosis.

Using such assays, it has also been shown that the basal TSH level is a good predictor of the TSH response to TRH stimulation.

7. "In vitro" ^{131}I-T_3 Uptake by Resin/Red Cells

The methods is as per ***Hamolsky et al (1957).***
- A known amount of ^{131}I-T_3 is added to a standard volume of serum from a patient.
- The amount of ^{131}I-T_3 which binds to the serum proteins varies inversely with the endogenous thyroid hormones already bound to serum proteins (TBG).
- Residual free ^{131}I-T_3 is then adsorbed by resin/sponge/sephadex/red cells, which is removed from the sample and then the adsorbed/bound ^{131}I is measured.

This method thus gives the measure of T_4 binding in the serum and not the actual level of thyroid hormones.

Interpretations

- *In normal subjects:* the value is 21 to 35%.

- *In hyperthyroidism:* saturation of binding of TBG with endogenous T_4 and T_3 is greater than normal, hence little of tracer $^{131}I\text{-}T_3$ can bind to TBG and more $^{131}I\text{-}T_3$ will be free to be adsorbed by resin/sponge. ***The resin uptake in hyperthyroidism will be greater than 35%.***
- *In hypothyroidism:* the reverse will occur. The proportion of $^{131}I\text{-}T_3$ taken up by the resin is ***inversely reduced*** and less than 21%.
- Resin uptake of $^{131}I\text{-}T_3$ also gets influenced by drugs, hormones, pregnancy, etc.

Note: Thus, **false high result** may occur in:

- hypoproteinaemic states,
- nephrotic syndrome and
- androgen therapy as TBG is decreased. Similarly, **false low result** may occur where TBG is increased as
- in pregnancy,
- oestrogen therapy and
- women on oral contraceptive pills.

8. *Plasma Tyrosine Level*

Rivlin et al (1965) studied plasma tyrosine level in normal subjects and in thyroid disorders.

Interpretations

- *Normal level:* was found to be 11.8 ± 0.4 µg/ml.
- *In hyperthyroidism:* plasma tyrosine level was found to be ***elevated*** in more than 70% cases.
- *In hypothyroidism:* the ***decreased*** level of plasma tyrosine was observed (average 8-9 µg/ml).

Mechanism of Increased Tyrosine Level in Hyperthyroidism

It is suggested that excess thyroid hormones has inhibitory effect on hepatic and tissue ***tyrosine transaminase.*** As a result, tyrosine catabolism is reduced thus increasing plasma tyrosine level. ***Rivlin et al*** proposed the use of ***tyrosine loading test*** for hyperthyroidism and claimed that it is not influenced by age, sex, pregnancy or by previous iodides/radioisotope administration. Using "tyrosine loading test" the authors observed markedly increased plasma tyrosine level in cases of hyperthyroidism.

III. TESTS BASED ON METABOLIC EFFECTS OF THYROID HORMONES

These tests are of much use where facilities for isotope techniques are not available.

1. *Basal Metabolic Rate (BMR)*

The test is helpful in diagnosis and is of particular value in assessing the severity and prognosis. At least two estimations consecutively after proper sedation and physical/mental rest will be helpful.

Interpretations

- A BMR between –15% and + 20% is considered as ***normal.***
- *In euthyroid states:* –10% to + 10% of normal.
- *In hyperthyroidism:* + 50% to + 75% is usually found
- *In hypothyroidism:* value below –20% is suggestive (usually –30% to –60% seen in hypothyroid states).

2. *Serum Cholesterol Level*

It is ***useful in assessment of hypothyroidism, where it is usually high.*** Not of much value in hyperthyroidism, though it is usually low. **Baron** has shown that 90% of hypothyroidism cases have serum cholesterol greater than 260 mg%. He found poor correlation with severity as judged by BMR. In hypothyroidism, the synthesis of cholesterol is impaired, but its catabolism is reduced more, leading to high cholesterol level.

3. *Serum Creatine Level*

Griffiths advocated the estimation of serum creatine level for diagnosis of hyperthyroidism, who considered a serum level greater than 0.6 mg% is diagnostic. He compared serum creatine with BMR. A raised serum creatine, between 0.6 and 1.6 mg% may or may not be accompanied by increased BMR. ***He considered a normal serum creatine and normal BMR excludes thyroid dysfunction*** and held that when symptoms of thyroid disorders is present, a raised serum creatine is highly significant even though BMR is normal.

4. *Serum Uric Acid Level*

Serum uric acid has been found to be increased in myxoedematous males and post menopausal women, ranging from 6.5 to 11.0 mg%.

5. *Serum CK Level*

Serum CK level are often raised in hypothyroidism but the estimation does not help in diagnosis. CK levels are also raised in thyrotoxic myopathy.

6. *Hypercalcaemia*

It is very rarely found in severe thyrotoxicosis; there is an increased turnover of bone, probably due to direct action of thyroid hormones.

IV. THYROID SCANNING

Scintiscans provide visualization of the distribution of radioactive iodine in the gland and also permits characterization of its anatomical features.

Advantages/Uses of Scintiscan

- Readily distinguishes the diffuse glandular activity from the patchy pattern seen in nodular goitres.
- The scan also permits functional classification of nodules as:
  - **'Hot' or 'warm'** areas of increased uptake. **Hot nodules** suggest increased thickness of the gland in those regions/ or due to functioning adenoma or carcinoma; and
  - **'Cold' nodules** are due to reduced/or absent uptake. It may be due to cysts, haemorrhagic nodules, degeneration in an adenoma or carcinoma.

  In association with thyroid suppression regimes, helps to determine the TSH dependant or autonomous nature of the 'hot'/warm nodules.
- Scanning also provides useful information regarding size, shape and position of the gland.
- Facilitates identification and localization of functioning thyroid tissues ***in "ectopic"*** or ***"metastatic" sites,*** e.g. in lungs and bones.

Use of 99^m Technetium Pertechnate

Recently, 99^m technetium pertechnate has been used. It has similar properities as iodine. Thyroid follicles "trap" pertechnate ions, similar to iodine.

Advantages

- Radiation effect is low.
- Has very short half-life of 6 hours.
- Virtual absence of particulate radiations.

Limitations

- Remains unaltered in the gland.
- Cannot demonstrate retrosternal extension of thyroid, if any, due to attenuation of low energy γ-radiations passing through sternum.
- Fails to identify functioning metastasis from differentiated carcinomas of thyroid due to short half-life and lack of fixation of 99^m Tc by the functioning metastasis.

IMMUNOLOGICAL TESTS FOR THYROID FUNCTIONS

1. *Determination of Antithyroid Autoantibodies*

Antithyroid autoantibodies are found in a variety of thyroid disorders, as well as, in other autoimmune diseases and certain malignancies. These autoantibodies are directed against several thyroid components and thyroid hormone antigens. They are:

- Thyroglobulin (Tg)
- Thyroid microsomal antigen

- TSH receptor
- A non-thyroglobulin (non-Tg) colloid antigen
- Thyroid stimulating hormone (TSH) and
- Thyroxine (T_4).

Of these antibodies, only anti-Tg (antithyroglobulin) and antimicrosomal autoantibodies are commonly used in evaluating thyroid status and function.

Anti-Tg autoantibodies are directed against thyroglobulin (Tg), a major constituent of thyroid colloid. Several different techniques are available and used in clinical laboratory to detect and quantify Tg-autoantibodies in blood.

They are mainly:

- Agargel diffusion precipitation (Fig. 4.1)
- Tanned red cells haemagglutination test (TRCH Test);
- Enzyme-linked immunoabsorbent assay (ELISA)
- Immunofluorescence of tissue sections;
- Radioimmunoassay (RIA) method.

Most widely used method is based on haemagglutination.

A. *Tanned Red Cells Haemagglutination Test (TRCH Test)*

Principle

In TRCH test, an aliquot of patient's serum is mixed with erythrocytes that have been treated/coated with tannic acid and then coated with purified human Tg-antigen.

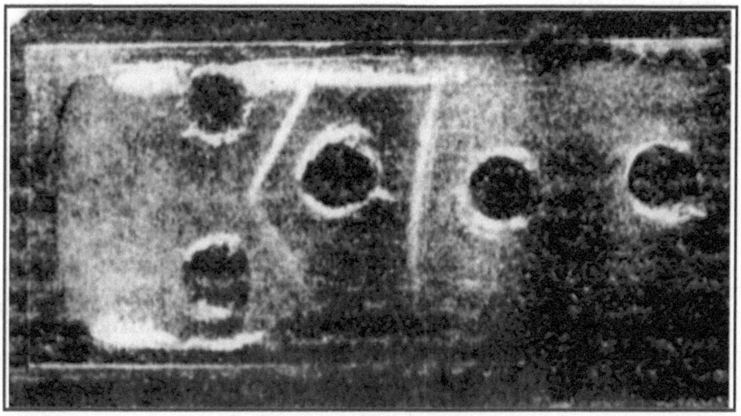

Gel diffusion precipitation test. Unstained positive result.

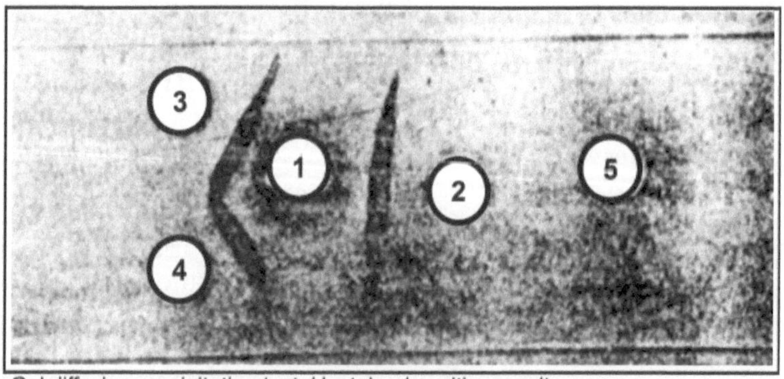

Well No. 1 – Test serum
Well No. 2 – Antigen 1/3 dilution
Well No. 3 – Antigen 1/6 dilution
Well No. 4 – Antigen 1/9 dilution
Well No. 5 – Negative control serum

Gel diffusion precipitation test. Unstained positive result.

Fig. 4.1: Thyroid antibodies in thyroid diseases by gel diffusion

When antibodies, if present in patient's serum, combine with tanned red cells coated with antigen, agglutination occurs which is visible as a 'carpet' at the bottom. Lack of agglutination is indicated by setting of the cells at the bottom as a compact button or ring.

Note: Use of Tg-coated erythrocytes makes this agglutination reaction much more sensitive than a simple antigen-antibody reaction.

Procedure

- Prior to testing, patient's serum is inactivated at 56°C × for ½ hour.
  Note:: Heating is important for inactivation of complement and thyroid binding globulin (TBG), which otherwise would interfere with the assay.
- A dried Perspex tray with wells is taken. Serial double dilutions of the patient's inactivated serum is made to establish Tg-antibody titre.
- A suspension of tanned-red cells coated with Tg-antigen is put in the each well.
- Tray is shaken and then kept in 4°C undisturbed for overnight.
- Reading is taken next morning.

Interpretation

- Titres are usually considered negative at less than 1 in 10 dilution ratio.
- The reported result is the highest dilution that causes agglutination ***(carpet of red cells at bottom of the well).***
- The test is not highly specific and about 5 to 10% of the normal population may have a low titre of Tg-autoantibodies with no symptoms of the disease.
- Reactivity occurs more frequently in Hashimoto's thyroiditis. It is positive in very high titre in more than 85% of the patients.
- In Graves' disease (thyrotoxicosis) a high titre even greater than 1600 are common in more than 30% of patients.
- Positive responses with high titre also observed in spontaneous adult myxoedema (primary) in more than 45% of cases. In another 30% cases titres may be low but positive.
- Weakly positive and low titres may also be found in patients with non-toxic goitre, thyroid carcinoma and pernicious anaemia.

B. ELISA and RIA Methods

These methods have been developed for measuring anti-Tg antibodies. Correlate well with agglutination tests but are generally more sensitive and specific for thyroid autoimmune diseases. Some assays also allow identification of subclasses of Tg-antibodies. The clinical significance of these subclasses is still not clear.

1. Determination of Antimicrosomal Antibodies

Antimicrosomal antibodies are directed against a protein component of thyroid cells microsomes. These antibodies can be measured using:

- complement fixation test (CFT)
- immunofluorescence of tissue sections
- passive haemagglutination test similar to TRCH
- ELISA techniques
- Radioimmunoassays (RIA) method.

2. Tanned Red Cells Haemagglutination Test—Using Microsomal Antigen

Tanned erythrocytes agglutination method uses red cells coated with tannic acid and with microsomal antigen isolated from human hyperplastic thyroid glands. The procedure is simple and is easily carried out in clinical laboratory.

Interpretation

- ***Positive reactivity*** occurs in nearly all adult patients with Hashimoto's thyroiditis and in nearly 85% of patients with Graves' disease.
- Low titres may, however, be seen in 5 to 10% of normal asymptomatic individuals.

- When compared with TRCH test of Tg-antibody (as described above), the ***result of microsomal antibody is more frequently positive for thyroid autoimmune diseases and usually titres are much higher.***

3. Complement Fixation Test (CFT)

CFT is used also in clinical laboratory but not routinely as compared to TRCH Test

Limitations of anti-microsomal assays

- Limited availability of human thyroid tissue
- Contamination of microsomal preparations with Tg.
- Presence of irrelevant thyroid antigens and autoantibodies.

Approximate positivity reactions of TRCH (Tg) and CFT in normal and various thyroid disorders and other autoimmune disorders as reported in a study group are shown in the box below.

IV. NEWER TESTS

Recently the following newer techniques have been put forward

- Determination of antithyroid peroxidase antibody (anti-TPo antibodies)
- Determination of thyrotropin-receptor antibodies (TRab)

a. Determination of Antithyroid Peroxidase Antibody (Anti-TPo Antibody)

In recent years, TPo has been identified and claimed as the main and possibly the only autoimmune component of microsomes. Its purification by using affinity chromatography and its production by recombinant technology has led to the development of ELISA and RIA methods for measuring anti-TPo antibodies.

Methods are easy to perform, provide greater sensitivity and specificity as compared to TRCH Tests, and can be used for ***"screening"***.

A suitable "immunometric assay" has been developed.

Immunometric Assay

Principle: Immunometric assay is based on competitive inhibition of the binding of radio-iodinated TPo to an anti-TPo monoclonal antibody coated onto plastic tubes.

Advantages

- Easy to perform
- Assay is rapid (only 2-hours incubation period is required).

Result

The antibody concentration is expressed as units/ml.

Interpretation

- ***In normal healthy persons:*** the mean anti-TPo activity in serum is 69 ± 15 units/ml.
- Detectable concentration of anti-TPo antibodies are observed in nearly all patients with Hashimoto's thyroiditis, spontaneous adult myxoedema (idiopathic primary type) and in a majority of patients with Graves' disease.

Group	*TRCH*	*CFT*	*Remarks*
• Normal (control group)	< 10%	< 10%	% may increase with age and more often in females
• Thyrotoxicosis	50%	80%	
• Myxoedema (primary)	43%	35%	
• Autoimmune thyroiditis	71%	92%	
• Non-toxic goitres and carcinoma of thyroid	< 10%	< 10%	
• Collagen diseases and other autoimmune disorders	< 10%	< 10%	

Note: It is important to realize that autoantibody presence only in high titre should be taken indicative of autoimmune thyroiditis.

- The frequency of detectable anti-TPo autoantibodies found in normals and non-thyroid cases is similar.

b. *Determination of Thyrotropin-Receptor Antibodies (TRAb)*

- The first indication that autoantibodies to TSH receptor plays a role in the pathogenesis of Graves' disease came with the discovery of LATS (long-acting thyroid stimulator) in serum of some patients.
- Thyrotropin-receptor antibodies (TRAb) are group of related immunogobulin (Igs) that bind to thyroid cell membranes at or near the "TSH receptor" site.
- These antibodies have recently been demonstrated frequently in patients with Graves' disease specially and also in other thyroid autoimmune disorders.

Note

- These antibodies show substantial heterogeneity.
- Some cause thyroid stimulation.
- Some others may have no effect or decrease thyroid secretion by blocking/inhibiting action of TSH.

Types of Receptor Antibodies

Two types have been described:

- Thyrotropin binding inhibitory immunoglobulins (TBI)
- Thyroid stimulating immunoglobulins (TSIgs)

Methodology

At present these abnormal antibodies, Igs cannot be differentiated by chemical or immunological methods Their presence is determined by either:

(i) radioreceptor assays;
(ii) bioassays.

1. *Thyrotropin-binding Inhibitory Immunoglobulins (TBI)*

- Determined by direct radioreceptor assay.
- The method assesses the capacity of Igs to inhibit the binding of radioisotope labelled TSH to its receptors in human or animal thyroid membrane preparations.
- In this method, detergent-solubilized porcine TSH-receptors and ^{125}I-labelled TSH are used.
- The ability of a purified fraction of serum Igs to displace ^{125}I-labelled TSH from the receptors is measured.

Interpretation

- Normal immunoglobulin G (IgG) concentrates do not produce significant displacement, and produces only less than 10% inhibition.
- This method detects over 85% of patients with Graves' disease.

2. *Thyroid Stimulating Immunoglobulins (TSIgs)*

- 'In vitro' bio-assay utilised.
- The method assesses the capacity of the Igs (antibodies) to stimulate a functional activity of the thyroid gland such as adenyl cyclase stimulation leading to increase in cyclic-AMP formation.
- Measurement of increase in cyclic-AMP level can be done using human thyroid slices, frozen human thyroid cells culture or a cloned line of thyroid follicular cells.

Interpretation

- The effect of stimulation is expressed as a % of basal activity.
  In normal: range is 70 to 130%.
- ***TSIgs*** have been detected in 95% of patients with untreated Graves' disease. It has been claimed to be highly ***sensitive*** and ***specific*** technique in diagnosing Graves' disease.
- TSIgs measurement has also been found to be useful for predicting relapse or remission in hyperthyroid patients.
- Also found useful for predicting the development of neonatal hyperthyroidism.

Practical Implications of Immunological Tests

Thyroid autoantibodies detection is of importance in diagnosis of the following conditions:

- In nodular goitres, detection of thyroid autoantibodies in high titres make the possibility of goitres being due to carcinoma less likely.
- Primary hypothyroidism can be differentiated from obesity and other hypometabolic states.
- Autoimmune thyroiditis diagnosis is confirmed.
- In differential diagnosis of endocrine exophthalmos other ocular lesions can be excluded.
- Serological tests may provide choice of line of treatment in patients with Graves' disease.

ADDENDUM

PRINCIPLES OF CPBA, RIA AND ELISA TECHNIQUES

IN CPBA TECHNIQUE

- T_3 or T_4 is extracted from the serum by either organic solvent or by use of absorptive material.
- Extracted T_3 or T_4 is then allowed to interact with a standard quantity of TBG in presence of radioiodinated T_3 or T_4 as "tracer".
- Ratio of bound and free form of T_3 or T_4 is then determined and compared with standard curve prepared by interacting known quantities of T_3 or T_4 with standard solution of TBG and T_3/T_4 "tracer".

Note

CPBA technique is not good and accurate for T_3 as it has very low affinity for TBG. Moreover, it will be necessary to remove T_4 completely from serum. It is good for estimation of T_4.

RADIOIMMUNOASSAY METHODOLOGY AND INTERPRETATION

Summary of radioimmunoassay principle and procedure is as follows:

The general methodology of radioimmunoassay is, in theory, relatively simple. An outline of the steps required to establish a radioimmunoassay for a hypothetical human protein hormone "X" is given below.

- Antiserum to X is raised in heterologous species, e.g., rabbit or guinea pig.
- If the hormone X is itself non-immunogenic, i.e., a hapten, it is first coupled to a macromolecular carrier, e.g., bovine γ-globulin, and the hapten and carrier complex is then used to raise an antiserum.
- X is then radiolabelled, usually with I (•X).
- Labelled antigen •X reacts with enough antibody to bind about 70% of •X.
- Various known amounts of unlabelled hormone X are added to a mixture of •X and anti-X and compete for antibody combining sites.
- After an appropriate incubation period, labelled •X bound to antibody is separated from unbound X.
- From the amount of •X bound at various X concentrations (Fig. 4.2), a curve can be constructed which will allow computation of any unknown X concentration desired (Fig. 4.3).

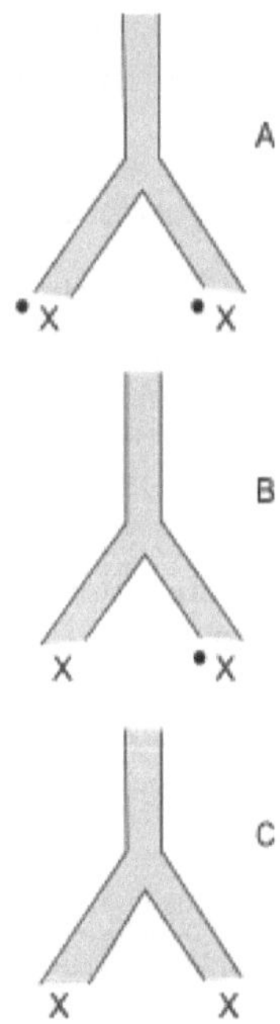

Fig. 4.2: A. No unlabelled X added and labelled •X. B. Approximately equal amounts of X and •X are added. C. Excess of X compared to •X displaces radiolabelled antigen

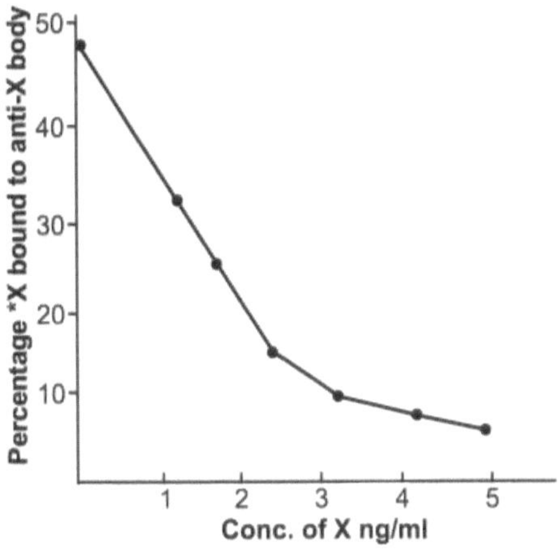

Fig. 4.3: Standard curve for radioimmunoassay of X

- Since the curve is linear over a relatively limited range, dilution of the sample containing an unknown amount of hormone X is necessary to adjust its concentration to within this measurable range.

ENZYME-LINKED IMMUNOSORBENT ASSAY (ELISA)

ELISA is based on the estimation of different antigens by allowing them to react specifically with the antibody to which an appropriate enzyme molecule has been coupled so that the enzyme activity would tell us how much Ag-Ab-E complex is present, and hence the Ag-concentration.

Two-types of procedures are used:

1. Competitive-Saturation analysis
2. Non-competitive.

- ***Competitive:*** The principle is the same as that of RIA, i.e., labelled and unlabelled antigen is incubated with the limiting amount of Ab.
  - ***Equilibrium techniques:*** Here all reagents are incubated together to achieve an equilibrium.
  - ***Sequential saturation or non-equilibrium technique:*** Here unlabelled Ag is incubated with Ab prior to the addition of labelled Ag.
- ***Non-competitive:*** Here, the labelled antigen behaves differently than the unlabelled one, i.e., binding of labelled Ag to the Ab results in steric hinderance to the enzyme activity so that enzyme activity is blocked or reduced. Therefore, labelled and unlabelled Ag need not be separated from the Ag-Ab complex, so-called homogeneous EIA.

Rest of the procedure is similar to that of RIA which is already described above.

Chapter 5

Adrenocortical Function Tests

INTRODUCTION

Adrenal glands are two semilunar or pyramidal structures one each on upper pole of both the kidneys—also called as suprarenal glands. Each gland consists of two developmentally and physiologically separate parts called,

(i) adrenal cortex; and
(ii) adrenal medulla, consisting 10% of the whole gland.

Adrenal cortex occupies outer peripheral portion and is histologically differentiated into three layers.

- Outer zona glomerulosa.
- Middle zona fasciculata.
- Inner zona reticularis.

All the three layers can produce glucocorticoids but mineralocorticoid synthesis is done by zona glomerulosa only. Adrenal cortex also produces the androgens. The chief gucocorticoid is cortisol. Cortisol secretion has a diurnal rhythm. Glucocorticoid secretion is stimulated by pituitary corticotropin ACTH which, in turn is regulated by hypothalamic corticotropin-releasing hormone (CRH). The secretion is controlled by ***"negative feed back inhibition"*** by high blood cortisol.

With the advancement of new techniques, e.g., radioimmuno assay and Enzyme-linked immunosorbent assay and new equipment e.g., fluorimeter, etc., a number of tests have been evolved to evaluate the function of adrenal cortex. Some tests measure the primary function of the gland, i.e., production of cortisol, aldosterone and androgens by adrenal cortex and by isotope dilution technique secretion rate of these hormones can be measured.

Tests have been evolved to measure the pituitary "reserve" ***by provocative tests.*** Tests are available to determine the integrity of hypothalamo-pituitary-adrenal axis.

Certain biochemical tests can find out the peripheral effects of the hormones. Lastly, availability of ^{131}I-labelled cholesterol has made possible the radioscanning of the adrenal cortex to delineate small adenomas/carcinoma. A classification of various tests based on the above is given below.

CLASSIFICATION

Tests for assessing adrenal cortical function can be divided under the following heads.

I. ***Tests based on cortisol production***
- Cortisol secretion rate
- Estimation of plasma cortisol level
  - i. RIA methods
  - ii. Chemical methods.
- Estimation of conjugated corticosteroids in urine
- Urinary cortisol estimation
- Estimation of urinary 11-OH corticoids.

II. ***"Provocative" tests***

ACTH stimulation tests:
- ACTH gel
- Aqueous ACTH

- Synacthen test
- Cortrosyn (Tetracosactrin test)
- IV ACTH test.

III. ***Tests of pituitary-adrenal function***
- "Stress" situations:
  - Insulin hypoglycaemia
  - Low plasma cortisol level
  - Metapirone (Metyrapone) test
  - Vasopressin Test.

IV. ***Tests using suppression or inhibition***
- Use of cortisone or cortisone-like acting steroids
- Dexamethasone suppression test.

V. ***Tests of hypothalamo-pituitary-adrenal function***
CRF test

VI. ***Tests based on aldosterone production***

VII. ***Tests based on androgen production***

VIII. ***Radioscan of adrenal cortex***

IX. ***Miscellaneous biochemical tests:***

X. ***Special Investigations***

Certain special investigations may be helpful to determine the cause of dysfunction in some cases.

They are:

1. If primary involvement of adrenals is suspected like some tumours then it may be helpful to do:
   - ***CT scanning*** of both the adrenals
   - Scanning can also be carried out with ^{131}I-labelled to do cholesterol which can differentiate hyperplasian adenoma and carcinoma.
   - ***Arteriography*** may be useful for differentiating adrenal hyperplasia and tumour.
2. Prior to above, one can perform radiological studies like:
   - X-ray skill
   - X-ray chest
   - X-ray lumbar spine
   - IV Pyelography with nephrotomography for renal stones and defection of adrenal enlargement.
3. In suspected pituitary tumour following can be helpful
   - Pituitary CT scan
   - Cerebral arteriography
4. In suspected case of ectopic ACTH syndrome
   - Tomography of lung can be helpful.
   - Oncogenic markers.
     Total and differential WBC count—shows lymphopenia and eosionopenia
5. ***Quantitative urinary estimations:*** Quantitative estimations of Na, K and uric acid in 24 hrs urine shows:
   - Decreased $Na^+ \downarrow$
   - Increased K^+ excretion (Kaliuresis)
   - Increased uric acid excretion $\uparrow$

   Measuring the peripheral effects of glucocorticoids/mineralocorticoids/androgens.

I. TESTS BASED ON CORTISOL PRODUCTION

Tests based on the measurement of cortisol and/or its metabolites in the plasma and urine are direct evidences for adreno-cortical function.

1. *Cortisol Secretion Rate*

Best method is to determine cortisol secretion rate but it is feasible if an isotope laboratory is available. It is determined by an isotopic dilution technique. Secretion rate provides an accurate measure of the total cortisol production over a period of 24 to 48 hours. This technique has proved invaluable in investigating adrenocortical function in man.

But the ***test is unsuitable for routine clinical use.***

Procedure

The method involves the following steps:

- Introduction into the patient of a small "tracer" dose of radiolabelled cortisol (^{14}C Cortisol).
- Collect all the urine passed during the following 24 to 48 hours.
- Tetrahydrocortisol or tetrahydrocortisone is then isolated from the urine by paper chromatography.

- Its specific activity is determined. Assumption is made that the "tracer dose" is metabolized by the same metabolic pathways as the endgenous cortisol, and that the same fraction of each will appear in the urine as these metabolites.

Calculation

Cortisol secretion rate is calculated from the equation

$$\text{Secretion rate} = \frac{\text{Dose}}{\text{M}}$$

Where,

Dose = the administered ^{14}C labelled cortisol expressed as counts/minute; and

M = the specific activity of the metabolite expressed as counts/minute/µg of the metabolite.

Interpretations

- ***Normal range*** of cortisol secretion rate observed = 6.3 to 28.6 mg/24 hours.
  Mean secretion rate=16 mg/24 hours.
- A marked rise in cortisol secretion rate is seen after ACTH stimulation test.

2. *Plasma Cortisol Level*

a. *Radioimmunoassay*

This is the best and most convenient method. RIA and immunoenzyme assay kits are available.

By this method:
Diurnal rhythm variation—
A.M.: 5 to 25 µg/dl (138-690 n mol/L)
P.M.: Approximately half of A.M. values.

b. *Chemical Methods*

The estimation is difficult in chemical methods. Earlier estimations are based on either

(i) Porter-Silber reaction for 17-OH corticoids, or
(ii) on the measurement of fluorescence of the individual steroids, after their separation by chromatography.

Porter and Silber reaction: The colour reaction which is given by 17-OH corticosteroids of the steroidal dihydroxyacetone group with a Phenylhydrazine-H_2SO_4 reagent was used by Porter-Silber. This method was modified by Paterson and used subsequently.

Disadvantages

- Requires 5 ml of plasma for a single estimation
- Time consuming and laborious for routine use.

c. *Fluorimetric Methods*

An advance of major clinical importance was made when simple but effective methods based on fluorescence were developed for estimation of cortisol in human plasma.

Principles: These methods depend on the fluorescence of certain steroids in conc. H_2SO_4 and only require 2 ml of plasma for each estimation. It measures 11-OH corticoids and the main 11-OH corticoids in human plasma is cortisol.

Advantages

- Requires lesser amount of plasma
- Specific test for 11-OH corticoids
- Synthetic analogues of cortisol and cortisone do not give fluorescence. Hence, it is possible to measure adrenocrotical activity in patients with these drugs.

Note

- Plasma 11-OH corticoid estimations only reflect adrenocortical activity at the time blood is taken. It is important to take this into account when interpreting the results.
- Basal levels must be measured in the morning to avoid the normal diurnal variation in plasma cortisol levels, which may be large.

Interpretations

- ***Normal value*** is in the range of 5.0 to 23.5 μg/100 ml, mean=14.5 μg/100 ml when the estimations are done in morning between 9 a.m. and 10 a.m.
- At midnight, lower values in the range of 0 to 6.0 μg/100 ml (mean = 3 μg/100 ml) are obtained. The estimations measure all the free or unconjugated 11-OH corticoids in the plasma.
- The total plasma 11-OH corticoid level is a reliable measure of adrenocortical activity except during:
  i. pregnancy, and
  ii. oestrogen therapy when the protein-binding is markedly increased.

  High levels in these patients do not necessarily indicate increased adrenal activity.
- Elevated 11-OH corticoid levels were found in women taking contraceptive pills.
- Other drugs known to interfere with these estimations are mepacrine and aldactone.

3. *Estimation of Conjugated Corticosteroids in Urine- (17-Oxosteroids)*

Cortisol metabolites are mainly conjugated with glucuronic acid and excreted as glucuronides in urine. Several tests have been developed which are based on the group estimation of these conjugated steroids in the urine. The **method** of **Gibson** and **Norymberski** is for the estimation of 17-oxogenic steroids, the steroids in which side chain on carbon atom C-17 can be removed by oxidizing agents to form 17-Oxosteroids. 17-Oxosteroids are estimated by the ***"Zimmerman reaction"*** in which colour is produced by the action of the steroids with m-dinitrobenzene in strong alkali.

Sources of 17-oxosteroids

In males, one-third of 17-oxosteroid is derived from testes and remaining two-third from adrenal cortex while ***in females*** mainly from adrenal cortex.

Interpretations

- ***Normal value:*** ranges from 6 to 22 mg/24 hours in adult males and 5 to 18 mg/24 hours in adult females.
- The values of 17-Oxosteroids are elevated in adrenocortical carcinoma, bilateral hyperplasia of the adrenal cortex and in testicular tumours (Leydig cells tumour).
- Decreased in Addison's disease, pituitary dwarfism, Simmond's disease, occasionally in anorexia nervosa, and in myxoedema.
- These estimations are of little value in assessing adrenocortical hypofunction during childhood, since the levels are so low below the age of puberty that only gross divergencies from normal can be detected.
- Estimations include steroid metabolities of cortisol and also its inactive precursors and these methods do not distinguish between them.
- Elevated levels do not necessarily indicate an increased production of cortisol but may be due to a block in the cortisol synthesis, resulting in an increased output of its precursors.
- The urinary output of these conjugated steroids is ***also dependant on renal function*** and may be seriously affected by alterations in the glomerular filtration rate (GFR). When renal function is impaired there is retention of these conjugated steroids in the body and a reduced output in urine.
- Neither of these methods is sufficiently accurate to distinguish between the low levels found in many debilitated patients from those occurring in patients with adrenal hypofunction.
- Drugs administered to patients do not interfere with these estimations except meprobamate.
- A serious source of error is the presence of glucose in the urine—glucose prevents the oxidation of 17-oxogenic steroids to 17-oxosteroids. ***Glycosuria can thus lead to underestimations.***

4. *Urinary Cortisol Estimation*

Less than 0.5% of the cortisol is normally excreted unchanged in the urine. This small amount can be measured by suitable techniques and has been found of particular value in the diagnosis of Cushing's syndrome.

Normal cortisol excretion has been found to be less than 10 to about 80 μg/24 hours (radioimmunoassay) with a mean value of 28.5 μg/24 hours.

Mean rise in Cushing's syndrome was found to be 8 to 9 times the normal.

- ***Estimation of Urinary 11-OH Corticoid***

Mattingly and her colleagues have used a rapid screening test for adrenocortical function which is based on the fluorescence of "free" unconjugated 11-OH corticoids in urine. A good correlation was found between these estimations and the cortisol secretion rate determined simultaneously. Most of the fluorescence in the urine extracts appears to be produced by free cortisol and its metabolites 20-OH cortisol.

Interpretations

- *Normal range:* varies from 78 to 370 μg/24 hours, when expressed as cortisol equivalents
- *In Cushing's syndrome:* the value ranges from 400 to 7000 μg/24 hours
- Glucose in urine does not interfere with these estimations
- Drugs which are known to interfere with the tests are mainly mepacrine and aldactone.

Note

- Mepacrine can produce abnormally high results which may persist for a month after even stopping the drug.
- Synthetic steroids do not fluoresce so that method can be used to measure the degree of adrenocortical suppression produced by these drugs.

II. PROVOCATIVE TESTS (ACTH STIMULATION TESTS)

A large number of ACTH stimulation tests have been described which differ in the:

- dose and preparation of ACTH employed;
- the route of administration and duration of the test; and
- the method used to determine the adrenocortical respose to stimulation.

Tests based on IV infusion of ACTH involves the risk of severe allergic reactions sometimes and have not been widely adopted. This is avoided by:

- Giving ACTH IM or by the use of ACTH gel; and
- Secondly by using synthetic preparations, viz. Synacthen and Tetracosactrin.

1. *Importance of ACTH stimulation tests*

ACTH stimulation tests are valuable in differentiating between hypoadrenocorticism due to Addison's disease and that due to hypopituitarism.

Procedure

- *Estimation of plasma 11-OH corticoids:* Plasma 11-hydroxy corticoids estimation (Mattingly, 1963) provides a simple and quick measure of the adrenal response to ACTH gel, the peak levels in normal subjects being reached between 4 and 6 hours after the injection.
- *ACTH gel:* Blood is taken for ***"basal"*** plasma 11-OH corticoids estimation between 9 a.m. and 10 a.m. The patient is then given an IM injection of 50 units of ACTH gel. A further blood sample is taken 5 hours later and the response is measured by the rise in plasma 11-OH corticoid level over the 5 hours.

There is a wide range of response to this test in patients with intact adrenal glands.

Interpretation

- *Normal range:* is 19 to 110 μg/100 ml with a mean rise of 45 μg/100 ml. This test can be completed within a few hours of admitting a patient to hospital.

2. Screening test

A quicker screening test has also been described (Maynard et al, 1966) which can be done in OPD by using aqueous ACTH. Patient is given a single IM injection of 25 units of aqueous ACTH. Plasma 11-OH corticoid level is measured immediately before and one hour after the injection.

Interpretations

- *Normal range:* is 11 to 48 μg/100 ml with a mean value of 25 μg/100 ml.
- No response is seen in patients with primary adrenal insufficiency.
- *IV ACTH test:*

On the day before the test, a 24-hour urine is collected and the quantities of 17-ketogenic steroids/or 17-OH corticoids excreted are determined. Subsequently, on three consecutive days, 25 units of ACTH in 1000 ml of 5% dextrose in normal or 0.45 (N) saline are infused IV over a period of exactly 8 hours. Daily 24-hour urine specimens are collected for 17-ketogenic steorids/or 17-OH corticoids.

Interpretation

- *Normally,* a three-fold or greater excretion occurs on the first day of the test, with a further increase on the second day and maximum excretion on the third day.
- A rise in steroid excretion of less than 100% of the control value is diagnostic of adrenocortical insufficiency.

Note
- The test is specific and sensitive for adrenocortical insufficiency.
- Risk of allergic reaction.

3. Synacthen Test

Reported by ***Wood et al, 1965,*** it is a simple test and can be performed in OPD. There is a rise in plasma 11-OH corticoid level 30 minutes after a single IM injection of 250 μg of synthetic "Synacthen" is given (dose is equivalent to 25 units of natural hormone).

- *Normal value:* ranges from 7.0 to 25 μg/100 ml with a mean increase of 16.5 μg/100 ml.

Note

Where facilities for plasma cortisol estimation are available, it can be estimated in place of plasma 11-OH corticoids.

4. Cortrosyn (Tetracosactrin) Test

It is a simple test and can be used for screening purposes.

Plasma cortisol level is determined from a blood sample drawn between 7 AM and 9 AM **("basal level").**

Cortrosyn in a dose of 0.25 mg is injected IM.

Plasma cortisol levels are then determined in blood samples drawn 30 and 45 minutes after the injection.

Interpretation

- *In normal subjects:* plasma cortisol levels rise by at least 7 μg/100 ml in 30 minutes, or the total value exceeds 18 μg/100 ml. Usually there is at least two-fold rise above the control value to 20 μg/100 ml or above. The plasma cortisol value at 45 minutes also found similar to 30 minute sample.
- A normal response excludes primary adrenocortical failure,
- A subnormal response showing no significant increase indicates adrenocortical failure and requires further investigations.

Remarks

Synthetic steroids have certain advantages and disadvantages over natural ACTH obtained from pituitary glands of animals.

Advantages

- Synthetic preparations are pure compounds.
- Not contaminated with foreign proteins
- Can be assayed by weight

- Shorter amino acid sequences.
- Purity and shorter amino acid sequence decreases likelihood of any allergic reaction.

Disadvantage

Major disadvantage is shorter duration of action. The action is over within 4 hours of IM injection. Thus its use in therapy is limited.

III. TESTS OF PITUITARY-ADRENAL FUNCTION

The provocative ACTH stimulation tests indicate only the degree of adrenal cortex atrophy and adrenocortical insufficiency. These tests do not give any indication regarding the ability of the anterior pituitary to produce and secrete ACTH.

A number of tests have been described for testing pituitary adrenal function, but none are entirely satisfactory. Ideal requirements for getting the satisfactory results are:

- The procedures should test the entire hypothalamic pituitary-adrenal system;
- Should be simple to carry out as routine test in clinical laboratory
- Should be reproducible; and
- Should be free from any side effects.

Stressful situations like insulin-induced hypoglycaemia and fever produced by bacterial "pyrogen" injection are potent stimuli to the neural mechanism controlling ACTH release. *The major drawbacks* with the latter are that it is not popular and not used widely as the response to standard dose is not predictable and vary from case to case and is associated with certain amount of risks. However, insulin-induced hypoglycaemia has been used.

1. *Insulin-Induced Hypoglycaemia*

Measurement of the plasma cortisol response to insulin-induced hypoglycaemia has become a useful test to measure the pituitary reserve in suspected ACTH lack.

Interpretations

- If ***Addison's disease*** (adrenocortical insufficiency) is not present, i.e., the adrenals can respond to ACTH, a peak plasma cortisol response less than 550 nmol/L (provided blood glucose has been lowered to less than 2.5 nmol/L for 30 minutes, indicates impairment of ACTH function.
- The test is of value in Cushing's syndrome. It is helpful in distinguishing the normal response in cases of psychosis with abnormal cortisol regulation from the absent response in "true" Cushing's syndrome.

Advantages

- The test is sensitive and simple.
- Though the risk of hypoglycaemia is there, it is safe in experienced hand.
- Easily combined with other assays to determine the full profile of pituitary reserve.

Precaution

Should be avoided in elderly patients and/or in those with history of cardiac ischaemia.

2. Low Plasma Cortisol Level

Principle A strong natural stimulus to ACTH release is provided by an abnormally low plasma cortisol level, which occurs after recovery from prolonged corticosteroid therapy. ***Robinson et al. (1962)*** tested the integrity of the pituitary-adrenal axis after prolonged corticosteroid therapy by following the spontaneous rise in plasma cortisol concentration after the sudden cessation of treatment.

Interpretation

If the pituitary-adrenal axis is intact, a rise in normal levels occurs within 48 hours of the last dose, after stopping of treatment.

Advantages

- It is a natural stimulus.
- Simple test and quick method
- Valuable in determining whether the pituitary has been completely destroyed by surgery or radioactive seeds in the treatment of carcinoma of the breast.

3. *Metyrapone (Metapyrone) Test*

The discovery that the insecticide DDT produces adrenal atrophy in animals, led to a search for other compounds which may interfere with adrenal function. A number of substances have been synthesized since then, but only one compound which has been accepted and widely used is ***"Metyrapone" (Metapyrone, SU 4885).***

Mechanism of action: Metyrapone produces inhibition of the enzyme *"11-β-hydroxylase"* in the synthesis of cortisol and corticosterone.

Principle As the enzyme ***11-β-hydoxylase*** is inhibited by metyrapone, cortisol/corticosterone synthesis suffers and their 11-deoxy precursors are produced. Plasma cortisol level falls rapidly to very low levels and the anterior pituitary promptly secretes more ACTH since the normal feedback control of ACTH release is thus removed. The elevated ACTH levels in blood increases adrenal steroid synthesis leading to accumulation of increased amounts of 11-deoxycortisol (compound S) and 11-deoxycorticosterone (DOC).

The above results in urinary excretion of 17-oxosteroids and 17-oxogenic steroids which increases during administration of the drug, the increase in latter fraction being largely due to presence of abnormal amounts of ***"tetrahydro-derivatives of 11-deoxycortisol"*** in urine.

Structure

Chemically Metyrapone is 2-methyl-1,2-bis-(3-pyridyl)-propanone.

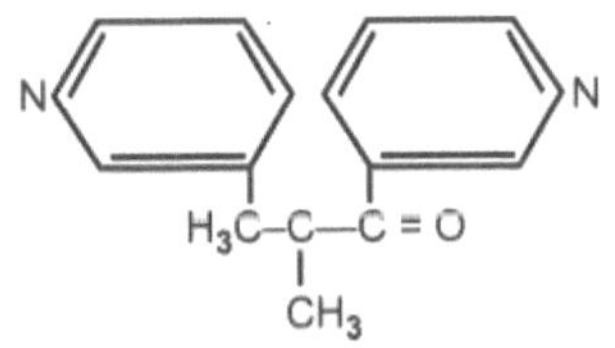

Procedure

- A non-toxic drug, metyrapone can be given preferably orally or intravenously. It is given in a dose of 750 mg every 4 hours, in 6 doses.
- Daily dosage of 4.5 gm usually produces 95% inhibition of the enzyme. Smaller dosage is less effective. Effect of a single dose lasts over 4 to 5 hours.

  Measurement of urinary excretion of 17-OH-corticoid: The pituitary-adrenal response to Metyrapone is determined by measuring the urinary excretion of 17-OH corticoids (or 17-oxogenic steroids) on the day before, during and on the day after Metyrapone administration. Peak levels are found on the day of administration but usually occur on the following day.
- The response is measured by the maximum rise in steroid excretion on either of these two days over the control day level.

Interpretation

- A range of 10 to 38 mg/24 hours, with a mean rise of 24 mg/24 hours is observed.
- A poor response to this test does not necessarily imply that the pituitary is incapable of secreting more ACTH, for the adrenal itself may be atrophied and unable to respond.
- Whenever an impaired response is obtained with this test, it should be followed by an ACTH stimulation test to exclude the above possibility.
- In pituitary dependent Cushing's syndrome, the mean rise in 17-OH corticoids is about three-fold, but about 5% of patients do not respond.

Side effects

- Sensation of light headedness or giddiness is most common. It lasts for about 30 minutes after taking the tablet. Incidence can be reduced if the drug is administered after food or with a glass of milk
- There is risk of precipitating acute adrenal insufficiency.

Precaution

Corticosteroids or exogenous ACTH will interfere with the Metyrapone test by suppressing ACTH secretion from the pituitary and should be discontinued at least three days before hand.

4. Vasopressin Test

Principle: When vasopressin, chemically related to the corticotrophin-releasing factor (CRF), is administered to humans in adequate doses it produces a rise in the plasma cortisol level, which is due to direct action on anterior pituitary.

Procedure

- Test is carried out in early afternoon.
- Synthetic "lysine-vasopressin" is used. Patient is given 10 pressor units of synthetic `lysine-vasopressin' IM.
- The test measures the ability of the anterior pituitary to secrete ACTH.
- Blood is drawn immediately before and after the injection of vasopressin.
- Blood samples are assayed for plasma 11-OH corticoids.

Interpretations

- *In normal persons:* There is quick and consistent rise in the plasma 11-OH corticoids which reaches a peak level one hour after the injection. Peak level is more than twice the control value.
- Also there is rise in plasma ACTH level.

Note

A similar but more complicated test using continuous IV infusion of lysine-vasopressin has been described recently.

IV. TESTS USING SUPPRESSION OR INHIBITION

1. Use of Cortisone or Cortisone-like Acting Steroids

Useful in distinguishing between hyperplasia and tumours. In adults, 100 mg of cortisone may be given daily.

Alternatively, 25 mg of prednisone or prednisolone or 10 mg of 9-α-fluorocortisol can be used.

Interpretation

- If 100 mg cortisone is given, about 40 mg of 17-oxogenic steroids are excreted while with 25 mg of prednisone only about 10 mg of 17-oxogenic steroids excreted.

  Note

  Prednisone is preferred due to low dosage of administration and as smaller amounts of metabolites are produced.
- In ***patients*** with ***congenital adrenal hyperplasia,*** a considerable fall in the excretion of 17-oxosteroids and 17-oxogenic steroids rapidly occurs, which may reduce values to normal or even subnormal levels within 2 to 3 days.

2. Dexamethasone Suppression Tests

In Cushing's syndrome, studies with the more potent inhibitor of pituitary ACTH, dexamethasone, are more useful. Both low and high dosages have been used.

a. Low Dosage Suppression Test

Liddle (1960) found that 8 doses of 0.5 mg dexamethasone given every 6 hours orally suppressed the adrenal cortex in normal patients but not in patients with Cushing's syndrome, whatever may be the cause.

b. High Dosage Suppression Test

A larger dose of 2 mg given similarly, suppressed when this condition is due to hyperplasia but rarely in tumour cases.

Urine samples are collected for 24 hours periods and then for two more specimens for further 24 hrs while the dexamethasone is being given and analyzed for total 17-OH corticoids mg/24 hours. In one study, **Grant** (1966) found the following results:

	Total 17-OH corticoids (mg/24 hours)	
	Control group	*Second day after dexamethasone*
• *Normal healthy adults*	3 to 12	< 2.5
• *Cushing's hyperplasia*	12 to 36	Decreased by 0.5 mg dose
• *Cushing's tumour*	19 to 60	No decrease even with 2.0 mg dose.

V. TESTS FOR HYPOTHALAMO-PITUITARY ADRENAL FUNCTION

1. *Corticotropin-Releasing Hormone (CRH) Stimulation Tests*

Corticotropin-releasing hormone, produced in the hypothalamus is a peptide having 41 amino acids and major regulator of ACTH secretion.

Its secretion is modulated by neuroendocrine, physical and emotional factors. Injection of CRH stimulates ACTH secretion in normal subjects within 60 to 180 minutes, glucocorticoids inhibits this effect.

Use

The test is used:

- In differential diagnosis of adrenal cortical hyperfunction and hypofunction, and
- Endogenous Cushing's syndrome and of secondary and tertiary ACTH deficiency.

Rationale

Exogenous CRH stimulates the secretion of ACTH from the anterior pituitary gland in normal subjects.

Cortisol level is an indicator of ACTH response.

Procedure

- Synthetic CRH/or human CRH can be used, the former preferred
- A dose of 1 µg/kg of body weight is given IV in bolus form either 0900 hours or 2000 hours.
- Blood samples for cortisol and ACTH assays are collected 15 minutes and immediately before. Samples are also collected 5, 15, 30, 60, 120 and 180 minutes after CRH injection.

Interpretations

- ***In normal subjects:*** plasma ACTH concentrations peak in 30 minutes after CRH injection is 80 ± 7 pg/ml at 0930 hour and 29 ± 2.6 pg/ml at 2030 hour, and serum cortisol peaks in 60 minute is 13 ± 1 µg/dl at 1000 hour, and 17 ± 0.7 µg/dl at 2100 hour.
- Patients with pituitary ACTH deficiency, (secondary adrenal insufficiency) have decreased ACTH and cortisol responses.
- Patients with hypothalamic disease have prolonged ACTH responses and subnormal cortisol responses.
- Most patients with Cushing's syndrome caused by adrenal tumours or non-endocrine ACTH producing tumours do not respond to CRH.
- Most patients with Cushing's disease respond with a normal or excessive increase in ACTH.
- Responses are usually normal in patients with depression.

VI. TESTS BASED ON ALDOSTERONE PRODUCTION

The daily production of aldosterone is only 1/100th that of cortisol and the measurement of such minute amounts presents great difficulties. No method is available at present for routine clinical use in laboratory. However, various immunoassay methods have now developed recently but require considerable skill and experience and can be done in few laboratories. Several non-isotopic enzyme immunoassays have been described for serum and urinary aldosterone ***using both monoclonal and polyclonal antibodies*** generated against aldosterone.

- ***Estimation of aldosterone secretion rate*** determined by isotope dilution using similar techniques employed for cortisol.
- ***Plasma and urinary aldosterone levels*** for which commercial kits are available and are estimated by direct radio-immuno assay.

Interpretation

- *In healthy adults:* plasma aldosterone levels range from 3 to 16 ng/dl (supine position) and 7 to 30 ng/dl (upright position).

  The urinary aldosterone levels range from 3 to 19 µg/24 hours urine.
- *High values of plasma aldosterone have been found in*
- Na-depleted patients,
- Patients with aldosterone secreting tumours, and
- Some patients with severe hypertension.

VII. TESTS BASED ON ANDROGEN PRODUCTION

The conjugated metabolites of the adrenal androgens are 17-oxosteroids, and form a major part of the total 17-oxosteroids excretion in the urine. "Group methods" for the estimation of urinary 17-oxosteroids have been widely used, but they are relatively "crude" index of adrenal androgen production.

These methods do not distinguish between the:

- metabolites of the androgens secreted by the adrenal cortex; and
- those derived from testes and ovary

More specific methods for the estimation of individual androgens and their metabolites in blood and urine are time consuming and laborious and not suitable for routine clinical laboratory use.

Interpretation

- During first 2 weeks of life, urinary 17-oxosteroids excretion may be 5 mg/24 hours.
- But after 2 weeks, it falls rapidly to less than 1 mg/24 hours until the child is between 6 and 10 years old,
- After that it rises slowly to reach adult levels after puberty.
- Maximum excretion occurs in both sexes around the age of 20.
- There is slow decline in the level after age of 50.
- *In normal young adult males,* the value ranges from 5 to 26 mg/24 hours while in *young adult females,* it ranges from 4 to 17 mg/24 hours.

The mean value in men is about 5 mg/day higher than the mean value in females. This difference is mainly due to additional 17-oxosteroids derived from testicular androgens.

Note

Low 17-oxosteroid levels are often found in chronically ill patients, particularly if renal function is impaired. Hence, these estimations will be misleading if taken as sole criterion for diagnosing adrenal hypofunction.

VIII. RADIO SCAN OF ADRENAL CORTEX

Recent production and availability of **^{131}I-labelled cholesterol** made it possible for gamma-camera imaging of the adrenal uptake, a day or two after injection. Adrenal uptake found to be sufficiently selective relative to nearby organs such as liver and kidney and delineates the adrenal cortex properly. This has potential application in Cushing's syndrome—unilateral uptake in that condition would strongly suggest autonomous adrenal adenoma with atrophy of the other adrenal gland. It can also show small adenomas in Conn's syndrome.

IX. MISCELLANEOUS BIOCHEMICAL TESTS

Glucocorticoids produce a number of important biochemical changes in the body. In hyper function, produces hyperglycaemia by increasing gluconeogenesis and cause insulin resistant diabetes. There is negative nitrogen balance and increased uric acid excretion. The number of eosinophils in peripheral blood is reduced. Urinary Na^+ excretion falls and there is K^+ diuresis. Prolonged administration of corticosteroids in large doses leads to osteoporosis and negative calcium balance.

Following investigations will be helpful:

1. *Absolute Eosinophil Count*

- ***In normal persons:*** the eosinophil count ranges from 100 to 300/cumm. The count tends to rise during the morning to a maximum at midday, falls in the afternoon and rises again in the evening.
- In patients with increased glucocorticoid formation, the value is usually below 50/ cumm.
- ***In hypofunction (Addison's disease),*** it is in upper normal range or above.

2. *Blood Sugar Estimation*

In hyperfunction shows hyperglycaemia and may cause insulin resistant diabetes.

GTT is impaired.

3. *Serum Electrolytes and CO_2—Combining Power*

- ***In hyperfunction:*** hypokalaemic alkalosis may be seen.
- ***In hypofunction (Addison's disease):*** evidence of sodium depletion, potassium retention and extrarenal uraemia may be observed.

Chapter 6

Pancreatic Function Tests*

1. FUNCTIONAL ANATOMY OF THE PANCREAS

The pancreas is ***both an endocrine*** and ***an exocrine gland.*** The flattened organ, weighing less than 100 g, is located posterior and slightly inferior to the stomach. The oblong gland, about 12.5 cm long and 2.5 cm thick, consists of head, body, and tail (Fig. 6.1). The endocrine function of the gland is due to 1-2 million tiny clusters of cells of endocrine tissue called pancreatic ***islets of Langerhans,*** scattered among the exocrine portions of the pancreas and contributing 1-1.5% of the pancreatic mass.

The ***islets are found throughout the pancreas but are more abundant in the tail region of the gland.*** The islets vary in size from 50 to 300 μm in diameter and are surrounded by clusters of cells (acini) that form the exocrine part of the pancreas (Fig. 6.2). Each islet contains on an average 2500 cells and is composed of four major cell types. Each cell type synthesizes and secretes a different hormone.

- ***α-cells:*** The α-cells are located toward the edges of the islet, forming a rim. They contribute about 20-30% of islet cells and ***secrete the hormone glucagon.***

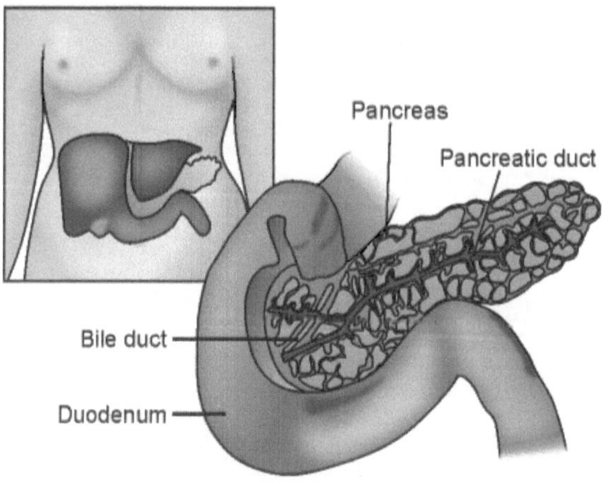

Fig. 6.1: Pancreas-gross anatomy

**Contributed by Professor R Chawla, MSc, DMRIT, PhD, Professor of Biochemistry , Faculty of Medicine, Addis-Ababa University, Ethiopia, ex-Professor of Biochemistry, Christian Medical College, Ludhiana (Punjab)*

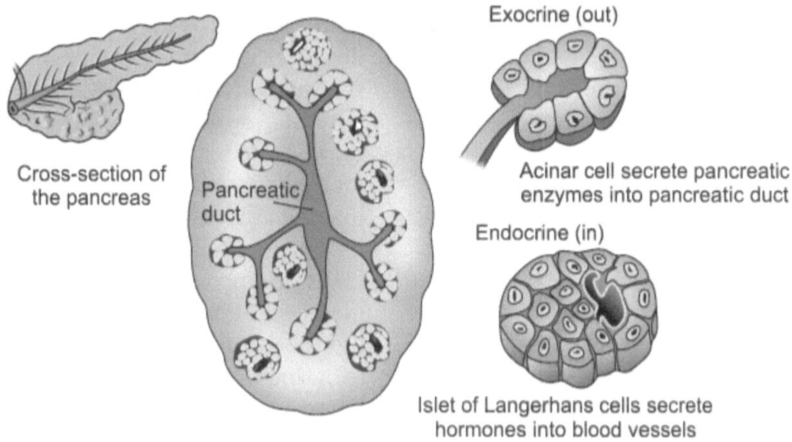

Fig. 6.2: Cross-section of Pancreas with Acinar and Islet cells

- *β-cells:* About 60-80% of the islet cells are β-cells that tend to be located more toward the centre of the islet. They are generally 10 to 15 μm in diameter, contain secretory granules that measure 0.25 μm and *secrete the hormone insulin.*
- *δ-cells:* δ-cells are scattered in between the rim of α-cells and core of β-cells. The make up 10% of the cells and *secrete the hormone* somatostain or *Growth Hormone Inhibiting Hormone (GHIH).* Somatostain can inhibit the secretion from both α-and β-cells.
- *F-cells:* Around 1% of the islet cells scattered between α-cells toward the edges of the islet are the cells known as F-cells. They *secrete pancreatic polypeptide.* The pancreatic polypeptide regulates the release of pancreatic digestive enzymes.

Pancreatic secretions pass from the secreting cells in the pancreas into small ducts. Smaller ducts unite to form two larger ducts that convey the secretions into the small intestine. The *larger duct* is called the *pancreatic duct (duct of Wirsung)* and the *smaller duct* is known as *accessory duct (duct of Santorini).* In most people, the pancreatic duct joins the common bile duct from the liver and gall baldder and enters the duodenum as a common duct called the ampulla of Vater (hepatopancreatic ampulla). The accessory duct leads from the pancreas and empties into the duodenum about 2.5 cm above the ampulla of Vater.

PANCREATIC FLUID AND ITS SECRETION

The control of pancreatic activity is under both nervous and endocrine control. Branches of the vagus nerve can cause secretion of a small amount of pancreatic fluid when food is smelt or seen, and these secretions may increase as the bolus of food reaches the stomach.

However, most of the pancreatic action is under the hormonal control of secretin and cholecystokinin (CCK-formerly called pancreozymin). **Secretin,** secreted in response to the acidic contents of the stomach reaching the duodenum, is responsible *for the production of bicarbonate rich and therefore alkaline pancreatic fluid* (Table 6.1), which protects the lining of the intestine from damage. It can also affect gastrin activity in th stomach. CCK, in the presence of fats and/or amino acids in the duodenum, is produced by the cells of the intestinal mucosa and is responsible for release of enzymes from the acinar cells into the pancreatic fluid.

More than 1200 ml of the pancreatic fluid reaches the duodenum everyday. The *fluid is*

highly alkaline (pH > 8.0), rich in sodium, chloride and bicarbonate (Table 6.1). The enzymatic component constitutes all the types of hydrolytic enzymes viz. • **proteolytic** that digest the different types of ingested dietary proteins; • **lipolytic** that hydrolyze the triglycerides, cholesterol esters as well as the membrane phospholipids; the • **amylolytic** ***enzyme α-amylase*** for the digestion of the polysaccharides; and the nucleases.

Table 6.1: Composition of the pancreatic fluid

Daily secretion	:	1200 to 1500 ml
pH	:	approximately 8.0
Cations	:	Na^+, K^+, Ca^{++}, Mg^{++}
Anions	:	HCO_3^-, $C1^-$, SO_4^-, HPO_4^-
Enzymes:		
Proteolytic	:	Trypsin, Chymotrypsin, Carboxypeptidase-A and B, Elastases
Lipolytic	:	Pancreatic lipase, Co-lipase, Phospholipase A2, Cholesterol esterase
Amylolytic	:	Pancreatic α-amylase
Others	:	Ribonuclease, Deoxyribonuclease

In this chapter, the discussion will be made on exocrine functions of pancreas. Endocrine functions will not be considered. For this refer to laboratory investigations or hyperglycaemia and hypoglycaemia.

TESTS FOR EXOCRINE PANCREATIC FUNCTION

The first line laboratory tests for the detection of pancreatic exocrine dysfunction are the ***estimation of the serum levels of the pancreatic enzymes*** viz. ***amylase*** and ***lipase.*** Raised levels of these enzymes indicate pancreatic pathology and can then be further invetigated in light of the clinical findings and history of the patient. It is easy to diagnose pancreatic insufficiency in the presence of the clinical triad of pancreatic calcification, diabetes and steatorrhea. Most pancreatic diseases, however, remain clinically silent until approximately 90% of the gland is destroyed. Lipase secretion appears to decrease earlier than trypsin secretion; hence, steatorrhea appears earlier than azotorrhea in patients suffering from pancreatic disease. Earlier recognition of pancreatic dysfunction may improve the management of the patient's disease and his/ her quality of life.

Other laboratory tests of pancreatic function include those used for detection of malabsorption (e.g., microscopic examination of stools for excess fat, starch and meat fibres, exocrine function (e.g. secretin, CCK, faecal fat, trypsin, and chymotrypsin), tests assessing changes associated with extra-hepatic obstruction (e.g. bilirubin), endocrine-related tests (e.g., gastrin, insulin, glucose, and cortisol) that reflect changes in the endocrine cells of the pancreas.

Exocrine Pancreatic function tests may be divided into ***two main groups:*** • direct ***(duodenal intubation)*** and • indirect (Table 6.2)

Table 6.2: Exocrine pancreatic function tests

A. ***Direct Invasive Intubation Tests***	• CCK/secretin stimulation • Lundh meal • ERCP and pancreatic aspiration
B. ***Indirect non-invasive tests***	• Stool fats and nitrogen • Stool trypsin and chymotrypsin • Breath tests • Oral function tests (bentiromide test and pancreolauryl test)
C. ***Blood determination***	• Pancreatic amylase • Lipase • Trypsinogen

A. Direct Invasive Intubation Tests

Tube tests require an oroduodenal tube that aspirates pancreatic secretion from the duodenum near the ampulla of Vater so that the response to stimulating factors can be measured.

The stimulants used are ***secretin, cholecystokinin*** and the ***Lundh test meal.*** The test performance requires the presence of a gastroenterologist because the accuracy of these tests can be compromised by ineffective tube placement and lack of success in aspiration. The ***collection period varies from 45 to 120 minutes.***

Direct evaluation of pancreatic fluid may include measurement of the total volume of pancreatic fluid, and the amount or concentration of bicarbonate and/or enzymes, all of which require pancreatic stimulation. Stimulation may be accomplished using a predescribed meal or administration of secretin, which allows for volume and bicarbonate evaluation, or secretin stimulation followed by CCK stimulation which adds enzymes to the pancreatic fluid evaluation.

The advantage of these teste is that the chemical and cytologic examination are performed on actual pancreatic secretions. Cytologic examination of the fluid can often establish the presence or at least the suspicion of malignant neoplasm, although precise localization of the primary organ of involvement (i.e., pancreas, biliary system, ampulla of Vater, or duodenum) is not possible by duodenal aspiration. Because of advances in imaging techniques, these stimulation tests are used less often.

None of the tests has proven especially useful in diagnosis of mild or acute pancreatic disease in which the acute phase has subsided. Most of the tests have found their usefulness for their negative predictive value for excluding the pancreatic disease.

The following pancreatic function tests will be reviewed briefly: ***the Lundh meal, secretin tests, faecal fat analysis, sweat chloride determinations,*** and ***amylase*** and ***lipase*** interpretation.

• Lundh Meal Test

A physiological stimulation test of the pancreas by a meal is called the Lundh test. It assesses the response of the pancreas to endogenous secretin and pancreozymin (or CCK) released in response to a test meal of 5% protein, 6% fat and 15% carbohydrates and 74% non-nutrient fibre. The concentration of trypsin and the volume of secretion are measured in samples obtained in the duodenal aspirate in 10 to 20 minute intervals over a period of two hours.

The ***advantage*** of this test is its relative simplicity and the fact that a natural physiologic stimulus is given. The Lundh meal is virtually always abnormal in pancreatic insufficiency but the ***major disadvantage*** is that abnormal results also occur when disease is present in the small bowel, liver, or biliary tree. A border-line zone of abnormal values is seen in these patients.

Many non-pancreatic factors can influence the results of a Lundh meal, including small bowel mucosal disease, rate of gastric emptying, and surgical interruption of gastroduodenal anatomy. Although this is a more physiological test, its senitivity and specificity are lower (70-80%) than those of direct hormonal stimulation.

• Secretin/Cholecystokinin Stimulation Test

The stimulation of the pancreas can be accomplished directly by infusing secretin alone or in combination with cholecystokinin. The combination allows the assessment not only of bicarbonate secretion (with secretin) but also of enzyme secretion, mainly trypsin. Therefore, the test is a direct determination of the exocrine secretory capacity of the pancreas. The test requires intubation of the duodenum and aspiration of pancreatic fluid without contamination by gastric fluid, which would neutralize any bicarbonate.

The test is performed after a 6-hour or overnight fast. Pancreatic secretion is stimulated by intravenously administered secretin in a dose varying from 0.25 to 1 U/kg of body weight followed by CCK administ-ration. If a simple secretin test is desired, the higher dose of secretin may be given alone.

Pancreatic secretions are collected at 30, 60, or 80 minutes or as single pooled collection. The pH, fluid volume, enzyme activities (e.g. trypsin, amylase, or lipase) and amount of bicarbonate are determined. The average amount of bicarbonte excreted per hour is about 15 mM per hour for males and 12 mM per hour for females. Assessment of enzymes must be take in view of the total volume output.

Interpretation

Dicreased pancreatic flow is associated with pancreatic obstruction and with an increse in enzyme concentrations. Low concentrations of bicarbonate and enzymes are associated with cystic fibrosis, chronic pancreatitis, Pancreatic cysts, calcification and oedema.

ERCP and Pancreatic Aspiration

Cannulation of the pancreatic duct during endoscopic retrograde cholangio-pancreatography (ERCP) has been combined with direct stimulation of the pancreas. This technique allows the measurement of pure pancreatic juice uncontaminated by biliary or intestinal secretions, but this method is possibly no more sensitive than other tests in the diagnosis of pancreatic disease.

B. Indirect Non-Invasive Tests

The intubation tests tend to be unpleasant for patients; they are also time-consuming and expensive and are performed mostly in specialized centres. Indirect tests of pancreatic function detect the result of pancreatic disease.

1. Oral Function Tests

There are primarily ***two oral function tests*** available for assessing pancreatic functions: the bentiromide test and the pancreolauryl test. Shilling's test may also be used for the purpose.

a. Bentiromide Test

Bentiromide, a synthetic compound attached to para-aminobenzoic acid (PABA), is hydrolyzed by pancreatic chymotrypsin in the duodenum. The bentiromide test is ***useful in distinguishing patients with pancreatic steatorrhea from those with normal fat absorption.*** Chymotrypsin hydrolysis of bentiromide liberates the para-aminobenzoic acid, which is absorbed in the proximal small bowel and is conjugated in the liver. The PABA conjugates are excreted in the urine and urine output of PABA reflects duodenal chymotrypsin activity.

Interpretation: The excretion of less than 50% of the ingested dose in six hours indicates pancreatic exocrine insufficiency. Falsely abnormal results occur in patients with intestinal mucosal, hepatic or renal disease as a result of abnormalities of absorption, conjugation or excretion of PABA. A two-stage test has therefore been proposed in which PABA excretion following bentiromide is compared with the urine recovery of an equivalent dose of free PABA given on a subsequent occasion. PABA may also be measured in plasma instead of urine, and the plasma test may be more reliable in identifying patients with pancreatic insufficiency. The greatest use of this test may be in excluding pancreatic disease as a cause of diarrhoea, steatorrhoea, or weight loss.

b. Pancreolauryl Test

The pancreolauryl test, using fluorescein dilaurate, has been extensively evaluated in Europe. It can detect only severe pancreatic insufficiency. This test is rarely used.

c. Schilling Test

Oral administration of radioactive ^{57}Co labeled vitamin B_{12} followed by intravenous injection of 'cold' vitamin B_{12} to wash-out the absorbed vitamin in urine constitutes the principal of Schilling test. The excretion of radioactivity in urine is a measure of the absorption of vitamin

B_{12} from intestine and hence is a function of duodenal pancreatic enzymes activity.

Chronic pancreatitis may give rise to an abnormal Schilling test, but rarely causes vitamin B_{12} deficiency. Vitamin B_{12} is released from food by gastric hydrochloric acid. This B_{12} is bound to an R factor that is present in the saliva and the gastric juices. In the upper intestine, pancreatic enzymes release the R factor from B_{12}, which is then bound to intrinsic factor; the complex is subsequently absorbed in the terminal ileum. The Schilling test is relatively simple, but unfortunately it is not predictably abnormal except in instances of obvious pancreatic insufficiency.

C. Pancreatic Enzymes—Blood Determination

a. Trypsinogen

Trypsinogen, a proteolytic proenzyme, is exclusively produced in the pancreas. This enzyme can be detected by radioimmunoassay. Elevated levels are found during an attack of pancreatitis and in renal failure; whereas the decreased levels are associated with severe pancreatic insufficiency, cystic fibrosis and insulin-dependent diabetes. Low levels are foud in about 60% of the patients with pancreatic insufficiency. Patients with pancreatic insufficiency who have ongoing inflammation may have normal or raised levels. This fact, in addition to low levels in non-insulin-dependent diabetes, casts some doubt on the usefulness of this test in diagnosing pancreatic insufficiency. It may be useful in patients with steatorrhoea that is due to non-pancreatic causes.

b. Amylase

Amylase is produced and released from a variety of tissues, including the salivary glands, intestine and genitourinary tract. Normal serum contains three types of isoamylases as indentified by isoelectric focusing. The pancreatic gland secretes one amylase at an isoelectric point of 7.0 that constitutes 33% of the total serum amylase. The parotid gland secretes several isoamylases with isoelectric points of about 6.4 and 6.0. Electrophoresis on polyacrylamide gel can separate five isoamylases on the basis of electrode mobility. Amylases originating in the fallopian tubes, tears, mucus and sweat have the same mobility as salivary amylase. All amylases have similar molecular weight and amino acid composition, but vary in terms of their glycosylation or deamination.

Amylase is filtered through the glomerular membrane and is reabsorbed in the proximal tubule. In healthy individuals, the amylase clearance parallels creatinine clearance. During acute pancreatitis, there is an increase in amylase clearance as opposed to creatinine clearance. Although most of the physicians rely on serum amylase for the diagnosis of pancreatitis, it is not, however, a function test.

Interpretation

Amylase is ***particulary useful*** in the ***diagnosis of acute pancreatitis,*** for which the sensitivity of the test is about 75%. Amylase starts rising in serum within a few hours of the onset of disease, reaches a peak in about 24 hours and returns to normal within 3 to 5 days due to increased renal clearance.

Urinary Amylase

The increased renal clearance of amylase is reflected in increased levels of amylase in urine and for this reason many clinicians consider the ***urinary amylase as a more sensitive indicator of acute pancreatitis than serum amylase.***

Determination of the renal clearance of amylase is useful in detecting minor or intermittent increase in the serum concentration of this enzyme. To correct for diminished glomerular function, the most useful expression is the ratio of amylase clearance to creatinine clearance.

$$\% \frac{\text{Amylase clearance}}{\text{Creatinine clearance}} = \frac{\text{Urinary amylase}}{\text{Serum amylase}} \times \frac{\text{Serum creatinine}}{\text{Urinary creatinine}} \; 100$$

Normal Range	:	*1.0 to 3.1 %*
Acute Pancreatitis	:	*4.0 to 12%*

Although this ratio was once thought to be specific to acute pancreatitis, other conditions that produce hyperamylasemia (Table 6.3) may demonstrate a similar elevation.

Table 6.3: Non-pancreatic causes of hyperamylasemia

- Diabetic ketoacidosis
- Burns
- Renal failure
- Perforated duodenal ulcer
- Gall stones
- Malignancy
- Ovarian cyst
- Macroamylasemia
- Ruptured ectopic pregnancy

Occasionally, the serum amylase may be markedly increased in the absence of pancreatic or salivary diseases, whereas the urinary amylase is normal. In this instance, one must suspect either renal disease or macroamylasemia. In the latter condition normal serum amylase is bound by an IgA globulin, forming a complex that is too large to be filtered by the glomerulus. Affected individuals have an elevated serum amylase and a low to normal urinary excretion rate.

Frequently, physicians are faced with a patient who has no overt salivary gland disease but has hyperamylasemia and no specific abdominal findings. As a rule, the level of amylase in pancreatitis is usually elevated to greater than 3 times the upper limit of normal and returns to normal within 2 to 10 days. If the amylase continues to be elevated in the absence of pancreatic complications, other causes (such as malignancy and macroamylasemia) should be investigated.

A rapid rise and fall in serum amylase in a patient with abdominal pain suggests the passage of a stone through the ampulla of Vater. When the serum amylase remains elevated for several days, the gallstone disease is usually complicated by pancreatitis.

Macroamylase consists mostly of salivary amylase complexed with globulins, being therefore too large to be filtered at the glomerulus. Therefore, these individuals have elevated serum amylase and low urinary amylase, with a low amylase-to-creatinine clearance ratio.

c. Lipase

Normal values for serum lipase are 5–208 U/I, In acute *pancreatitis,* lipase levels are very high, often 2 to 5 times the normal amount. Slightly high lipase values may occur in other conditions such as renal insufficiency, salivary gland inflammation, peptic ulcer or malignancy. The rapid and sharp rise of lipase in the blood within hours after the beginning of an attack, and the decline after about 4 days, usually indicates acute pancreatitis. Serum lipase levels may also be used for the diagnosis and follow up of *cystic fibrosis, celiac disease,* and Crohn's disease.

Low lipase levels often mean pancreatic tissue damage/destruction and hence are associated with diabetes mellitus. Lipase-deficient people may also have high cholesterol and/or high blood triglycerides, high blood pressure, difficulty losing weight, and varicose veins.

While the amylase levels in serum and urine are usually used as a measure of acute pancreatitis, measurements of lipase may be more specific and sensitive than total serum amylase. The assay of lipase is as accurate as the pancreatic isoamylase assay, and is likely to replace the amylase assay. Sensitivity of Amylase and Lipase tests for the detection of acute pancreatitis is 91% and 94% respectively. Measuring both, although a routine practice, offers no advantage.

OTHER INDIRECT NON-INVASIVE TESTS

2. Screening Tests for Faecal Fat

The standard indirect test is the 72-hour faecal fat determination. Individuals on a lipid-free diet will still excrete 1 to 4 g of lipid in the faeces in a 24-hour period. Normal faecal lipid is composed of about 60% fatty acids; 30% sterols and higher alcohols, carotenoids; 10% triglycerides; and small amounts of cholesterol and phospholipids. Faecal lipids are derived from four sources: • unabsorbed ingested lipids, • lipids excreted into the intestines (predominantly in the bile), • lipids shed by the cells into the intestines, and • metabolism of intestinal bacteria. Eve with a lipid-rich diet, the faecal fat will not normally exceed about 7g in a 24-hour period.

Although significantly increased faecal fat can be caused by biliary obstruction, severe steatorrhoea is almost always associated with exocrine pancreatic insufficiency or disease of the small intestines.

The patient is placed on a 100 g/day fat diet and the stool is collected daily for three days. ***Individuals with normal pancreatic functions excrete less than 7% of the total amount of fat ingested, whereas those with pancreatic insufficiency excrete more than 20%.*** Although steatorrhoea occurs in mucosal malabsorption, it is not as great as that encountered with pancreatic insufficiency.

Limitations

The major limitations of the stool fat tests are the ***lack of specificity*** and the ***inconvenience of collecting and analyzing the specimens.*** Attempts to screen for steatorrhoea with less offensive tests (such as urine oxalate levels, ^{14}C-triolein/^{3}H-oleic acid assimilation test tripalmitate or palmitic acid breath tests) are promising but not generally accepted.

The screening for the faetal fat is of vital importance for the diagnosis of pancreatic malabsorption syndrome and steatorrhoea. Digestive activity of the pancreatic secretion is essential for the proper absorption of dietary fats. In the case of pancreatic exocrine dysfunction, the content of undigested/unabsorbed fats in the stools validates the diagnosis. The digestion of the dietary fats could still be partially carried out by the intestinal bacteria.

A. Qualitative Test

The qualitative test for faecal fats involves the visualisation of the fat droplets/free fatty acids under the microscope using fat-soluble stains viz. Sudan III, Sudan IV, Oil Red 0, or Nile blue sulphate, etc.

Triglycerides and many other lipids stain yellow-orange to red with Sudan III but free fatty acids do not stain appreciably unless the specimen is heated in the presence of the stain with 36% acetic acid. The number of stained fat droplets is counted. Faecal sample is mixed on the slide with 10% alcohol and stained with eosin to visualise the muscle fibres. The muscles appear as rectangular cross-striated fibers.

Normal faeces can have up to 40 or 50 small (1-5 μm) neutral lipid droplets per high-power microscope field. Steatorrhoea is characterized by an increase in both the nuber and size of the droplets, often with some fat globules in the 50-to 100-μm range.

B. Quantitative Test

The quantitative faecal fat estimation is the confirmatory test for steatorrhoea. The patient is put on high fat (50 to 100 g fat/day) diet at least two days prior to the start of faecal collection and is asked to collect the complete stool for 72-hour (sometimes even five days stool collection is advised).

The total faecal fat can be analyzed by ***two methods*** viz. • Titrimetric method and • gravimetric method.

- ***The titrimetric method*** involves the saponification of faecal lipids with hydroxide and then conversion of salts of the fatty acids to free fatty acids with acid treatment. The titration methods obviously measure only saponifiable fatty acids and, consequently, render results about 20% lower than those from gravimetric methods. Since the titration methods depend upon the equimolar concentration of the reactants at the end point, they give the results in molar concentrations which then have to be converted to grams for final interpretation.

- ***The gravimetric method*** on the other hand involves the extraction of the total faecal lipids in an organic solvent followed by their physical measurement by a sensitive balance. Before extraction, calcium and magnesium soaps of fatty acid are converted to free fatty acids. The organic solvent is evaported so that the lipid residue can be weighed.

The faecal fat is generally reported as gram excretion per day. Although the total volume/ weight of the faeces have a huge patient to patient variation, expressing the faecal fat per dry weight or wet weight of the stools improves the sensitivity or specificity or the test.

Normal healthy individuals excrete about 1-7 gram of fats per day.

2. Sweat Electrolyte Determinations

The ***primary molecular defect in cystic fibrosis*** is a ***mutation in the gene*** that ***encodes the electrogenic Cl- channels*** in the apical plasma membranes of the acinars cells (Fig. 6.3). As a result of this mutation, the number of Cl^- channels inserted into the plasma membrane is drastically reduced. The decreased transport of Cl^- into the acinar and duct lumens impairs the co-transport of water and electrolytes. Consequently, in cystic fibrosis, the acini and ducts of the pancreas and the small airways of the lung become clogged with mucus and subsequently the acinar cells and duct system of the pancreas are destroyed. In many infants with cystic fibrosis, pancreatic exocrine function may be irreversibly damages *in utero*. Because of the almost complete absence of pancreatic enzymes, infants with cystic fibrosis frequently have severe digestive difficulties, especially in the digestion and absorption of fats.

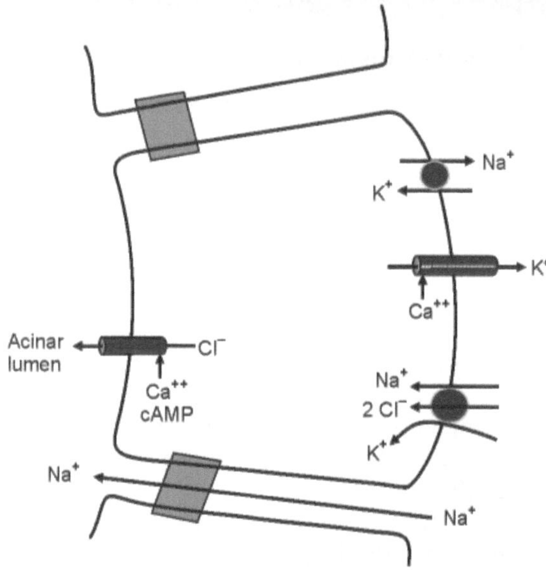

Fig. 6.3: Postulated ionic mechanisms for secretion of NaCl-rich fluid by the pancreatic acinar cells and perhaps by the cells of the intercalated ducts also

One of the ***major features*** of the disorder is ***excretion of large quantities of electrolytes through the skin,*** therefore, ***estimation of sweat electrolytes is helpful in the diagnosis of the disease.*** Significantly elevated concentrations of both these ions occur in more than 99% of affected individuals. The ***two to five fold increases of sweat sodium and chloride are diagnostic of cystic fibrosis*** in children. Even in adults, no other condition will cause increases in sweat chloride and sodium above 80 mEq/L. Sweat potassium is also increased, but less significantly so, and is not generally relied upon for diagnosis.

It is widely accepted that sweat chloride concentration in children greater than 60 mmol/L is diagnostic of cystic fibrosis. In females, sweat sodium and chloride concentrations undergo variations with the menstrual cycle and reach a peak 5 to 10 days prior to the onset of menstruation but the values are never as high as seen in cystic fibrosis.

D. Other Tests of Pancreatic Function

The pancreatic malabsorption has to be differentiated from the gastrointestinal malabsorption syndrome. The tests that are used to achieve this goal are discussed in detail in the chapter on gastric function tests. Nevertheless, a brief summary is provided here.

Although the primary effect of the pancreatic exocrine dysfunction is that the pancreatic digestive enzymes do not reach the intestine, measurement of the proteolytic activity in the faeces does not provide a good parameter. ***Firstly,*** the enzyme protein might be hydrolyzed by the intestinal bacteria; ***secondly*** bacteria themselves synthesize and excrete the proteolytic enzymes and contribute to the overall activity. Still, the test may be used with limited reliability for the detection of cystic fibrosis.

Among the absorption tests, • ***Starch tolerance*** and • ***D-xylose*** tests can provide useful information but are rarely used.

• ***Starch tolerance test:*** Pancreatic amylase deficiency in the intestine should compromise the hydrolysis of the carbohydrates and hence after an oral ingestion of starch, the rise in the blood glucose levels should be lower than the normal individuals. This is the principle of the Starch Tolerance Test (STT) performed on the pattern of the standard glucose tolerance test (GTT) and is interpreted with reference to the latter. The problem is with the specificity of the test. Although the pancreatic malabsorption patients show a flatter STT curve, the majority of the intestinal malabsorption patients also show abnormal STT as well as GTT patterns.

• ***D-xylose absorption test*** relies on the fact that D-xylose, being a pentose sugar, does not require pancreatic enzymes for absorption. Therefore, in a patient of malabsorption syndrome, a normal D-xylose indicates pancreatic insufficiency.

In case of pancreatic carcinoma, clinical features can be seen with • ***ultrasonography*** by the time they appear; but insulinomas, glucagonoma would require the • ***estimation of respective hormones*** with radioimmunoassay/enzyme immunoassays or chemiluminescence immunoassays. Other pancreatic tumours might be diagnosed with the help of a range of • ***tumour markers*** with variable efficacy. The tumour markers would be discussed in a separate chapter in the book.

Finally, the clinical presentation, signs and symptoms on examination as well as the clinical history of the patient remain the most reliable parameters for the diagnosis of the pancreatic disorders. The imaging modalities like chest and abdominal X-rays, ultrasound, duodenography, computerized tomography, endoscopy and angiography provide sufficient information to make at least a provisional diagnosis. The pancreatic biopsy will be the ultimate test to confirm the diagnosis. Therefore, the laboratory tests for the pancreatic exocrine dysfunction have only a supplementary role to play, although the estimations of serum amylase and lipase levels are included in the routine protocol of clinical investigation.

Part Two

Laboratory Investigations

Chapter 7

Hyperglycaemia

INTRODUCTION

Hyperglycaemia is characterized by the presence of elevated blood glucose levels above normal in fasting or postprandial subjects. It is a common finding, particularly in the postprandial period. The main clinical concern is fasting hyperglycaemia and the possibility of diabetes mellitus. Diabetes mellitus is a clinical syndrome associated with an abnormally high plasma glucose concentration, either when fasting or after ingestion of carbohydrates and is often accompanied by the presence of glucose in urine. There are also a number of "temporary" causes of hyperglycaemia.

CAUSES

The causes can be grouped conveniently into two categories.

a. Postprandial—oral/IV

b. Fasting

- ***Diabetes mellitus:*** This is the most important and common cause of elevated blood glucose level. This is of two Types:
  - Insulin-dependant diabetes mellitus (IDDM) or Type I
  - Non-insulin dependant diabetes mellitus (NIDDM)—Type II—Maturity onset diabetes.
- *Endocrine causes*
  - Cushing's syndrome
  - Acromegaly
  - Thyrotoxicosis
  - Pheochromocytoma
- *Pancreatic disorders*
  - Pancreatectomy
  - Haemochromatosis
  - Chronic pancreatitis
  - Carcinoma of pancreas.
- ***"Stress reactions:*** This produces temporary hyperglycaemia.
  - Acute myocardial infarction
  - Cerebrovascular accidents (CVA)
  - Trauma/shock/infection
  - Burns
- *Effects of drugs (Iatrogenic)*
  - Prolonged administration of steroids
  - Oral contraceptives/oestrogens
  - Thiazides
  - Salicylates

Note

- About 60% of the 'stress' hyperglycaemias, 5% of all admissions are for acute myocardial infarction, subsequently have been shown to be due to primary diabetes mellitus.
- In cases of 'stress' and drug-induced hyperglycaemia, it is necessary and must to reinvestigate the patient after the stress has resolved or cessation of drug administration.

LABORATORY INVESTIGATION

From the laboratory investigation point of view, **oral glucose tolerance test (OGTT)** is the most crucial test. Besides oral GTT, there are a number of other laboratory investigations which may be useful in the assessment of a case of hyperglycaemia.

- Urine—Glucose and ketone bodies
- Plasma—Insulin assay
- Plasma C—Peptide assay
- Estimation of glycosylated Hb (Hb A_1 c)
- Estimation of lactic acid.

In addition to above, depending on the clinical circumstances, tests for endocrine functions may be indicated in certain cases.

- Thyroid function tests
- Tests for adrenal cortex and pituitary function
- Tests for adrenal medulla

An insulin tolerance test may be carried out in selected cases where indicated.

• *Oral Glucose Tolerance Test (OGTT)*

The main aim of this test is to investigate the glucose tolerance of subjects who have equivocal symptoms and signs of diabetes mellitus and who do not have a fasting plasma glucose concentration greater than 156 mg% (7.8 m Mol/L) on at least two occasions.

Note

- Glucose determinations performed on plasma or serum are preferable to those performed on whole blood sample. Plasma and serum methods are not dependent on the haematocrit value and are suitable for use in autoanalyzers.
- Plasma and serum glucose levels are usually the same, but they are usually 15% higher than those obtained from whole blood.
- Glucose estimation **by enzymatic method *(glucose oxidase)*** is preferable so that 'true' glucose value is obtained and other reducing substances are eliminated.
- Venous blood should be used throughout. Capillary blood by finger prick may be convenient for children. Values tend to be higher (10-30 mg% or more) in capillary blood than in venous blood.

In ***performing GTT all samples should be venous blood*** or ***capillary blood.***

1. Standard Oral GTT

Indication

- In patients with symptoms of DM but with no glycosuria and normal fasting blood glucose level.
- In patients with transient or sustained glycosuria who have no clinical symptoms of DM with normal fasting blood glucose and postprandial blood glucose.
- In patients with or without symptoms of DM showing one abnormal value.
- In persons with ***strong family history but no "overt" symptoms.***
- In patients with glycosuria associated with thyrotoxicosis, infections/sepsis, liver diseases, pregnancy, etc.
- In patients with neuropathies or retinopathies of undetermined origin.
- In women with characteristically large babies 9 pounds or individuals who were large babies at birth.

Pre-requisites of the Test

Precautions to be taken on the day of the test and prior to it are as follows:

- The individual takes usual supper at about 20.00 hours and does not eat or drink anything after that. Early morning, if so desires, a cup of tea/or coffee may be given ***without sugar or milk.*** No other food or drink is permitted till the test is over (overnight fast for 10 to 14 hours).
- ***Should be on normal carbohydrates diets at least for three days prior to test*** (aproximately 300 gm daily) otherwise false high curve may be obtained.
- Complete mental/and physical rest
- No smoking prior to or during test.
- Should not be on drugs that tend to elevate blood glucose/or interfere with the laboratory determination of glucose.

- All samples of blood should be venous preferably. If capillary blood from "finger prick" is used, all samples should be capillary blood.

Procedure

- A fasting sample of venous blood is collected in a fluoride bottle *(fasting sample)*
- The bladder is emptied completely and urine is collected for qualitative test for glucose and ketone bodies (fasting urine sample)
- The adult individual is given 75 gm of glucose dissolved in water about 200 to 250 ml to drink. Lemon can be added to make it palatable and to prevent nausea/vomiting.

  In children, 1.75 gm/kg body weight not exceeding a total of 75 gm.

  In gestational pregnant diabetes 100 gm is recommended.
- A **total of five specimens** of venous blood and urine are collected every 30 minutes after the oral glucose administration, viz. 30, 60, 90, 120 and 150 minutes. May be extended to 3 hour in some cases, specially in pregnancy.
- Glucose content of **all the six (including fasting sample) samples** of blood are estimated by glucose oxidase method and corresponding urine samples are tested qualitatively for presence of glucose by Benedict's qualitative test and ketone bodies by Rothera's test.
- A curve is plotted which is called as *"Glucose Tolerance Curve"* (GTC) (Fig. 7.1).

Glucose Tolerance Curves (GTC)

1. *A Normal GTC*
   - Fasting blood glucose within normal limits of 60 to 100 mg% "true" glucose
   - The highest peak value is reached within 60 minutes
   - The highest value does not exceed the renal threshold, i.e., 160 to 180 mg%

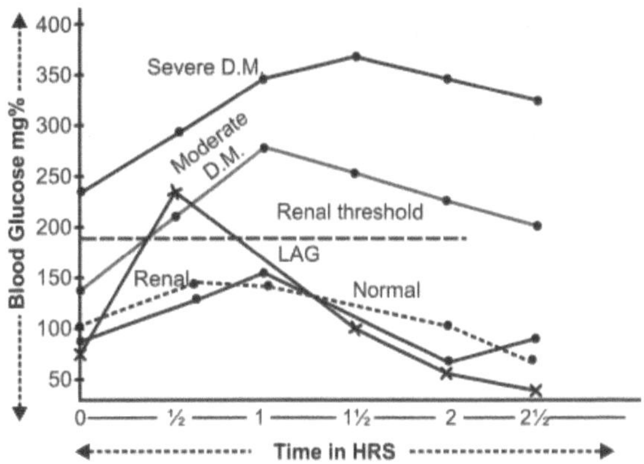

Fig. 7.1: Showing different glucose tolerance curves

   - Fasting level is again reached by 150 minutes (2½ hours)
   - No glucose or ketone bodies are detected in any specimens of urine.

   A typical response is shown below:

	Fasting	Minutes after 75 gm glucose administration 30	60	90	120	150
Blood glucose	75	130	150	100	65	76
Urine	-	-	-	-	-	-

2. *Diabetic Type of GTC*
   - Fasting blood glucose is definitely raised 110 mg% or more ("true" glucose)
   - The highest value is usually reached after 60 to 90 minutes
   - The highest value exceeds the normal renal threshold
   - ***Urine samples always show presence of glucose.*** Urine may or may not contain ketone bodies depending on the type of diabetes and severity
   - ***Blood glucose does not return to the fasting level within 150 minutes, the most characteristic feature of DM.***

According to severity GTC may be
- Mild diabetic curve;
- Moderately severe diabetic curve; and
- Severe diabetic curve.

Typical examples of GTC in DM are shown below:

	Minutes after 75 gm glucose administration					
	Fasting	30	60	90	120	150
(a) Moderate diabetic GTC						
Blood glucose	130	200	280	260	220	170
Urine glucose	—	++	++	++	++	±
(b) Severe diabetic GTC						
Blood glucose	230	300	345	365	350	330
Urine glucose	++	+++	+++	++++	+++	+++

Interpretations

- ***Diagnosis of DM by GTT (WHO recommendation)***

In 1980, WHO Expert Committee on DM, has proposed raising the degree of hyperglycaemia necessary for the diagnosis of DM and created a new category ***"impaired glucose tolerance" (IGT)*** which is not regarded as diabetic but must be recognized as at **"RISK"** of large vessel disease and probably of coronary heart disease. For diagnosis of DM, new proposals state the following criteria.

a. ***In patients with symptoms***
   - A fasting venous plasma concentration of 144 mg/dl (8 mmol/l) or ***greater*** is diagnostic of DM and no GTT is required.
   - If the concentration is below 108 mg/dl (6 m.mol/l) ***the diagnosis of DM is excluded.***

ii. Patients with results in intermediate zone, i.e., 108 to 144 mg/dl (6 m.mol/L) to 8 m.Mol/l) should be given a 75-gm of oral glucose load and GTT performed
   - if the 2 hour venous plasma concentration is greater than 198 mg/dl (11 mmol/L) ***the test is diagnostic of DM;***
   - if it is less than 198 mg (11 mmol/L) but greater than 144 mg/dl (8 mmol/L) ***the diagnosis should be IGT.***

b. ***In patients without symptoms***
   - The criteria require an additional abnormal value after 75 gm glucose load e.g. an one-hour plasma concentration of 198 mg/dl (11 mmol/L) or greater
   - Should subsequent tests confirm either a raised fasting more than 144 mg/dl (8 mmol/l) or 2 hours value less than 198 mg/dl (11 mmol/L) may also be classified as diabetic.

Criteria for Impaired Glucose Tolerance (IGT)

In adults **three criteria** must be met:

- A fasting venous plasma concentrations less than < 144 mg/dl (8 mmol/L)
- The glucose concentration 120 minutes after glucose administration must be greater than 144 mg/dl (8 mmol/L) and less than 198 mg/dl (11 m.mol/L).
- The value, between the 30 and 120 minutes sample, must be unequivocally elevated.

Gestational Diabetes and OGTT

Gestational diabetes is a temporary condition that occurs during pregnancy and is ***defined as any degree of glucose intolerance with onset or detection during pregnancy.*** Almost 1,35,000 pregnant women get the condition every year, making it one of the top health concerns related to pregnancy. If a woman had gestational diabetes during pregnancy, there is ***an increased risk of developing diabetes for both mother and the child.*** In most cases, gestational diabetes is managed by diet and exercise, and goes away after the baby is born.

Gestational diabetes, ***present in approximately 7% of pregnancies,*** is important to diagnose early because of the increased perinatal morbidity associated with poor glycemic control. The prevalence increases up to 33% in the high risk women. Criteria for the diagnosis of this condition remain controversial because the glucose thresholds for the development of complications in pregnancies with diabetes remain poorly defined.

Screening for gestational diabetes: is performed routinely between 24 and 28 weeks of gestation. If the woman is at high risk, however, screening should be performed at an earlier stage. For routine screening of gestational diabetes, the American Diabetes Association recommends that ***a random 50 gram oral***

glucose load be administered. This screening test is administered regardless of the timing of previous meals. The test is considered abnormal if the 1 hour post-load glucose level is ≥ 140 mg/dl (7.8 mmol/l), identifying 80% of women with gestational diabetes. Approxi-mately 90% of women with gestational diabetes show a 1 hour post-load glucose level of >130 mg/dl (7.2 mmol/l).

Diagnostic Test

If the screening test is abnormal, the diagnosis of gestational diabetes should be confirmed ***using a formal OGTT.*** The OGTT should be performed after an overnight (8-14 h) fast. It is Generally recommended that the woman ingest ***at least 150 grams of carbohydrate/day for the 3 days prior to testing to prevent false positive results.*** The necessity of this preparatory diet in normally nourished women, however, has been challenged.

The preferred diagnostic test for gestational diabetes is the ***100 gram 3 hour OGTT.*** The American Diabetes Association recently ad-opted more stringent cut-off values when compared to the older recommendations from the National Diabetes Data Group.

The American Diabetes Association, using the original work of **O'Sullivan and Mahan** and the **Carpenter and Coustan** modifications, suggests that ***at least 2 of the following 4 venous plasma glucose levels must be attained or exceeded.***

Table 7.1: Diagnosis of gestational diabetes with 100 g oral glucose load

100 g glucose load test	*American Diabetes Association*	*National Diabetes Data Group*
Fasting glucose	≥95 mg/dl (5.3 mmol/l)	≥105 mg/dl (5.8 mmol/l)
1 hour glucose	≥180 mg/dl (10.0 mmol/l)	≥190 mg/dl (10.6 mmol/l)
2 hour glucose	≥155 mg/dl (8.6 mmol/l)	≥165 mg/dl (9.2 mmol/l)
3 hour glucose	≥140 mg/dl (7.8 mmol/l)	≥145 mg/dl (8.1 mmol/l)

If the 3rd hour glucose is omitted, the sensitivity of this test is lowered by 13%. This "2 tiered" approach (1 hour 50 gram glucose load screening test followed by the 3 hour 100 gram OGTT in women with abnormal screen results) has been endorsed by the National Diabetes Data Group, the American College of Obstetricians and Gynaecologists, and the American Diabetes Association, and has been shown to be cost-effective.

The 75 gram OGTT is advocated by the World Health Organization in the "one-tiered" approach but is less well validated than the 100 gram test. The World Health Organization uses cutoffs of fasting plasma glucose ≥ 126 mg/dl (7.0 mmol/l) or 2 hour post-load glucose ≥ 140 mg/dl (7.8 mmol/l). The American Diabetes Association, in contrast, requires that at least 2 of the 3 venous plasma glucose levels be attained or exceeded to diagnose gestational diabetes as shown in Table 7.2.

Table 7.2: Diagnosis of gestational diabetes with 75 g oral glucose load

75 g glucose load test	*American Diabetes Association*	*World Health Organization*
Fasting glucose	≥95 mg/dl (5.3 mmol/l)	≥126 mg/dl (7.0 mmol/l)
1 hour glucose	≥180 mg/dl (10.0 mmol/l)	
2 hour glucose	≥155 mg/dl (8.6 mmol/l)	≥140 mg/dl (7.8 mmol/l)

Postpartum Testing

The incidence of abnormal glucose tolerance one-year after gestational diabetes has been reported to be quite variable (7-57%). Women at the highest risk are those who had more severe gestational diabetes and who have multiple risk factors. The American Diabetes Association recommends testing women at least 6 weeks after delivery. Recommended studies include a fasting plasma glucose level or a 75-g oral glucose tolerance test. Women with normal results should be re-tested every 3 years of sooner; and subjects with impaired fasting glucose or impaired glucose tolerance be re-tested on a yearly basis.

Value of urine analysis in GTT: The qualitative estimation of the urine glucose and ketone bodies are commonly performed procedure and many patients with DM are identified in this manner. For qualitative tests of glucose, Benedict's qualitative test is performed and for ketone bodies—Rothera's test.

These are not a necessary part of OGTT but can provide useful informations:

- It will identify those patients who have renal glycosuria but not DM; and
- It provides some rough approximate indication in the diabetic subject, of the blood glucose level and is of importance in determining the insulin dose, if plasma glucose estimation is not done.

- ***Plasma Insulin and C-peptide***

C-peptide is a 31 amino acid peptide that is cleaved off from the pro-insulin during processing in the beta cells. The enzymatic cleavage results in release of the dimeric insulin molecule. C-peptide circulates independently from insulin and is mainly excreted by the kidneys, therefore, the levels are elevated in renal failure. Standardization of different C-peptide assays and their clinical application is still sub-optimal. The major use of C-peptide measurements is in the evaluation of hypoglycaemia and to measure the endogenous insulin synthesis in Type I diabetics or in Type II diabetes patients switching from dietary to insulin support.

In Type 1 diabetes, there is progressive loss of C-peptide with progressive destruction of the beta cells in the islets of the pancreas, until eventually levels are extremely low of undetectable. ***In Type 2 diabetes,*** there is also a progressive loss of beta cell function over many years, with progressive loss of insulin secretory capacity and decreasing C-peptide levels. Fasting and glucose-stimulated C-peptide levels have been used to distinguish Type 1 from Type 2 diabetes with limited success and poor discrimination. Some workers have been successful in detecting the onset of diabetes in younger individuals (LADA) with C-peptide and Glutamic acid decarboxylic acid antibodies (GAD ab).

C-peptide stimulation using glucagon or a mixed meal such as **Sustacal** has also been used to help differentiate between Type 1 and Type 2 diabetes, and to determine the need for insulin therapy in Type 2 diabetes. In the glucagons stimulation test, glucose, insulin and C-peptide levels are measured 6 and 10 minutes after the intravenous injection of 1 mg of glucagon. Normal stimulation of C-peptide is a 150-300% elevation over basel levels. In the mixed meal tolerance test, Sustacal (6 mg/kg up to a maximum or 360 ml) is ingested over 5 minutes, and glucose and C-peptide are measured 90 min after oral ingestion. A basal C-peptide value of <0.2 pmol/ml and stimulated level of<0.5 pmol/ml can be used to confirm the presence of Type 1 diabetes.

These tests have had limited general clinical utility since they do not reliably discriminate between patients who require insulin therapy. The tests have been used in research studies and in the evaluation of patients after pancreatectomy and pancreatic transplantation.

Note

Plasma insulin and C-peptide assays are of immense use in the evaluation of hypoglycaemia.

- ***Plasma lactic acid and ketone bodies***

These are useful in the evaluation of diabetic coma and other causes of a high anion gap metabolic acidosis.

- ***Estimation of glycosylated Hb (Hb A_{1C})***

A single glucose measurement in an OPD clinic is not necessarily representative of a patient's control over any length of time. An increased blood glucose concentration leads to an increased rate of glycosylation of various blood proteins, including most commonly glycosylation of HbA leading to formation of glycosylated Hb (Hb A_1c).

In normal adult, about 90% of Hb is Hb A and glucose is able to combine fairly rapidly but **reversibly,** with the α-NH_2 group of the valine residue at N-terminus of the β-globin chains to form an aldimine (Schiff base) intermediate, which is labile, but can undergo a slow, irreversible Amadori rearrangement to form a ***stable ketoamine derivative known as HbA_1c. The reaction is non-enzymatic.***

It is formed continuously throughout the 120-day life span of the average red cell, and thus provides an index of the "average" plasma glucose concentration over the preceding 2 to 3 months.

Methods

Various methods are available for estimation of HbA_{1C}.

- ***Colorimetric method Fluckiger and Winterhalter:*** described a method for measuring ketoamine-linked hexoses which hydrolyzed to 5-hydroxy methylfurfuraldehyde (HMF) when heated with oxalic acid. Reaction with 2-thiobarbituric acid produces a coloured compound which is measured.
- **Other methods are:**
  - cation exchange chromatography;
  - electrophoresis and electroendosmosis;
  - affinity chromatography;
  - high pressure liquid chromatography (HPLC);
  - isoelectric focusing; and
  - immunoassay.

HPLC and isoelectric focussing both are specific but not suitable for routine use in clinical laboratory.

Interpretation

- ***In normal adult:*** It is present in concentration of 3 to 5% of total Hb.
- ***In patients with DM:*** It may be increased as much as 6 to 15% or more of total Hb.

Clinical Importance

The ***level of*** HbA_{1C} ***appears to be an index of the levels of blood sugar for a period of several weeks prior to the time of sampling.*** Once the RBCs glycosylated, these remain so for the remaining lifespan. Thus, it is ***useful:***

- In detection of DM and hyperglycaemia; and
- In assessment of diabetic control.
  Levels correlate with mean blood glucose levels as given in Table 7.3.

Table 7.3: Correlation of HbA1c with the average blood glucose levels

Hemoglobin A1c (%)	*Blood Glucose (mg/dl)*
6	120
7	150
8	180
9	210
10	240
11	270
12	300
13	330
14	360

Note:

Depending upon the assay method being used, certain hemoglobinopathies may interfere with results. This problem is highly method-dependent. Inaccurate results may also be obtained in the presence of salicylates, chronic alcohol or opiate use, hyperbilirubinemia, iron deficiency, vitamin C, vitamin E, hypertriglyceridemia and lead poisoning, and when there are conditions of increased red blood cell turnover, such as in hemolytic anemia and renal disease.

Use of HbA1c test for the diagnosis of diabetes is not recommended but high HbAlc levels in the absence of above mentioned conditions, particulary abnormal red cell turnover, could be useful. The major benefit of the use of HbA1c for the diagnosis of diabetes is that the test is easy to perform, dose not have to be performed in the fasting state, and does not require any special preparation. HbA1c has been shown to have high specificity (97.4%) but a moderate sensitivity (63.2%) as a screening test for un-diagnosed diabetes. The sensitivity may improve if the test is used in the high-risk group.

Fructosamine and Diabetes Mellitus

Fructosamine (FA) symbolizes the oligosaccharide residues attached to the different plasma proteins (albumin). Since albumin has a short half-life (14-20 days), this test indicates average blood glucose levels over the past few weeks and therefore, is ***considered to be an index of the short-term control of hyperglycemia.*** It represents a clinically accessible measure of non-enzymatic glycation of proteins in the same compartment as plasma glucose compared to HbA1c, which is intracellular and might not vary along with extracellular (plasma) glucose when faced with diabetic complications like nephropathy. The test may be affected by hypertriglyceridemia, hyperbilirubinemia, and hemolysis as well as by low serum protein and albumin levels, but it is unclear if fructosamine results should be corrected for serum albumin or protein levels (Table 7.4).

Table 7.4: Relation between fructosamine levels and the average blood glucose concentration over a period of three weeks

SNo	*Fructosamine (μmol)*	*Blood Glucose (mg/dl)*
1	200	90
2	250	120
3	288	150
4	325	180
5	363	210
6	400	240
7	438	270
8	475	300
9	513	330

There is a lack of studies demonstrating the usefulness of the fructosamine assay in predicting the development of diabetes-related complications. Since the clinical usefulness is not well established, fructosamine testing is generally recommended in situations where HbAlc testing is expected to be inaccurate, such as in the presence of hemoglobinopathies.

The point of care instruments for the measurement of fructosamine, either independent or combined with glucometers, are available and are destined to become more popular for the home/self monitoring of the glycemic control.

Autoantibodies in Diabetes Mellitus

Progressive beta cell destruction and ultimately beta cell failure have been attributed to the development of autoantibodies against the islet cells and their intracellular compoments.

The ***islet cell autoantibodies can be detected*** early in the development of type 1 diabetes, and are considered markers of auto-immune beta cell destruction. The autoantibodies for which ***specific immunoassays*** are available include the ***65-KDa isoform of glutamic acid decarboxylase (GAD65), insulin autoantibodies (IAA), islet cell antigen 512 autoantibodies (ICA512)*** and ***autoantibodies to the protein tyrosine phosphatases 1A-2 and IA-2b. ICA512 are autoantibodies to parts of the IA-2 antigen.*** The presence of high levels of 2 or more antibodies is strongly predictive of type 1 diabetes mellitus. These antibodies may be detected before the onset of type 1 diabetes and at the time of diagnosis, and have been primarily used in screening for type 1 diabetes in research studies related to its early detection. These assays have recently been standardized and the cut-offs are being defined. Diabetes Antibody Standardization Program and a Proficiency Testing Service have been developed by The Immunology of Diabetes Society and The Centers for Disease Control and Prevention.

With the advent of human insulin preparations, particularly engineered 'humanized insulin', incidence of anti-insulin antibodies (IAA) has decreased but insulin therapy can trigger the formation of other autoantibodies, thus restricting the use of these tests during insulin therapy. ***GAD65 antibodies*** ane frequently observed early in the course of type 1 diabetes. They are also present in the rare neurological disorder, **Stiff-man syndrome,** and in some patients with **polyendocrine autoimmune disease.** The GAD65 assay is considered more sensitive than the ICA assay for the detection of early type 1 diabetes in adults, whereas **IAA are more common in young children who develop type 1 diabetes.** It has been suggested that GAD65 and IA-2 positivity show high diagnostic specificity for type 1 diabetes and along with C-Peptide, they may be helpful in determining which type 2 diabetes patients require insulin therapy. Starting the insulin therapy in autoantibody positive non-insulin dependent patients has been suggested to have a protective role against the beta cell destruction and might facilitate the regener-ation of the islet tissue.

Non-Diabetic Causes of Abnormal Glucose

A fasting hyperglycaemia, otherwise unexpl-ained, is virtually diagnostic of DM particularly in a patient with a family history of DM.

Similarly, it holds true for an OGTT which is clearly abnormal and diabetic curve is obtained. But in doubtful cases, the final decision depends on the exclusion of non-diabetic causes of impaired glucose tolerance (IGT).

Major non-diabetic causes of an abnormal OGTT are:

- ***Inadequate dietary preparation.*** If carbohy-drates excluded from diet for a couple of days before test
- Malnutrition and starvation
- Hepatocellular diseases
- Chronic diseases and prolonged physical inactivity (bed rest)
- **"Stress"** due to myocardial infarction, su-rgical operations, CV accidents, febrile illnesses.
- Chronic renal disease and uraemia.
- Iatrogenic (drug therapy): administration of steroids for prolonged periods, women on oral contraceptive pills, diuretics, nicotinic acid.
- Alimentary hyperglycaemia following gastrectomy
- Endocrinopathies:
  - Hyperactivity of anterior pituitary (acromegaly);
  - Hyperactivity of adrenal cortex—Cushing's syndrome;
  - Hyperactivity of thyroid (thyrotoxi-cosis); and
  - Glucagonomal, pheochromocytoma.

Investigations

- An abnormal GTT found in any of above mentioned conditions should be considered non-diabetic until proved otherwise, provi-ded the ***fasting blood glucose is normal***
- Adequate dietary preparation and inclusion of carbohydrate (300 gm) for 3 days prior to OGTT is a must
- Patients having hyperglycaemia after 'Stress', must be retested with an OGTT after stressful situaiton is over and recovery has taken place/and normal physical activity is resumed
- IVGTT may be helpful in differentiating bet-ween alimentary hyperglycaemia and DM
- In suspected endocrinopathies, special 'tests' pertaining to the endocrine glands, have to be carried out. An insulin tolerance test may be helpful.

• *Insulin Tolerance Test*

This test is mainly used in investigating patients with endocrinopathies.

Procedure

- The patient should be put on a diet con-taining at least 300 gm of carbohydrates daily for 2 to 3 days before the test is carried out
- No food is allowed in the morning before the test is done
- Blood is taken for the fasting blood sugar
- Insulin is then injected intravenously in an amount of 0.1 unit/kg body weight

- Further, blood samples are taken 20, 30, 45, 60, 90 and 120 minutes after the insulin administration. Blood sugar is estimated on these samples.

Interpretation

- *Normal response* fall of the blood sugar to approximately 50% of the fasting level in about 3 minutes, followed by a steady rise back to the normal fasting limits which are reached within 90 to 120 minutes.
- *Abnormal responses* Two types of abnormal responses have been recognised.
  a. Insulin resistant type
  b. Hypoglycaemia unresponsiveness.

a. ***Insulin resistant type:*** In this type, there is a relatively slight or delayed fall in blood sugar. This may be obtained:
- In some cases of DM
- Cushing's syndrome (adrenal cortical hyperactivity)
- Acromegaly (anterior pituitary hyperfunction)
- Sometimes in early stages of rheumatoid arthritis.

b. ***Hypoglycaemia unresponsiveness:*** In this type, the blood sugar falls as in the normal person, or even to lower levels, but in which the subsequent rise is delayed or even does not occur. This type of response is seen in **hypoactivity of endocrine glands,** viz:
- Anterior pituitary hypofunction (Simmond's disease)
- In adrenal cortical hypofunction, (Addison's disease)
- In hyperinsulinism
- in hypothyroidism, the return to a normal blood sugar occurs more slowly than in normal persons.

IGT vs DM

There are certain clinical conditions in which the fasting blood sugar is normal but the OGTT is abnormal and it becomes difficult to decide whether the glucose intolerance is a reflection of the clinical condition/disease or as the result of co-existing DM. The following clinical conditions require special considerations.

- ***Pregnancy:*** Criteria for diagnosis of gestational diabetes already discussed above.
- ***Chronic liver diseases:*** Hepatocellular disease may produce an abnormal OGTT *but fasting hyperglycaemia is rarely seen.* Usually the glucose intolerance disappears when the patient recovers from hepatic disease and LFT returns to normal. No test is available that can differentiate GTC of hepatic disease and of DM.
- ***Obesity:*** An abnormal OGTT in an obese individual must be considered an evidence of DM and treated.
- ***Degenerative vascular diseases:*** Cardiovascular accidents (stroke and intracerebral haemorrhages) and coronary infarction are commonly associated with transitory hyperglycaemia. Unless the diagnosis of DM is unequivocal, a final decision as to whether or not such patients are diabetic should be postponed until complete recovery has taken place. Such patients should be again reviewed and OGTT performed after complete recovery and when physical activity is resumed.
- ***Hyperlipoproteinaemias: Type III, IV and V*** familial hyperlipoproteinemias are often associated with abnormal glucose tolerance. Patients with hyperlipoproteinaemias and glucose intolerance should be treated as associated DM with standard regimes like weight reduction and carbohydrate restriction.
- ***Gout and hyperuricaemia:*** Usually associated with higher incidence of glucose intolerance as compared to general population. Usual criteria for the diagnosis of DM are applicable in such cases.

Flow Chart for investigation of a case of hyperglycaemia is given on next page:

Flow Chart for Investigation of Hyperglycaemia

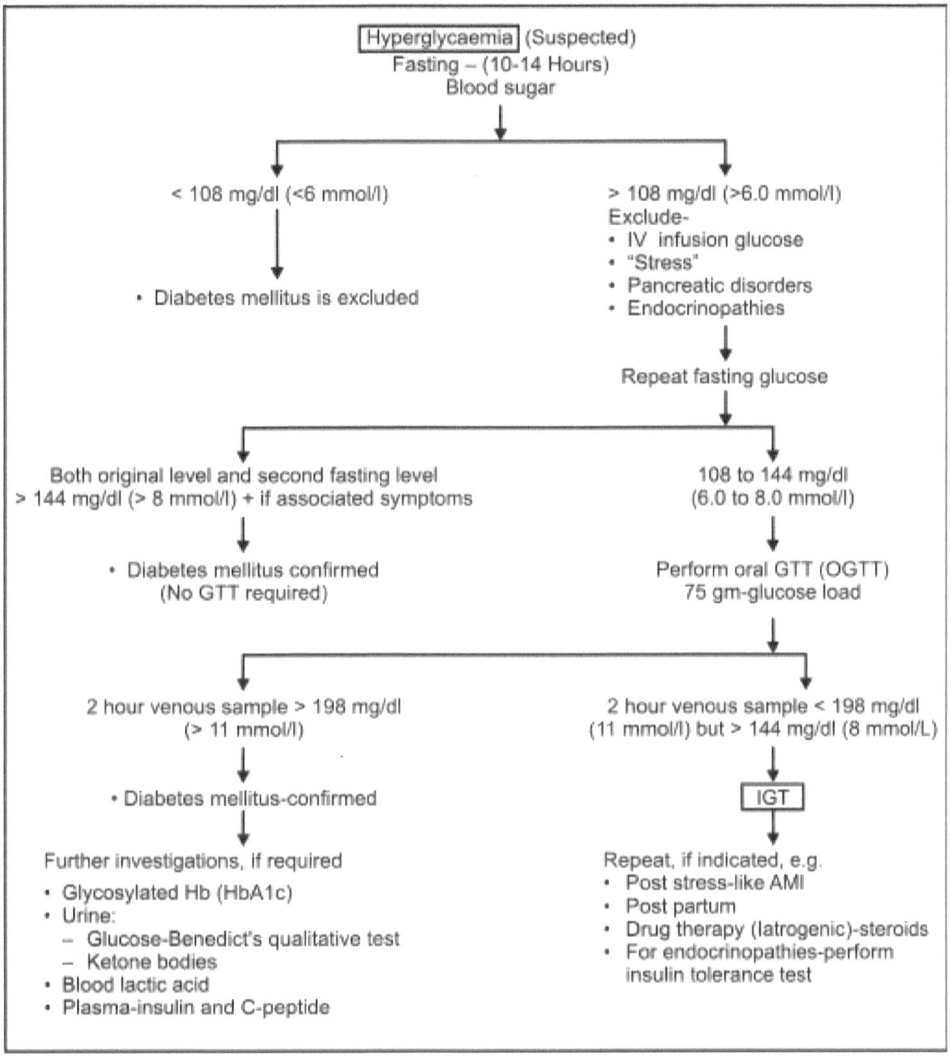

Chapter 8

Hypoglycaemia

INTRODUCTION

Hypoglycaemia may be **defined biochemically as occurring when the blood glucose level ("true" glucose) is less than 40 mg/dl (2.2 mmol/l) and it may occur without clinical manifestations.**

The symptoms and signs of hypoglycaemia may be present without biochemical hypoglycaemia, especially when there is a rapid fall from a previously high level. Individuals who for some reasons maintain a generally low blood glucose may not become clinically hypoglycaemic until it falls below 30 mg/dl (1.65 mmol/l).

CLINICAL FEATURES

The symptoms and signs can be divided into **two groups, acute** and **chronic.**

- ***Acute***

These mainly reflect adrenergic effects (due to stress). The symptoms are largely due to catecholamine release and can be corrected promptly by correction of hypoglycaemia. The acute **symptoms and signs include:**

- A sensation of not feeling well.
- Anxiety, sweating and faintness.
- Restlessness, hunger, palpitation.
- Headache, nausea and vomiting.

The above may be accompanied by loss of consciousness and even coma. ***Children may develop convulsions.***

- ***Chronic***

These occur if the condition has been present for some time, when the fall in glucose level is slow and prolonged.

Neuroglycopenic symptoms occur, viz.

- Headache
- Restlessness
- Loss of intellectual function
- Reduction in spontaneous conversation and activity
- Mental confusion
- Psychotic symptoms and abnormal behaviour

A definitive diagnosis of hypoglycaemia must include the following:

- Symptoms and signs of hypoglycaemia
- Low blood glucose concentration, less than 40 mg/dl ("true" glucose)
- Relief of symptoms with glucose administration (oral/IV)

CAUSES

The causes of hypoglycaemia are mainly of three types:

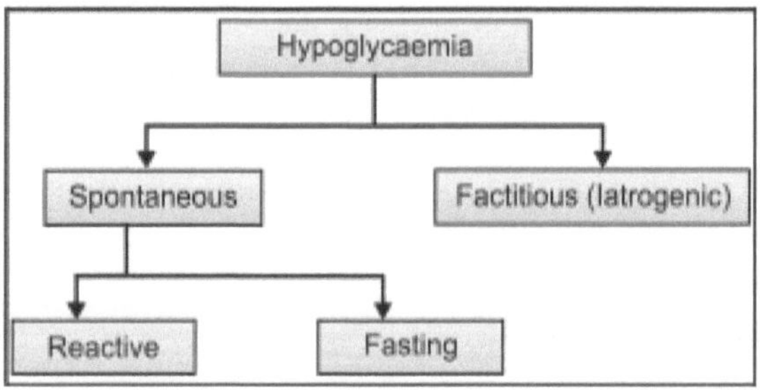

1. Reactive Hypoglycaemia

• *Reactive Functional Hypoglycaemia*

This is one of the most common cause of hypoglycaemia in adults and follows 2 to 4 hours after eating glucose or a meal containing carbohydrates. There occurs rapid decline in blood glucose concentration but the symptoms usually subside spontaneously within half an hour after their onset. It stops short of loss of consciousness or convulsions.

Predilection, to occur in individuals who are emotionally unstable.

Mechanism: Not exactly known, it is thought to be caused by excessive insulin response to glucose.

Note

Reactive functional hypoglycaemia does not predispose to the subsequent development of diabetes mellitus.

• *Post Gastrectomy Hypoglycaemia (Alimentary Hypoglycaemia)*

This type of hypoglycaemia is found in 5 to 10% of patients who have undergone partial to complete gastrectomy or gastroenterostomy, but rarely, it can occur in individuals who have not undergone gastric surgery. Symptoms usually occur 1½ to 3 hours after meals, corresponding to the time when blood glucose levels are low.

Mechanism: Because of gastrectomy, glucose rapidly reaches small intenstine and swift absorption of glucose along with hyperglycaemia stimulates β cells to produce more insulin leading to hypoglycaemia.

Note

- High blood insulin level has been found before hypoglycaemia.
- Excessive vagal activity may be another cause. More pronounced in subjects with peptic ulcers. May stimulate the islets, and there may be an abnormal insulin secreting response.

• *Reactive Hypoglycaemia Secondary to Early/Mild/Diabetes Mellitus*

Reactive hypoglycaemia secondary to mild or early DM is another common type of hypoglycaemia found in adults. It is present with spontaneous hypoglycaemia 3 to 5 hours after a meal. A family history of diabetes mellitus may be obtained.

Mechanism: Exaggerated plasma insulin response in mild or early diabetes.

• *Hereditary Disorders*

a. Galactosaemia
b. Fructose intolerance
c. von Gierke disease

a. Galactosaemia

It is an ***autosomal recessive*** inherited disorder of galactose metabolism.

Enzyme defects

- Usually in classical type deficiency of the enzyme, *"galactose-1-P uridyl transferase."*
- Minor type *"galactokinase"* deficiency.
- Sometimes associated *"epimerase" deficiency.*

Clinical features

Infants appear normal at birth but later develop:

- Intolerance to milk.
- Failure to thrive
- Lethargic and may vomit
- Hypoglycaemia.

If the child survives, later on due to deposition of galactose-1-P, develops cirrhosis liver, mental retardation and cataract.

Mechanism: Due to enzyme deficiency galactose cannot be converted to glucose. Increased galactose level in blood stimulates β-cells and increased insulin secretion ***(insulin-induced hypoglycaemia).***

Points in Favour

- Hypertrophy and hyperplasia of pancreatic islets reported in galactosaemic patients.

Points Against

- Insulin assays have recently shown that galactose does not stimulate insulin secretion.
- Excessive accumulation of galactose-1-P inhibits the enzyme ***"Phosphoglucomutase"*** which would inferfere with hepatic gluconeogenesis/and glycolysis.

b. Fructose Intolerance

Patients with familial fructose intolerance may produce postprandial reactive hypoglycaemia following ingestion of fructose containing foods, specially to cane sugar (table sugar). It is an inherited disorder of fructose metabolism and deficiency of enzyme ***"Aldolase-B"***.

- Nausea and vomiting (which may be haemorrhagic) and profuse sweating are seen.

Mechanism: It may provoke an insulin-induced hypoglycaemia and may be due to excessive accumulation of fructose-1-P inhibiting the enzyme ***"phosphoglucomutase"***.

c. von Gierke Disease

It is also an inherited autosomal recessive disorder associated with glycogen metabolism and enzyme deficiency of ***"glucose-6-phosphatase."*** Liver cells, intestinal mucosa and cells of renal tubular epithelium are loaded with glycogen which is normal in structure but metabolically not available.

Clinical and Biochemical Features

- Children with this disease develop hypoglycaemia, since glucose is not available from glycogenolysis.
- Glucose-6-P cannot be converted to glucose due to deficiency of the enzyme ***"glucose-6-phosphatase"***.
- Fat is utilized as source of energy which leads to ***lipaemia, acidaemia*** and ***ketosis.***
- Excess acetyl-CoA is diverted for ***cholesterol synthesis*** leading to an increase in cholesterol level in blood which produces ***xanthomas.***
- Increased fatty acids synthesis can produce ***fatty infiltration of liver.***
- Hypoglycaemia inhibits insulin secretion ↓ which, in turn, inhibits protein synthesis ↓ causing stunted growth (dwarfism).
- Hypoglycaemia stimulates catecholamine secretion ↑ which causes muscle glycogen to break down, producing lactic acid and lactic acidosis.
- Increased blood lactic acid competes with urate excretion by kidneys leading to increased blood uric acid ↑ level producing gout (there may be increased synthesis of uric acid also).

2. Fasting Hypoglycaemia

- ***Pancreatic Islet Cell Disease***

Symptoms of hypoglycaemia, due to islet cell tumours and insulinomas are produced by excessive secretion of insulin. It has been reported that:

- Of the total insulinomas, 10% insulinomas may be malignant and 80% benign, remaining 10% doubtfully malignant;
- About 50% of benign adenomas are multiple;
- Insulinomas may be solitary or multiple and may be either macroscopic or microscopic in size.

Multiple islet-cell tumours are sometimes associated with multiple endocrine adenomatosis as part of ***"pluriglandular syndrome"***, in which multiple endocrine tumours, functioning and non-functioning co-exist. Sometimes, the pancreatic islet-cell diseases are associated with peptic ulceration ***(Zollinger-Ellison syndrome).***

Most frequently persons between 30 and 55 years of age suffer. Benign and malignant insulinomas may occur at any age. There is an equal sex distribution and a family history of diabetes in 25% of patients with insulinoma.

Clinical Features

- Hypoglycaemic symptoms develop insidiously but tends to increase in intensity and severity later on.
- Most attacks occur early morning before breakfast, and sometimes late afternoon hours.
- Excessive sweating which is usual with hypoglycaemia, is conspicuously absent.

Note

The diagnosis which is often delayed for years should be considered in the presence of unexplained or bizarre mental or neurologial changes, psychosis, epilepsy, focal neurological signs or signs of motor neurone-disease.

- ***Islet-cells Hyperplasia***

a. ***Islet-cell hyperplasia and hypertrophy*** of β-cells may be a prominent feature in the pancreas of the infants of diabetic and prediabetic mothers. Such infants may have abnormally low blood glucose levels, immediately after their birth.

Mechanism: It may be due to abnormal stimulation of foetal pancreas by maternal hyperglycaemia, and/or, due to an antagonist to insulin, crossing the placenta from the mother.

b. ***Obstruction of the pancreatic ducts:*** may cause hyperplasia of cells of islets of Langerhans and severe clinical hypoglycaemia may occur.

- ***Leucine Sensitivity***

Leucine-induced hypoglycaemia is a rare disorder in adults but is not an uncommon cause of fasting hypoglycaemia in children below the age of 4 years. Leucine sensitivity implies a rapid and significant fall in blood glucose to less than 50% from the initial level within 20 to 40 minutes after oral administration of leucine 150 mg/kg body weight.

- ***In normal persons*** there may not be fall or a mild decline in blood glucose may be seen.
- Plasma insulin levels rise after leucine administration to susceptible children
- It may not be a specific entity.
- Recently, it has been shown that a ***significant percentage of patients with insulinomas are leucine sensitive.*** The removal of the neoplastic tissue abolishes the sensitivity.
- Administration of leucine may produce hypoglycaemia in those who are on sulphonylureas.

- ***Liver Diseases***

Hypoglycaemia may occur in severe, diffuse liver diseases, viz. fulminating hepatitis, hepatic necrosis due to toxic agents, cirrhosis liver, etc., and also in some patients with hepatomas.

- ***Alcohol-induced Hypoglycaemia***

Ethyl alcohol, free of other toxic contaminants, may induce hypoglycaemia usually in chronic alcoholics, who are poorly nourished and eating no or little food. Hypoglycaemia follows 8 to 12 hours or more after alcohol ingestion. Occasionally, following a 2 to 3 day fast, the ingestion of alcohol may produce hypoglycaemia in a young, healthy person. Patients with hypopituitarism or adrenocortical insufficiency exhibit increased sensitivity to the hypoglycaemic effects of alcohol. In ethanol-induced hypoglycaemia, a rapid clinical improvement is observed with IV glucose infusion.

- ***Malnutrition***

Hypoglycaemia is relatively common in children suffering from Kwashiorkor (protein energy malnutrition).

Note

In adults, even severe protein depletion and malnutrition rarely produces hypoglycaemia.

- ***Non-pancreatic Neoplasm***

Severe fasting hypoglycaemia may occur in the presence of certain non-pancreatic tumours, e.g.

fibrosarcomas or *leiomyosarcomas* specially when they are large. ***Also seen in fibromas, mesotheliomas.*** The fibrosarcomas are either, intra-abdominal (usually retroperitoneal), or intrathoracic in origin. Adrenocortical tumours and primary carcinomas of the liver are rare but well-established causes of spontaneous hypoglycaemia.

Mechanism: Cause exactly not known but it may be due to:

- ***excessive utilization of glucose by the tumour cells*** in liver carcinomas and adrenocortical tumours, and
- *fibrosarcomas* may either ***stimulate the pancreas to release insulin,*** or increase the tissue sensitivity to insulin, or even produce a substance with insulin-like activity.

- ***Endocrine Disorders***

Fasting hypoglycaemia may occur in patients with hypopituitarism or Addison's disease. It is rather a relatively uncommon finding in these disorders. Clinical features and findings will readily point to endocrine cause.

- ***Idiopathic Hypoglycaemia of Infancy***

Hypoglycaemia of unknown causes can occur in neonates which has been described as a syndrome, ***"familial idiopathic hypoglycaemia in infants."*** It occurs before the age of 2 years and disappears after a few years. Syndrome probably represents a heterogenous group of unrelated entities and in some cases, there is a failure of the normal adrenaline response to hypoglycaemia. Baby responds to ACTH treatment. After a successful response, usually within a week, the baby is weaned from ACTH. Surgery of the pancreas is not advisable.

3. Factitious or Iatrogenic Hypoglycaemia

Hypoglycaemia may be produced in diabetics by overdoses of insulin. ***It is one of the commonest cause and must be suspected in a case of diabetes mellitus.***

- ***Sulfonylureas*** may induce hypoglycaemia especially in the presence of renal failure or the use of alcoholic beverages.
- Hypoglycaemia may also be induced by *salicylates in large amount*, or *MAO (monoamine oxidase) inhibitors*, or *barbiturates* and other drugs.

LABORATORY INVESTIGATIONS

Laboratory investigations can be discussed under two heads.

I. ***To establish the presence of hypoglycaemia***

II. ***To establish the causes and type of hypoglycaemias.***

I. TO ESTABLISH THE PRESENCE OF HYPOGLYCAEMIA

A good history and clinical features as discussed above along with a blood sugar estimation showing blood glucose level less than 40 mg/dl will establish that hypoglycaemia is present.

II. TO ESTABLISH THE CAUSES OF HYPOGLYCAEMIA AND ITS TYPE

The following laboratory investigations will help in diagnosing the causative factors.

1. Five Hour Oral GTT

A five hour glucose tolerance test is essential and mainstay for the diagnosis of reactive hypoglycaemia. GTT is performed in the usual way, but blood samples are collected every half hour for 5 hours for plasma/blood glucose level.

Interpretations

- ***In reactive functional hypoglycaemia:*** The fasting blood sugar levels is normal. The GTT curve shows rise in half to one hour sample after glucose load, but shows abnormally low blood glucose values, 50 mg/100 ml or less, between the second and fourth hours of the test.

- ***In reactive hypoglycaemia*** secondary to mild diabetes mellitus, the GTT curve generally shows slightly elevated fasting blood glucose level, hyperglycaemia at the peak value and at second hour; but low blood glucose levels 50 mg/100 ml or less during the third and fifth hours.
- ***In alimentary hypoglycaemia,*** the GTT curve reveals a normal fasting blood glucose level, peak hyperglycaemia at half to one hour, normal glucose concentration at second hour and fall in blood glucose level shortly thereafter.

2. *Intravenous GTT*

Normally, not indicated, but it can be useful in differentiating alimentary hypoglycaemia.

Once oral GTT is performed and reactive hypoglycaemia is ruled out, the following procedures should be adopted for evaluation of patients with suspected fasting hypoglycaemia.

3. *Prolonged Fast Test*

The prolonged fast test is extremely valuable and virtually diagnostic of insulinomas. It must be performed in hospital under strict supervision so that prompt treatment is available. Blood samples are taken at regular intervals for blood glucose estimations and serial EEG when available are advantageous. The test is interrupted if coma occurs, or when the fast has continued for a minimum of 72 hours, without development of hypoglycaemia.

Simultaneously, it will be useful to perform plasma insulin assay:

- Initially determine, on at least two or three occasions, the blood glucose and insulin levels after an overnight fast. Blood glucose values of 50 mg per 100 ml or less together with plasma insulin levels, exceeding 40 μu/ml occurring in association with clinical features of hypoglycaemia are virtually diagnostic of insulinomas.
- If the blood glucose and insulin levels are not diagnostic, the overnight fast should be extended for 4 hours and the blood glucose and insulin assay determinations are repeated at regular intervals.
- If the results are still inconclusive, the fast may be extended for another 48 to 72 hours. Only unsweetened fluids may be permitted and the patients should be encouraged to exercise strenuously. As soon as low blood glucose level and hypoglycaemia features are noted, the test is terminated.

Interpretations

In patients with insulinomas blood glucose concentration normally falls below 30 to 50 mg/100 ml sometime during the fast. ***Hypoglycaemia of this severity is uncommon in patients who do not have insulinomas.***

4. *Plasma Insulin Assay*

Measurement of plasma insulin levels in association with blood glucose concentrations is extremely valuable in diagnosis of insulinomas.

Increased plasma insulin levels in association with low fasting blood glucose levels confirm the diagnosis of insulinomas.

Diagnostic changes in plasma insulin levels in the diagnosis of insulinomas, when performed alone are:

- High fasting insulin levels with spontaneous fluctuations, when blood is taken at 20 minutes intervals during the fast.
- An excessive rise in plasma insulin after IV tolbutamide. Samples of blood should be taken at 10 minutes interval for half hour.
- An excessive rise in plasma insulin after L-leucine.

Note

- Not all patients with islet-cell tumours show fasting hyperinsulinaemia.
- High fasting plasma insulin levels are not always pathognomonic, when performed alone, as they may sometimes occur in obese persons without fasting hypoglycaemia.

- Also in children with idiopathic hypoglycaemia and rarely seen in patients with non-pancreatic tumours.

5. "PROVOCATIVE" TESTS

The tests that can induce the secretion of insulin are called "provocative tests" and they ***are valuable in differential diagnosis of hypoglycaemia and insulinomas.*** The following provocative tests have been used and can be helpful in selected cases.

a. IV tolbutamide test
b. Leucine sensitivity test
c. Glucagon test.

In these tests, serial determinations of blood glucose and plasma insulin assays may be helpful after administration of the test substance.

(a) *IV Tolbutamide Test*

A promising adjunct in the diagnosis of insulinomas.

Procedure

After an overnight fast, 1.0 gm of sodium tolbutamide is give intravenously. Blood glucose and plasma insulin are estimated while fasting and then at half hourly intervals for 180 minutes, after the injection.

Interpretations

- Both normal subjects and patients with insulinomas show an initial fall in blood glucose which is maximal at 30 to 40 minutes after injection
- However, ***in normal persons,*** blood glucose soon rises and by 120 to 180 minutes reaches 70 to 80% of the initial level.
- ***In patients with insulinomas,*** blood glucose hardly rises after the initial fall and by 120 to 180 minutes remains less than 65% of the initial level, provided this was normal at the beginning of the test.

Note

- The test is invalid if fasting hypoglycaemia is already present.
- The plasma insulin concentration is elevated in patients with islet-cell tumours and the elevated concentration of insulin at 60 minutes is reported to be the most reliable discriminator.
- In various conditions such as liver diseases, malnutrition or renal insufficiency, blood glucose response to tolbutamide are indistinguishable from islet-cell tumours, but only patients with insulinomas exhibit exaggerated plasma insulin levels.

Criteria Used for Diagnosis of Insulinoma

- A decrease in blood gluocse of more than 65% or to levels below 30 mg% (1.7 mmol/l).
- Blood glucose of less than 40 mg% (2.2 mmol/l) presisting up to 180 minutes or longer.
- A significant increase in plasma insulin concentration.

b. *Leucine Sensitivity Test*

A leucine challenge can be given and response to blood glucose and plasma insulin is observed.

Procedure

- The patient is allowed to fast overnight.
- A fasting blood is taken for blood sugar estimation.
- ***Dose*** of 150 mg L-leucine per kg body weight, suspended in water, is given orally.
- Further blood samples for blood sugar estimations are taken at 15 minutes interval for one hour. Blood glucose is estimated on these samples.
- If facilities available, plasma insulin is also determined on these samples including fasting sample.

Interpretations

- Normal persons show a small fall in blood sugar level 5 to 15 mg/100 ml.
- A greater fall of at least 40%, usually occurs within half an hour in about 2/3rd of patients with an insulinoma and in idiopathic hypoglycaemia of children. A rise in plasma insulin occurs with the fall in glucose level.
- ***Negative results are obtained in reactive hypoglycaemia.***

(c) *Glucagon Test*

Procedure

- The patient is asked to fast overnight and the blood sample is taken for fasting blood sugar level next morning.
- A dose of 1.0 mg glucagon is given intramuscularly to the fasting patient, if adult. For children, 30 μg/kg body weight not exceeding 1.0 mg is recommended.
- Further blood samples for blood glucose estimation are collected half hourly for 3 hours.
- Blood sugar is estimated in all these samples.

Interpretations

- ***In normal persons:*** blood glucose rises, 30 to 90 mg/100 ml, and falls to normal or just below normal in 2 to 3 hours.
- A greater initial rise is seen in patients with an insulinoma and the subsequent fall is to hypoglycaemic levels.
- A smaller rise may be shown by patients with hypoglycaemia due to glycogen storage diseases (GSDs), liver diseases, and endocrine disorders.

Note

- All the three provocative tests should be performed in suspected islet-cell disease, as an abnormal response may be obtained with one test but not with the other.
- False positive results may occur with the tobutamide test in patients with malnutrition, non-pancreatic causes of hypoglycaemia, renal insufficiency with uraemia.
- False positive results may also occur with leucine tests in individuals on sulfonylureas.
- Glucagon test appears to be the most reliable provocative test.

Plasma C-Peptide Level

If facilities are available for plasma C-peptide levels determination, it can help to differentiate insulinoma from factitious (iatrogenic) insulin overdosage.

Interpretation

- If the C-peptide level is low in the presence of high concentration of circulating insulin, it can be assumed that the insulin is exogenous in origin (insulin overdose).
- On the other hand, if the C-peptide levels are elevated, the implication is that the insulin is secreted endogenously and is pointer to insulinoma.

Thus, blood glucose estimation, plasma insulin assay and C-peptide levels, if done simultaneously can differentiate insulinoma, insulin overdosage and hypoglycaemic drug abuse.

	Insulinoma	*Insulin abuse (overdosage)*	*Oral hypoglycaemic (drug abuse)*
• **Hypoglycaemia**	+	+	+
• **Plasma insulin**	high ↑	high ↑	high ↑
• **Plasma C-peptide**	high ↑	low ↓	high ↑ (History of taking drug will be available)

Flow Chart for laboratory investigation of a case of hypoglycaemia—as per age groups

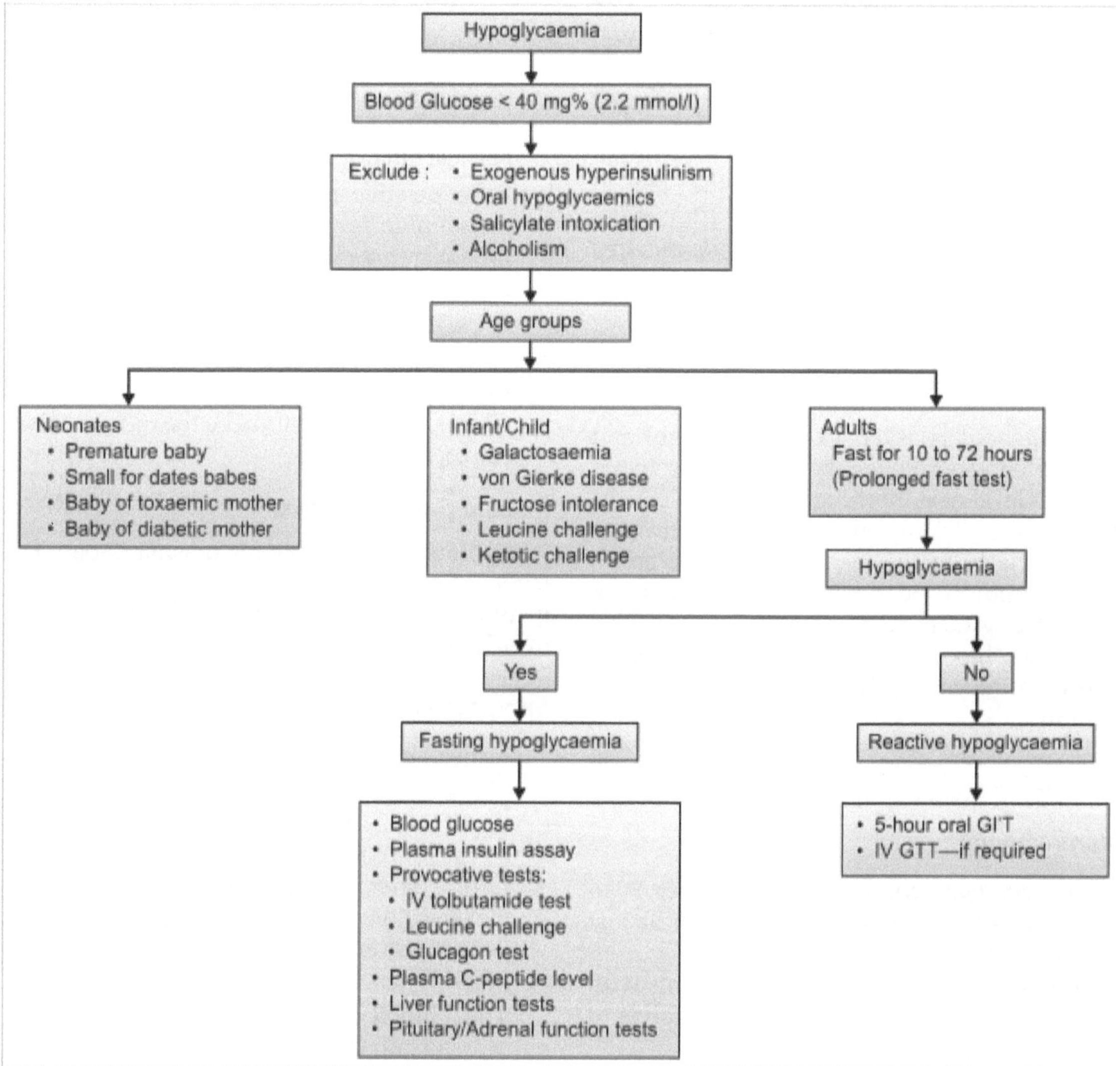

Note

One should remember the commonest cause of hypoglycaemia is ***drug therapy*** (Insulin injection, oral hypoglycaemics, alcohol, salicylates), if these are excluded one should then consider functional hypoglycaemia, early diabetes mellitus and finally insulinoma in that order.

Special Investigations

- ***Once the diagnosis of insulinoma is made based*** on above tests, ***additional investigations may be required*** viz:

a. Serum calcium and phosphorus determinations.

b. X-ray skull to rule out multiple endocrine adenomatosis.

  c. Arteriography to localize the tumour.
  d. A liver scan to rule out metastatic carcinoma.
  e. Pancreatic scan.
  f. "Oncogenic markers", to rule out liver carcinoma metastatic.
- ***For extra pancreatic neoplasm*** to rule out particularly in elderly individuals.
  a. X-ray of chest and abdomen.
  b. IV pyelography.
  c. Contrast studies of GI tract.
- ***Hypoglycaemia associated with diffuse liver diseases***
  a. Clinical picutre will help.
  b. Liver function tests may show abnormalities.
- ***Diagnosis of alcohol hypoglycaemia***
  a. History and clinical examination.
  b. A fall in blood glucose level after infusion of ethanol.
    - Determination of blood alcohol.
    - Serum γ-GT.

- **FACTITIOUS (IATROGENIC) HYPOGLYCAEMIA**

The following may help:

- Careful history and clinical examination
- Blood levels of sulfonylureas
- Serum insulin antibody level
- Examination of urine for tolbutamide excretion products
- Leucine sensitivity test.
- Plasma C-peptide level.

Note

- ***Drug induced hypoglycaemia is the commonest cause of a low blood glucose.*** Thus, in all cases of hypoglycaemia, drugs such as insulin, oral hypoglycaemics, alcohol, salicylates should be considered before any further investigations are initiated.
- After iatrogenic factors excluded reactive functional hypoglycaemia is considered as the next most common cause of hypoglycaemia.

Chapter 9

Hypercalcaemia

INTRODUCTION

Normal serum calcium level is 9 to 11 mg/dl. When the serum calcium level exceeds 11.0 mg/dl it is called as hypercalcaemia. ***Hypercalcaemia is coming up as an even more complex diagnostic problem than it was in the past.*** In routine biochemical profile/screening, serum calcium is included as a parameter. Elevations of the serum calcium level are found in about 1% of routine biochemical screens. Physicians come across with hypercalcaemia commonly in clinical practice—it can occur in an asymptomatic patient or in association with severe illness.

The prevalence of hypercalcaemia in the hospital population is around 5%, of which ***40% will have a malignancy*** and 20% primary hyperparathyroidism.

Primary hyperparathyroidism has been found to be the most common cause of hypercalcemia in outpatient's clinic whereas malignancy is the most common cause in hospitalised indoor patients. These two disorders together account for 90 to 95% of all cases.

Mechanisms of Hypercalcaemia

- Hypercalcaemia may occur when flux of calcium into ECF is greater than the efflux of calcium out of this compartment, e.g., when resorption of bone mineral occurs in excessive amount as in malignancies.
- When the capacity of the kidneys to excrete filtered calcium is exceeded.
- It can also be due to increased intestinal absorption of calcium, e.g., in hypervitaminosis D (vitamin D intoxication).
- Enhanced renal retention of calcium, e.g., in administration of diuretics like thiazide;
- Increased skeletal resorption, e.g., prolonged immobilization.
- It can also be due to combination of several of these mechanisms as occurs in primary hyperparathyroidism.

Thus pathogenesis, clinical presentation and differential diagnosis may vary widely from case to case.

CAUSES

From the mechanisms as discussed above it is apparent that causes may be multiple hence the diagnosis may be difficult. Sometimes the diagnosis can be established only by observation of the patient over a period of time. The various known causes of hypercalcaemia can be classified as follows.

1. Malignancy

This is the most important cause for hospital inpatients. Hypercalcaemia in malignancy may be due to the following factors:

- ***Humoral Factor***

No direct skeletal involvement **(HHM—humoral hypercalcaemia of malignancy)**

- PTH-related protein (PTH_rP).
- *Growth factors:* Tumour growth factor (TGF), epidermal growth factor (EGF), platelet derived growth factor (PDGF).

- ***Direct Skeletal Involvement of the Tumours***
  - Direct erosion of bone by tumour.
  - Production of PGE_2 by the tumour which can produce bone resorption.

- ***Haematological Malignancies***
  - Production of cytokines
  - Interleukin-1.
  - Tumor necrosis factor (TNF).
  - Lymphotoxin.
  - Production of 1, 25, -$(OH)_2D_3$ by lymphomas.

2. Primary Hyperparathyroidism

This is the most common cause for outpatients (OPD cases). It may be of the following types:

- Familial.
- Hyperplasia.
- Tumour like adenoma or multiple adenomas.
- *"Ectopic" hyperparathyroidisms:*
  - multiple endocrine neoplasia type I (MEN I) with pituitary and pancreatic tumours.
  - multiple endocrine neoplasia type II (MEN II)—medullary carcinoma of thyroid and pheochromocytoma

3. Other Endocrine Causes

- Hyperthyroidism.
- Hypothyroidism.
- Acromegaly.
- Acute adrenal insufficiency.

4. Granulomatous Diseases

- Tuberculosis.
- Saccoidosis.
- Berylliosis.
- Coccidiomycosis.

5. Overdosage of Vitamins

- Vitamin A intoxication.
- Hypervitaminosis D.

6. Drug-induced Hypercalcaemia (Iatrogenic)

- Thiazide diuretics.
- Spironolactone.
- Milk-alkali syndorme.

7. Miscellaneous Causes

- Idiopathic hypercalcaemia of infancy ***(William syndrome).***
- Familial hypocalcinuric hypercalcaemia.
- Prolonged immobilization.
- Increased serum proteins.
  - Hyperalbuminaemia—haemoconcentration.
  - Hyperglobulinaemia—due to multiple myeloma.
- Renal failures
  - Acute renal failure—diuretic phase.
  - Chronic renal failure.
  - Postrenal transplantation

CLINICAL FEATURES

It is obvious from above that causes of hypercalcaemia are many and as such presentation may be varied. Frequently, an asymptomatic patient is found to have an elevated serum calcium on routine biochemical screening. As malignancy and hyperparathyroidism are the most common causes (95% cases), causes and clinical presentation of hypercalcaemia in primary hyyperparathyroidism will be discussed first, followed by malignancy.

1. Primary Hyperparathyroidism

Excessive and inappropriate secretion of parathormone (PTH) is the cause of hypercalcaemia.

Causes

It is mainly due to:

- Solitary adenoma in 80 to 85% cases.
- Multiple adenomas in 2% cases.

- Chief cells hyperplasia involving all four parathyroid glands found in 15% cases.
- Parathyroid carcinoma in less than 1% cases.
- Inherited diffuse abnormality as in MEN Type I and II.

Clinical Features

Presentation changed as compared to past. ***Osteitis fibrosa cystica is not common as used to be earlier.***

By routine screening detection of hypercalcaemia is easier.

Signs and symptoms are non specific of hypercalcaemia, but presence of one or a number of them should alert a physician to the possibility by this diagnosis. In general higher the serum calcium, the more profound are the signs and symptoms.

Most common and vague symptoms are related to ***"neuromuscular system".***

1. • With serum calcium less than 12 mg/dl (3.0 mmol/l) there may be fatigue, malaise, muscle weakness generalized or involving shoulder/hips, and anorexia/ nausea.
   - With higher levels of serum calcium greater than 12.0 mg/dl and if prolonged, definitive symptoms may be present, e.g. depression, apathy and inability to concentrate may be prominent.
2. Hypercalcaemia may induce a mild ***"nephrogenic diabetes insipidus".*** Thus there may be:
   - thirst, polydipsia and polyuria may be present; and
   - nocturia may be the earliest symptom.
3. If hypercalcaemia is prolonged and chronic in type:
   - renal stones can produce renal colic; and
   - evidences of metastatic calcification may be in vascular tissues and eyes—cornea/ conjunctiva.
   - if nephrocalcinosis is present slow development of renal failure may be seen.
4. ***Osteitis fibrosa cystica is not common as used to be earlier.*** Such patients have severe "bone pain", may have osteoporosis and can have pathological fractures. Radiologically, cystic bone lesions may be seen.

2. Malignancy vs Hypercalcaemia

Up to 10 to 20% of patients with malignancy can have hypercalcaemia. In these cases rise in serum calcium is more rapid.

Tumours which are commonly associated with hypercalcaemia are:

- squamous cell carcinoma lungs, head and neck, cervix
- renal carcinoma (hypernephroma)
- Carcinoma of pancreas
- Breast carcinoma
- Multiple myeloma, leukaemias and lymphomas.

It has been estimated that 5% of hypercalcaemic malignancies have co-existent primary hyperparathyroidism also.

Clinical Features

Signs and symptoms in these patients are often associated with the malignancy. Those due to hypercalcaemia *"per se"*, are similar to those observed in other hypercalcaemic conditions as discussed above.

Certain symptoms are more common in malignancy as there occurs relatively rapid developemnt of hypercalcaemia. These are:

- weakness, lethargy;
- obtundations and
- nausea and vomiting.

These symptoms are more prominent when there is a rapid rise in serum calcium.

Signs in Hypercalcaemia

The physical examination may show no abnormalities, if hypercalcaemia is slow to develop and of short duration or if the serum calcium level less than 12 mg/dl. If hypercalcaemia is prolonged and serum calcium is more than 12 mg/ dl, certain signs are important. They are:

- ***Marked weight loss*** may be seen in patients with malignancy.

- ***Elevated systolic blood pressure*** with or without elevated diastolic pressure is a common finding.
- Skin lesions, viz. petechiae, purpura and echymosis may be present. There may be ***recurrent intermittent urticaria.***
- Bone or muscle tenderness on pressure. There may be proximal or generalized muscle weakness.
- An enlarged liver, or spleen, and lymphadenopathy may be present.

Machanisms of Hypercalcaemia in Malignancy

The following mechanisms may be operating in malignancy to produce hypercalcaemia.

- ***Humoral Factor***

Greater than 50% are, ***humoral hypercalcaemia of malignancy (HHM) syndrome***. This syndrome is defined as production of a humoral factor by the tumour which is secreted in circulation and stimulates bone resorption. Principal humoral factor has been delineated as **PTHrP** ***(parathormone related peptide),*** which can bind to PTH receptors in target tissues.

PTHrP

Also called humoral hypercalcaemic factor of malignancy (HHFM). PTHrP is a peptide containing 141 amino acids. Amino acid sequence on first 13 is same (8 of 13 are homologous) from N-terminus. It is produced by a number of tumours specially squamous cell carcinomas of lungs, oesophagus, head and neck, etc. ***Factor can bind to PTH receptor and can mimic the action of parathormone.*** Target tissues are bone and kidney and produces hypercalcaemia, hypophosphataemia and increases urinary cyclic AMP similar to parathormone.

It is produced by a gene on chromosome 12 which is distinct from PTH gene located on chromosome 11, serum levels of PTHrP are *low* or absent in normal healthy persons and in patients with primary hyperparathyroidism but ***it is high in majority of patients in malignancy and responsible for HHM.***

Note

Determination of PTHrP is becoming an important diagnostic tool in evaluation of hypercalcaemia.

- ***Direct Skeletal Erosion***

Invasion of bone by metastatic tumours. Tumour cells probably produce local factors capable of stimulating osteoclastic resorption of bone.

- ***Prostaglandins***

Production of PGE_2, which is a potent stimulator of bone resorption.

- ***Other Factors Responsible for Hypercalcaemia in Malignancy***
  - Transforming growth factors (TGF).
  - Cytokines, interleukin-1 (IL-1) and tumour necrosis factor (TNF).
  - Production of 1,25-$(OH)_2D_3$.

Note

- Multiple myeloma and other haematological malignancies are frequently associated with hypercalcaemia. Cytokines like interleukin 1 and tumour necrosis factor (TNF) have been incriminated as important mediators of bone resorption in these tumours (previously known as ***"osteoclastic activating factor").***
- Certain lymphomas associated with HIV and HTLV-1 infection in which hypercalcaemia develops have been found to be associated with very high serum concentration of 1,25-$(OH)_2$-D_3. Hence, determination of 1,25-$(OH)_2$-D_3 can be a useful diagnostic aid.

LABORATORY INVESTIGATIONS

Laboratory investigations can be discussed under two heads:

A. To establish the presence of hypercalcaemia.

B. To establish the cause (aetiology) of hypercalcaemia.

A. TO ESTABLISH THE PRESENCE OF HYPERCALCAEMIA

As discussed above, if the serum calcium level increases slowly or rapidly, certain symptoms and signs would point to hypercalcaemia, but many cases may be asymptomatic.

Laboratory tests that will be useful to establish hypercalcaemia are discussed below.

1. Serial Determination of Serum Calcium and Phosphorus

Determination of total serum calcium by a standard method is the most widely available means. ***It must be done several times along with estimation of serum phosphorus to establish that hypercalcaemia is present,*** these should be done while the patient is not on excessive intake of phosphate because this ion may reduce the serum calcium levels.

A careful review of all of the patient's medications and diet to be looked into. All durgs that are not essential or that are known to influence serum calcium level, e.g., calcium, vitamin D, thiazide diuretics, spironolactone should be withheld prior to tests.

2. *Estimation of Serum Albumin*

Serum calcium estimation must be done concomitantly with estimation of serum albumin (preferably on the same sample). Serum calcium must be corrected in cases of any deviation of serum albumin from normal. Serum calcium may be high with associated hyperalbuminaemia and low with hypoalbuminaemia. ***One gram of albumin per 100 ml of serum binds approximatley 0.8 mg/dl of calcium.*** Common formula for correction is—

Corrected serum calcium =	Serum calcium observed value + 0.8 (4.0 + serum albumin)

If facilities available, ***estimation of "free" calcium ("ionic" Ca^{2+})*** would provide a more specific and correct assessment of calcium status, specially in patients with altered proteins, pH, anions and so on.

Note

Hypercalcaemia must be documented more than once in a particular case before embarking on further biochemical testing.

3. *Urinary Calcium Excretion*

Hypercalcaemia ***per se*** usually results in an increased urinary calcium excretion rate.

PTH increases renal tubular calcium reabsorption and the 24-hour urinary excretion rate is normal in up to 25% of patients with hyperparathyroidism.

In malignant hypercalcaemia the excretion rate is usually high greater than 40 mg (10 mmol) per day, but it is not a useful test for distinguishing between the two conditions.

Note

The ***most useful application of urinary calcium excretion rate is the diagnosis of familial hypocalciuric hypercalcaemia.*** This disorder is characterized by decreased urinary calcium excretion, the hypercalcaemia in this disorder is associated with an excretion rate less than 25 mg (6.25 mmol) per day.

4. *Renal Calcium: Creatinine Ratio*

The Calcium: Creatinine clearance ratio is:

$$\frac{\text{Urine [Ca]} \times \text{Plasma [Creatinine]}}{\text{Urine [Creatinine]} \times \text{Plasma [Ca]}}$$

Determination of renal calcium creatinine clearance ratio ***may be useful in familial hypocalciuric hypercalcaemia.*** The ratio is less than 0.010 in this condition; whereas in other causes of hypercalcaemia the renal calcium: creatinine clearance ratio is greater than 0.010.

B. TO ESTABLISH THE CAUSE/AETIOLOGY OF HYPERCALCAEMIA

Once the hypercalcaemia is established, then one should proceed to find out the cause of hypercalcaemia. The aetiology of hypercalcaemia, in most cases be determined by a thorough clinical examination and radiological examinations, and evaluation of routine biochemical tests, by a process of elimination. As malignancy is the commonest cause, it is wise in cases of obscure aetiology, to hold this diagnosis until it is proved otherwise. In practice, the clinical examination is usually sufficient to determine whether it is malignant or non-malignant, non-parathyroid causes being usually obvious. However, in rare cases, it may be difficult to decide between primary hyperparathyroidism and hypercalcaemia of an ***"occult" (hidden) malignancy.***

Diagnosis of primary hyperparathyroidism can be done in addition to clinical findings, by ***concomitant determination of serum Ca and PTH on the same sample of serum*** as well as by assessment of the effect of PTH on the target tissues by laboratory examination. Certain laboratory tests and special investigations that can be useful or have been used for the evaluation of patients with hypercalcaemia for aetiological diagnosis can be discussed as under:

- ***Routine laboratory tests*** like Hb and haematocrit value, total and differential leucocyte count, ESR, etc.
- ***Routine biochemical tests*** like serum albumin, inorganic phosphate, alkaline phosphatase (ALP), serum electrolytes, serum magnesium, serum protein electrophoresis, urine protein electrophoresis.
- ***Determination of immuno-reactive PTH.***
- ***Indirect tests of PTH activity,*** e.g., plasma chloride: Po_4 ratio, renal tubular Po_4 reabsorption, urinary cyclic AMP excretion.
- ***Steroid suppression test.***
- ***Special investigations*** e.g. serum 1,25-$(OH)_2D_3$, determination of PTHrP, radiological investigations, and localization techniques.

1. Routine Laboratory Tests

Routine laboratory tests like Hb, haematocrit determinations, WBC and differential counts may give some relevant information.

- ***Anaemia***

Slight anaemia may be associated with patients of hypercalcaemia. But if anaemia is severe or moderately severe, it is usually seen in patients with leukaemias, myeloma, malignancy and secondary renal diseases.

- ***WBC and Differential Counts***

This may not be of much help except in leukaemia and sometimes occasionally in myeloma.

- ***ESR***

ESR is frequently normal in primary hyperparathyroidism but may be elevated markedly in leukaemias, myeloma and other malignancies.

It may also be elevated in patients with PTH hormone secreting non-endocrine tumours ***("ectopic" hyperparathyroidism)*** and sometimes in vitamin D intoxication.

2. Routine Biochemical Tests

Certain routine biochemical tests may be helpful in differentiating hypercalcaemia due to primary hyperparathyroidism and hypercalcaemia due to malignancy.

- ***Serum Albumin Determination***

As already discussed above, the concentration of serum albumin influences the calcium level in blood. About 40 to 60% of the circulating calcium is bound to albumin and other proteins and thus a high serum albumin level (as may occur in haemoconcentration) can result in hypercalcaemia.

Necessary correction may be done to get the correct serum calcium level or alternatively the serum calcium estimation should be repeated when albumin level is normalised with treatment.

- ***Serum Phosphate Estimation***

Increased activity of PTH increases urinary phosphate excretion thus lowering the serum phosphate level. Hence, ***a case of primary***

hyperparathyroidism with PTH overactivity is usually associated with hypophosphataemia. On the other hand, other causes of hypercalcaemia are usually associated with a normal or high serum phosphate (hyperphosphataemia).

Explanation: increased serum calcium concentration produces decrease in renal phosphate excretion (phosphaturia).

Note

This test is not reliable in differentiating these two types of hypercalcaemia because:

- some cases of hypercalcaemia of malignancy produces PTH related peptides, PTHrP, hummoral factor which increases urinary phosphate excretion lowering the serum phosphate level in blood; and
- prolonged hypercalcaemia of primary hyperparathyroidism, may induce renal insufficiency which, in turn, may decrease urinary phosphate excretion producing hyperphosphataemia in such cases.

- ***Serum Alkaline Phosphatase (ALP) Determination***

Serum alkaline phosphatase may be normal in the presence of hypercalcaemia. Elevation of this enzyme suggests the bone disease of hyperparathyroidism. Patients having hypercalcaemia due to malignancy, may also have high alkaline phosphatase level, but ***the serum alkaline phosphatase activity in malignancy is usually much higher than that found in hyperparathyroidism.***

Note

In hypercalcaemic patients with multiple myeloma the serum alkaline phosphatase activity is usually normal, and this often provides a clue to the diagnosis.

- ***Serum Electrolytes Determination***

Serum [Na^+] and [K^+] may be normal or reduced in primary hyperparathyroidism-Serum [Cl^-] is frequently, but not always, elevated in primary hyperparathyroidism being greater than 107 mEq/l (107 mmol/l), whereas in other causes of hypercalcaemia the chloride level is much lower.

In patinets with adrenal crisis, the serum sodium and chloride may be normal or reduced in association with elevated calcium and phosphorus levels. Increased PTH activity induces renal bicarbonate [HCO_3] wastage, whereas the reverse occurs in other causes of hypercalcaemia.

- ***Serum Magnesium Estimation***

Serum magnesium is usually normal or may be decreased in primary hyperparathyroidism.

- ***Routine Serum/Urinary Protein Electrophoresis***

Routine serum protein electrophoresis is of immense help to exclude multiple myeloma and sarcoidosis. Urine protein electrophoresis should also be carried out to identify the rare patient who may have an abnormal protein in the urine that is not detectable by serum protein electrophoresis.

- ***Estimation of Calcium, Phosphorus and Creatinine in 24-hour Urine***

A 24-hour urine collection (with the patient on a normal phosphate intake) for calcium, phosphorus and creatinine determinations may be useful. ***Hypercalciuria and hyperphosphaturia are commonly seen in primary hyperparathyroidism or in "ectopic" hyperparathyroidism.***

Note

May also occur in multiple myeloma, sarcoidosis and vitamin D intoxication. In benign familial hypercalcaemia, the 24-hour urinary calcium level is usually less than 150 mg. Usefulness of urinary calcium estimation and renal calcium: creatinine ratio ***in diagnosing "benign familial hypocalcuric hypercalcaemia"*** has already been stressed.

3. Determination of Immunoreactive PTH

Direct determination of concentration of intact PTH is the best test of parathyroid function.

Serum PTH level is probably the best single test for differentiating between hyperparathyroidism and hypercalcaemia due to other diseases. Various assays are available for PTH, and it is imperative that a modern "two-site" intact PTH assay be used. ***Serum calcium should be determined in the same sample in which PTH is determined. An elevated PTH level in the presence of hypercalcaemia generally establishes the diagnosis of primary hyperparathyroidism.***

Note

The hypercalcaemia of malignancy may be due to "ectopic" production of PTH like hormone, PTHrP, which can result in high serum PTH levels.

4. Indirect Tests of PTH Activity

These tests include the plasma/serum phosphate levels, urinary calcium (both discussed above), plasma/serum chloride: phosphate ratio, tests of renal tubular handling of phosphate and urinary excretion of cyclic AMP.

- ***Serum Chloride: Phosphate Ratio***

As discussed above increased PTH activity is associated with low serum phosphate concentration and an increased serum chloride level; the reverse occurring in decreased PTH activity. ***A plasma/serum chloride: phosphate ratio has been claimed to be useful. In 96% cases of primary hyperparathyroidism the chloride: phosphate ratio greater than 33 (if mg:mg) or 102 (if mmol:mmol) have been observed.***

On the other hand, in 92% of patients with hypercalcaemia due to other causes, the ratio has been found to be less than 30 (mg:mg) or 93 (if mmol:mmol).

- ***Tubular Phosphate Reabsorption***

PTH lowers renal Tm PO_4. Hypophosphataemia is thus commonly seen in primary hyperparathyroidism. Other causes of hypercalcaemia are associated with increased phosphate reabsorption thus producing hyperphosphataemia.

Note

Hypophosphataemia may be found in hypercalcaemic cancer patients as well, probably because of increase in the filtered calcium load and PTHrP lowers the Tm PO_4.

- ***Biocarbonate Reabsorption***

PTH alters acid-base status in as much as it lowers the tubular maximum of HCO^-_3 (Tm HCO^-_3). ***In PTH excess, a mild hyperchloraemic metabolic acidosis may be noted.*** On the other hand, in other hypercalcaemic conditions, a mild hypochloraemic metabolic alkalosis may be observed.

- ***Urinary Cyclic AMP Excretion***

PTH is considered to elicit its biological effect, viz. intermediary action of cyclic AMP. ***Excretion of cyclic AMP in urine has been used as a biological index of PTH secretion.*** The mean excretion rate of urinary cyclic AMP in patients with primary hyperparathyroidism is higher than in normal subjects, although much overlap occurs. In general, cyclic AMP excretion in urine is low in hypercalcaemia of most other causes.

Note

- Urinary cyclic AMP levels are elevated in primary hyperparathyroidism if renal function is normal.

  A decrease level of urinary cyclic AMP virtually excludes primary hyperparathyroidism in presence of normal renal function.
- Urinary cyclic AMP may be elevated in Humoral hypercalcaemia of malignancy (HHM) and is thought to be related to production of PTHrP by the tumour.

5. Steroid Suppression Test

Principle: The administration of a steroid, like dexamethasone, lowers the serum calcium level of patients with hypercalcaemia of non-parathyroid origin. In primary hyperparathyroidism the level remains elevated.

Procedure

A steroid test can be carried out to determine whether calcium suppression can be induced. Dexamethasone 1 mg three times a day for 7 days is administered. The serum calcium is determined before and after the test periods.

Interpretation

- ***Suppression of the calcium level usually does not occur in primary hyperparathyroidism*** and serum calcium level remains elevated.
- On the other hand, suppression occurs in hypercalcaemia of other causes and serum calcium level is lowered.
- The test may be ***useful in differentiation of malignant hypercalcaemia from hyperparathyroidism,*** but it is not specific, some patients with hyperparathyroidism show suppression and some patients with malignancy do not suppress.

6. Special Investigations

- ***Estimation of Serum 1,25,-$(OH)_2D_3$***

Principle: PTH is a major trophic factor in the production of 1,25,-$(OH)_2D_3$ by the kidney, by stimulating the enzyme ***"1α-hydroxylase".*** Hence, determination of this metabolitc of vitamin D may be useful in evaluating hypercalcaemia.

Serum 1,25,-$(OH)_2D_3$ can be estimated by radioimmunoassay.

Interpretations

- Serum concentrations of 1,25,-$(OH)_2D_3$ (calcitriol) are usually elevated in primary hyperparathyroidism.
- On the other hand, it is low normal or suppressed in other hypercalcaemic states, in which endogenous PTH secretion is suppressed and it is lower than normal.

Note

There are two exceptions:

- Lymphomas associated with 'AIDS' (acquired immune deficiency syndrome) or HTLV-1 infection (human T-cells lymphotropic type-1) usually have hypercalcaemia along with high serum cencentration of calcitriol. The source of calcitriol in these cases is not known.
- Patients of sarcoidosis may have hypercalcaemia with elevated levels of calcitriol. ***The source of calcitriol is pulmonary alveolar macrophages.***

- ***Estimation of Serum PTHrP***

A number of RIA methods have been developed and used for measuring PTHrP in sera. Methods are available to measure both N-terminal (1–34 a.a.) and C-terminal (109–138) by competitive RIA methods. ***But usually N-terminal assay is preferred, reason being C-terminal fragments of PTHrP may be elevated in renal failure.***

Interpretations

- ***In normal subjects:*** serum level ranges from 0 to 5 pmol/l.
- Level is also undetectable or normal in majority of malignancies which are not associated with hypercalcaemia, in primary hyperparathyroidism,hypoparathyroidism and other causes of hypercalcaemia.
- ***PTHrP levels found to be elevated in 60 to 90% patients of HHM*** (humoral hypercalcaemia of malignancy).
- It is ***found to be elevated in a wide variety of malignancies:***
  - specially in squamous cell carcinomas.
  - also in adenocarcinomas of lungs, kidneys.
  - in carcinomas of breast, renal cell, pancreas, prostate, colon, liver, ovary.
- Less frequently ***elevated in patients with haematological malignancies*** like lymphomas, leukaemias and multiple myeloma.

7. Radiological Investigations

Radiological investigation may provide the following information (in selected cases).

- *X-ray of chest* may show the presence of a hilar or peripheral lung lesion. The distal portion of clavicles should be examined for evidences of subperiosteal resorption.
- *X-ray of hands* may be normal or may demonstrate evidence of osteoporosis.
- *X-ray of lumbar spine* may reveal osteoporosis or the lytic lesions of multiple myeloma or both. In addition, nephrolithiasis and urinary tract stones may be observed.
- *X-ray of skulls* may demonstrate osteoporosis or presence of pituitary tumour or both. Occasionally intracranial calcification suggestive of sarcoidosis may be seen.

Note

- ***Subperiosteal resorption of bone is pathognomonic of hyper parathyroidism.***
- ***Osteoporosis*** is perhaps the ***most common radiologic finding in hyperparathyroidism.***

8. Localisation Techniques

A CT Scan of the cervical area, ultrasonography of the thyroid glands, and thyroid scanning may be useful if primary hyperparathyroidism is suspected.

9. Oncogenic Markers

Oncogenic markers may be useful for certain malignancies.

Table 9.1: Differentiation of hypercalcaemia of primary hyperparathyroidism and hypercalcaemia of malignancy and other causes

	Primary hyperparathyroidism hypercalcaemia	*Hypercalcaemia of malignancy, and other causes*
1. **Hypercalcaemia**		
• Severity	Usually <14 mg/dl not severe	Usually severe >14 mg/dl
• Rate of increase in calcium level	Slow rate, takes months	Rapid rate, in days/weeks.
2. **Metastatic calcification**	Common, renal calculi	Not common.
3. **Routine biochemical parameters**		
• *Serum* $[PO_4^{2-}]$	Normal or low ↓	Normal or high ↑ May be low if PTHrP production.
• *Serum ALP*	Normal or slight increase (<300 U/l)	Usually increased ↑ >300 U/l Much higher than that found in hyperparathyroidism.
• *Serum* $[CL^-]$	Elevated ↑ >107 mEq/l	Low ↓ <107 mEq/l
• *Serum* $[CL^-]:[PO_4^{2-}]$	>33 (mg:mg)	<30 (mg:mg)
• *Urinary* Ca^{2+}	Increased ↑ urinary Ca^{2+} rate with hypercalcaemia. May be normal up to 25% of cases	Usually high ↑ >40 mg /day. In familial hypercalciuric hypercalcaemia it is low ↓
4. **Plasma PTH**	Usually increased ↑ (diagnostic) (may be normal in some.)	Usually suppressed (may be high if PTHrP produced).
5. **Urinary cyclic AMP**	May be normal but usually high **N.B** *Low urinary cyclic AMP excludes primary hyperparathyroidism*	Low ↓ may be elevated if PTHrP production +
6. **Steroid suppression test**	No suppression, serum Ca^{2+} level remains elevated.	Usually suppression, serum Ca^{2+} level is lowered.
7. **Serum 1,25-$(OH)_2D_3$ (calcitriol)**	Elevated usually	Low, normal or suppressed.
8. **Serum PTHrP**	Undetectable	Elevated in patients of HHM (producing PTHrP)
9. **Radiology (bone)**	Subperiosteal bone resorption	Normal, In multiple myeloma, osteolytic lesions may be found

Flow Chart of laboratory investigation of a case of hypercalcaemia is given below

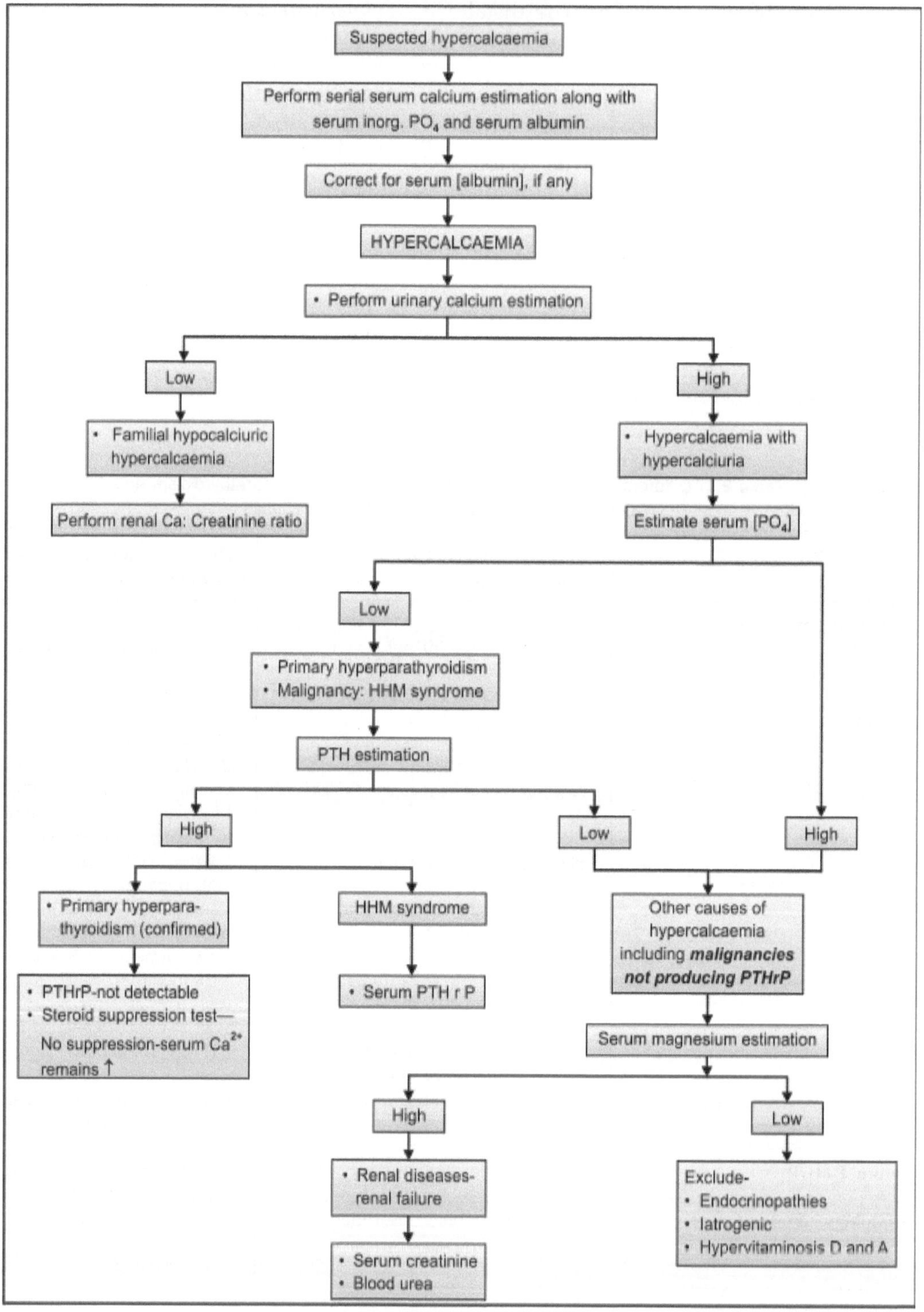

CONCLUSIONS

- In most cases of hypercalcaemia, proper history with clinical exmination along with routine biochemical tests and radiological examination would provide the aetiological diagnosis of hypercalcaemia without the necessity of performing further specialized investigations. Most of the specialized investigations are not available in hospital laboratory and help of special reference laboratory will be required in selected cases.
- **Plasma PTH estimation is the best single test** in presence of normal renal function for differnetiating between primary hyperparathyroidism and hypercalcaemia of other causes.
- If hyperparathyroidism is considered as the most probable cause of hypercalcaemia, other associated endocrine abnormalities should be considered. These include pituitary tumour, pheochromocytoma, medullary carcinoma of thyroid, islet-cell tumour, etc. Acromegaly is sometimes associated with hypercalcaemia and may occur in the presence of multiple endocrine neoplasia.
- Urinary calcium estimation should be performed on all cases of hypercalcaemia and if it is found associated with hypocalcinuria, possibility of "familial hypocalciuric hypercalcaemia" should be considered.

Table 9.1 gives the essential biochemical tests for differentiation of hypercalcaemia of hyperparathyroidism and hypercalcaemia of malignancy and other causes.

Flow Chart of laboratory investigation of a case of hypercalcaemia is given on page 116.

Chapter 10

Hypocalcaemia

INTRODUCTION

Hypocalcaemia is said to exist when serum calcium value is less than 8.5 mg/dl, as determined by a standard method. Total serum calcium may be low owing to a reduction in either:

- the albumin bound, or
- the "free fraction.

A reduction in the "free" serum calcium is usually due to impairment in physiological processes by which this fraction of serum calcium is maintained.

CAUSES

The commonest cause of hypocalcaemia is hypoalbuminaemia closely followed by renal failure. The other most common cause of hypocalcaemia is surgically induced hypoparathyroidism. Hence, if a thyroidectomy scar is present, the diagnosis usually becomes obvious. The various causes of hypocalcaemia can be grouped as listed below.

1. ***Reduction in serum albumin (Hypoalbuminaemia)***
   - Malnutrition
   - Malabsorption states
   - Nephrotic syndrome
   - Chronic liver diseases and liver failure.
2. ***Hypoparathyroidism***
   - May be surgically induced—partial or complete
   - Idiopathic: may be autoimmune
   - Bioinactive parathyroid hormone (PTH)
   - Transient hypoparathyroidism of infancy—may be partial.
3. ***Renal diseases and renal failure***
   - Renal tubular dysfunction
   - Acute tubular necrosis
   - Chronic renal failure
4. ***Pseudohypoparathyroidism***
5. ***Hypoparathyroidism in association with other disease states, which may be familial***
   - Addison's disease
   - Pernicious anaemia
   - Fungal disease like candidiasis
6. ***Other miscellaneous causes***
   - Acute pancreatitis: haemorrhagic or oedematous
   - Osteomalacia and rickets due to viatamin D dificiency or resistance
   - Medullary carcinoma of the thyroid, with or without associated endocrinopathies
   - **"Healing phase"** of bone disease of treated hyperparathyroidism, hyperthyroidism and haematological malignancies ***("hungry bone" syndrome)***
   - Magnesium deficiency
   - Iatrogenic—administration of ***foscarnet.***

• Reduction in Albumin Level (Hypoalbuminaemia)

Hypoalbuminaemia, as stated above, is the most common cause of reduction in the concentration of total serum calcium. Common clinical conditions, to be considered, which are associated with low serum albumin concentration include:

- chronic liver diseases/liver failure;
- nephrotic syndrome; and
- malnutrition and malabsorption states.

A correction for serum calcium in terms of low serum albumin should be made (Refer to laboratory investigation of hypercalcaemia). Under such clinical conditions, associated with hypoalbuminaemia, the 'free' fraction of calcium is normal and no therapy for hypocalcaemia is indicated.

2. Hypoparathyroidism

In 90% cases, the hypoparathyroidism is secondary to destruction/removal of parathyroids during neck surgery for thyroidectomy (accidental removal), or parathyroidectomy and head and neck malignancies. In 10% cases, hypoparathyroidism is primary idiopathic autoimmune type. May be associated with other familial autoimmune diseases, e.g. Addison's disease, hyperthyroidism, pernicious anaemia, etc.

3. Hypocalcaemia in Chronic Renal Failure

Chronic renal failure is also frequently associated with hypocalcaemia. Contributing factors for low serum values are:

- Hyperphosphataemia,
- Impaired synthesis of 1,25-$(OH)_2D_3$ due to inadequate renal mass due to disease process or tubular damage;
- Skeletal resistance to the action of PTH.

Note

Hypocalcaemia in chronic renal failure may not be associated with 'tetany'. Renal failure is associated with 'acidosis', in acidosis, ionization of calcium is not suppressed and ***ionic clacium is not lowered, hence there may not be any tetany.***

4. Pseudohypoparathyroidism

It is biochemically similar to hypoparathyroidism and characterised by low serum calcium level. Patients show peripheral resistance to PTH and **usually associated with elevated levels of circulating PTH.** The condition is associated with somatic abnormalities such as:

- Short stature, short neck, round face;
- Abnormally shortened metacarpals and metatarsals (Albright's hereditary osteodystrophy); and
- Mild mental retardation (diminished intelligence).

Mechanism: Molecular basis of this disorder appears to be a **defect in "G-protein"**—there is a **reduction in the amount of "guanosine nucleotide regulatory protein", (Ns)** in the adenylate cyclase enzyme system. Endorgan resistance to PTH owing to a defect in the interaction of PTH with cellular G-protein.

5. Hypocalcaemia in Acute Pancreatitis

Acute pancreatitis, haemorrhagic or oedematous, is frequently found to be associated with hypocalcaemia. Mechanism of hypocalcaemia is not clear. Following factors may be implicated:

- Impaired PTH secretion or PTH resistance
- Deposition of calcium in the necrotic peripancreatic fat
- If the pancreatitis is secondary to alcoholism, then deficiency of magnesium may be an additional contributory factor.

6. Hypocalcaemia in Osteomalacia/Rickets

Osteomalacia or rickets ***secondary to vitamin D deficiency*** may also be associated with hypocalcaemia. It may be due to:

- Partly to impaired intestinal absorption of calcium
- Skeletal resistant to PTH and thereby, limits calcium resorption from bone.

7. Healing Phase of Bone Diseases

Acute symptomatic hypocalcaemia may be noted in hospitalized patients undergoing surgical treatment for hyperthyroidism or primary hyperparathyroidism or in patients receiving therapy for haematological malignancies. In such conditions there may be rapid mineralisation of bones, which may precipitate a drop in serum calcium level producing hypocalcaemia *("Hungry-bone syndrome")*.

8. Hypocalcaemia in Magnesium Deficiency

Magnesium deficiency may be associated with hypocalcaemia—it is another common clinical cause.

Mechanism: Magnesium deficiency impairs PTH secretion as well as the action of PTH on bone and kidneys.

9. Iatrogenic

Foscarnet given for the therapy of cytomegalovirus retinitis in patients with acquired immune deficiency syndrome (AIDS) has also been reported to result in hypocalcaemia.

CLINICAL FEATURES

- Symptoms of hypocalcaemia usually occur when the serum calcium level is below 7.5 mg/dl, but sometimes occur at higher levels when there has been a rapid decrease in serum calcium concentration.
- Symptoms of hypocalcaemia are most commonly:
  - neuromuscular hyperexcitability such as "latent" tetany with Chvostek's sign and Trousseau's sign being positive; and
  - spontaneous tetany with carpopedal spasms and muscle cramps, paraesthesia/and seizures.

Note

- ***The neuromuscular excitability depends on level of ionic (free) calcium.*** Patients of chronic renal diseases have such symptoms infrequently because of coexisting metabolic acidosis. In acidosis ionized calcium may be normal though there may be hypocalcaemia.
- Patients with primary gastrointestinal disease may have remarkably few symptoms, complaining chiefly of weakness, weight loss, diarrhoea, increased frequency of stools and abdominal cramping.
- Children and adults with pseudohypoparathyroidism often complain of weight loss.
- Patients with rickets and osteomalacia (in adults) may have ***"bone pains"*** or problems related to growth of bone.
- Very low serum calcium concentrations may also be associated with:
  - hypotension; and
  - ECG abnormalities such as a prolonged Q-T interval.
- Chronic hypocalcaemia for prolonged periods (years) may be complicated by:
  - calcification of basal ganglia; and
  - cataract formation.

The presence of goitre may suggest medullary carcinoma of thyroid, thyroiditis or Graves' disease.

LABORATORY INVESTIGATIONS

This can be discussed under two heads:

- ***To establish the presence of hypocalcaemia.***
- ***To establish the cause of hypocalcaemia.***

A. TO ESTABLISH THE PRESENCE OF HYPOCALCAEMIA

Serial determinations of serum calcium should be carried out. All drugs that are not essential or that are known to influence serum calcium levels should be withheld. Simultaneously, on the same sample serum, inorganic phosphorus and serum albumin estimations should also be carried out. If there is evidence of hypoalbuminaemia, the necessary 'corrections' should be applied. Serum calcium may be corrected for any decrease in total serum albumin concentration (~4.0 g/dl), because ***one gm of albumin/100 ml of serum binds approximately 0.8 mg/dl of calcium.***

The following common formula is used:

Corrected serum calcium= Serum Ca + 0.8 (4.0 - Serum albumin)

Determination of "free" calcium (ionized calcium), provides a more direct and accurate assessment of calcium status of the body. Unfortunately, estimation of serum ionized calcium is not routinely available in most of the hospital laboratories. But an estimate of its level can be made using the following formula:

Adjusted serum [Ca] (mmol/l)	=	Measured serum [Ca^+] (mmol/l)	- (0.025 × [Albumin] (gm/l)	+ 1

B. TO ESTABLISH THE CAUSE OF HYPOCALCAEMIA

Once it is established that hypocalcaemia is present, then investigations should be done to establish the cause (aetiology). In most hypocalcaemic patients, the cause is evident from the history and clinical examination. If the cause is not readily apparent then there are a number of laboratory investigations which may help to clarify the diagnosis. The laboratory investigations that can help are listed below.

1. Routine laboratory tests

- Serum phosphate
- Serum alkaline phosphatase (ALP)
- Serum electrolytes
- Blood urea/creatinine/cholesterol

2. Special biochemical tests

- Serum PTH estimation
- Serum magnesium estimation
- Vitamin D studies
- Urinary cyclic AMP

3. Other special investigations depends on the suspected aetiology.

1. Routine Laboratory Tests

• *Estimation of Serum Inorganic Phosphorus*

Hypocalcaemia associated with a high serum inorganic phosphate concentration (hyperphosphataemia) occurs in:

- renal failure; and
- hypoparathyroidism syndrome.

On the other hand, hypocalcaemia and hypophosphataemia (decreased serum inorganic phosphate) is characteristically seen in ***"secondary hyperparathyroidism"***, e.g. vitamin D deficiency syndrome: rickets and osteomalacia. In these, the low serum clacium concentration stimulates PTH secretion which, in turn increases renal phosphate excretion.

Interpretation

When interpreting a patient's serum inorganic phosphate level, the age should be taken into consideration, normal infants and children have "higher" levels than those of normal adults as given below:

Serum inorganic *phosphate level* (range) in various age groups is given below:

- **Adults**—2.0 to 3.9 mg/dl (0.65 to 1.25 mmol/l)
- **Children**
  - Neonate: 3.7 to 8.7 mg/dl (1.20 to 2.80 mmol/l)
  - Less than 7 years: 4.0 to 5.6 mg/dl (1.30 to 1.80 mmol/l)
  - More than 7 years but less than 15 years: 2.2 to 3.8 mg/dl (0.70 to 1.20 mmol/l)

• *Estimation of Serum Alkaline Phosphatase (ALP)*

A high serum alkaline phosphatase (ALP) with reference to disordered calcium metabolism is indicative of increased osteoblastic activity. Vitamin D deficiency syndrome, e.g. in osteomalacia, hypocalcaemia is characteristically associated with high serum alkaline phosphatase level.

Note

When interpreting, it should be remembered that serum ALP levels in infants, children (growing) and adolescence are normally high as compared to normal healthy adults (up to 2½ times the normal adult upper reference limit).

• *Serum Electrolytes*

Renal failure is commonly associated with hypocalcaemia. Renal failure usually develops metabolic acidosis, the CO_2 combining power of the plasma is reduced (decrease in $[HCO_3^-]$.

In many patients with renal failure vomiting causes loss of EC fluid and electrolytes leading to depletion of body sodium and chloride. Na^+ and Cl^- continue to be lost in urine because tubular reabsorption is defective (plasma $[Na^+]$ ↓ and $[Cl^-]$ ↓; urinary $[Na^+]$ ↑ and $[Cl^-]$ ↑).

Hyperkalaemia $[K^+]$ ↑ is often found in the terminal stages when the urine volume falls.

- ***Blood Urea/Creatinine/Cholesterol Estimation***

Renal failure is a common cause of hypocalcaemia. High blood urea and creatinine concentration as well as a high serum phosphate level are found in such patients. A high blood cholesterol is found in nephrotic syndrome.

2. Special Biochemical Tests

- ***Serum PTH Assay***

Low serum PTH level and hyperphosphataemia are the hallmarks of primary hypoparathyroidism. Serum PTH level is increased ↑ in pseudohypoparthyroidism, in secondary hyperparathyroidism (vitamin D deficiency syndrome) and also in renal failure.

In pseudohypoparathyroidism

- Serum calcium is low; ↓
- Serum inorganic PO_4 is increased; ↑ and
- Serum PTH is increased ↑.

In secondary hyperparathyroidism Vitamin D deficiency syndrome, e.g. in osteomalacia/rickets, the biochemical profile is:

- Serum calcium is low; ↓
- Serum PTH high ↑ (secondary hyperparathyroidism due to the hypocalcaemia);
- Decreased serum inorganic phosphate ↓ (hypophosphataemia due to high PTH);
- High serum alkaline phosphatase (ALP) ↑; and
- Low serum 25-$(OH)_2$ D_3 ↓.

In renal failure: Serum PTH is increased alongwith hypocalcaemia.

- ***Estimation of Serum Magnesium***

Most hospitals and clinics do not usually offer serum magnesium determination as a routine and as a part of routine "screening" of biochemical profile. It must be specifically carried out if magnesium deficiency is suspected. ***Magnesium deficiency may also cause hypocalcaemia by:***

- Decreasing PTH secretion.
- Inactivating its activity at the bone level.

As it is known, severe hypomagnesaemia may cause clinical features similar to hypocalcaemia (like "tetany") and that these two conditions, i.e. hypomagnesaemia and hypocalcaemia may coexist in the same patient.

Note

Hence, if the clinical features of a patinet with hypocalcaemia do not respond to IV calcium administration, the possibility of magnesium deficiency must be considered.

- ***Estimation of Serum 25-(OH) D_3***

In vitamin D deficiency syndrome, due to malnutrition or malabsorption, the serum levels of 25-(OH) D_3 is usually decreased.

Note

Vitamin D deficiency syndrome associated with anticonvulsant or barbiturate therapy often have normal levels of serum 25-(OH) D_3, although the 1,25-$(OH)_2D_3$ level is usually low.

- ***Urinary Cyclic AMP Estimation***

In primary hypoparathyroidism, as serum PTH is low, urinary cyclic AMP excretion is decreased.

- On the other hand, ***in secondary hyperparathyroidism*** due to vitamin D deficiency syndrome and in pseudohypoparathyroidism the urinary cyclic AMP excretion is increased (due to increased serum PTH level).

Flow Chart for laboratory investigation of a case of hypocalcaemia

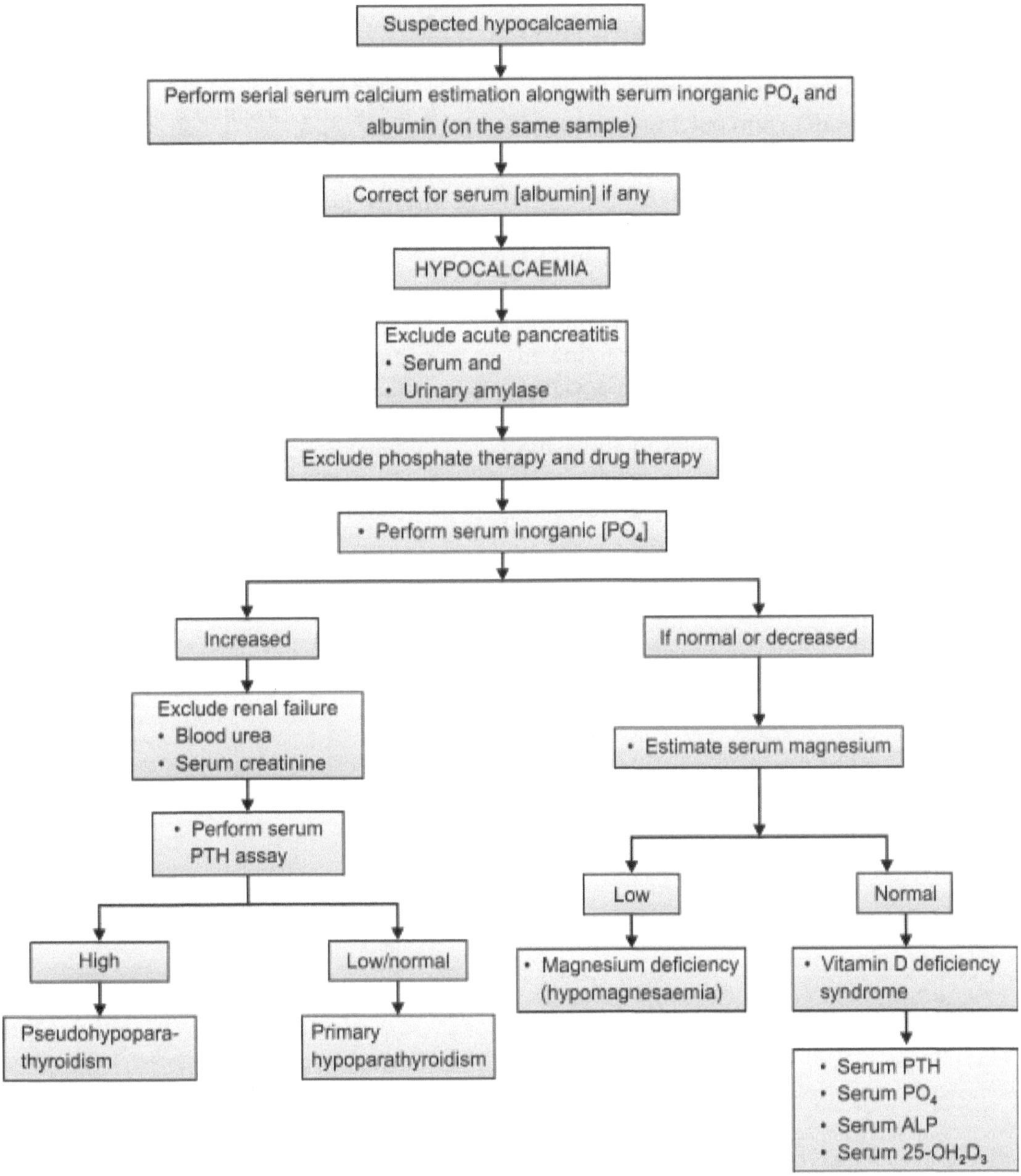

3. Special Investigations

In addition to above routine laboratory and special biochemical tests, certain special investigations may be required to establish aetiology/cause in a particular selected case.

1. If hypocalcaemia is suspected to be due to malnutrition/malabsorption, then certain special investigations will be required to establish the causative factor for malabsorption.

(Refer to Laboratory Investigation of Malabsorption Syndrome).

2. If the routine and speical biochemical test-point to primary hypoparathyroidism, certain additional tests may be required.
   - ***X-ray of skull*** to find out any evidence of intracranial calcification
   - ***Ophthalmoscopic examination*** for evidence of presence of cataract
   - ***ECG*** may demonstrate a defect in Q-T interval which may be prolonged
   - ***In suspected idiopathic hypoparathyroidism,*** the patient should be followed and studied, as indicated, for associated autoimmune disorders, if any, viz. Addison's disease, diabetes mellitus, hyperthyroidism, pernicious anaemia or polyglandular autoimmune disorders.
3. If a goitre is present then
   - RAI uptake,
   - scanning of thyroid gland, and
   - determination of autoantibody may be indicated.
4. ***If medullary carcinoma of thyroid*** is suspected, neck X-rays, urinary catecholamines, VMA and calcitonin assay and biopsy of thyroid gland may be indicated.
5. Other miscellaneous investigations include:
   - ***In case of suspected associated candidiasis*** fungus culture from throat swab, urine and blood may have to be carried out
   - ***In case of pseudohypoparathyroidism*** GTT may be abnormal, X-ray of long bones and hand may demonstrate ***brachydactylia***
   - ***In case of suspected acute pancreatitis,*** serum and urinary amylase may be helpful.

Chapter 11

Hypercortisolism

INTRODUCTION

Elevated levels of cortisol and/or other glucocorticoids above normal level in blood is called hypercortisolism. The recognised syndrome is called Cushing's syndrome. This syndrome results from excessive secretion of adrenal cortex.

CUSHING'S SYNDROME

CAUSES

The causes can be divided into **two groups.**

1. ACTH Independant Hypercortisolism

- ***Iatrogenic***

This is the most common cause in clinical practice and include:

Long-term therapeutic use of cortisol/other glucocorticoids in a variety of systemic inflammatory diseases, management of transplant recipients and autoimmune diseases.

In such long-term therapy, production of cortisol by patient's adrenals is suppressed, and when exogenous cortisol is stopped abruptly, adrenal insufficiency may develop.

Note

Discontinuation of cortisol therapy should be done gradually **("taper" the dose)** over several days to allow the patient's adrenals to begin to produce cortisol again.

- ***Adrenal Adenomas/and Carcinomas***

Hypercortisolism or Cushing's syndrome is also caused by primary lesions in adrenal cortex, viz. adrenocortical neoplasms: adenomas or carcinomas. These account for 20 to 25% cases of Cushing's syndrome.

It may be autonomous hyperplasia associated with low levels of ACTH. Dexamethasone fail to suppress cortisol production.

2. ACTH Dependent Hypercortisolism

- ***Cushing's Disease***

Pituitary based hypercortisolism accounts for 60 to 70% cases of Cushing's syndrome. The disease may be due to a solitary pituitary adenoma or multiple microadenomas. Some patients may not have the pituitary lesion suggesting primary hypothalamic dysfunction. Usually there is excessive secretion of ACTH by anterior pituitary leading to adrenocortical hyperplasia (may be bilateral). Plasma ACTH level is usually high and hypercortisolism is suppressed by high doses of dexamethasone.

- ***Ectopic ACTH Syndrome (Non-pituitary Tumours)***

It is caused by production of ACTH-like peptide or sometimes peptide similar to CRH by non-pituitary tumours and hypercortisolism.

This accounts for 10 to 15% cases of Cushing's syndrome.

Non-pituitary tumours may be:

- **Bronchogenic carcinoma** (60%)—most commonly 'Oat-Cell' type
- **Thymomas-malignant type** (15%)
- **Bronchial adenoma**
- **Pancreatic carcinoma** (10%)—usually islet cells tumours.
- **Other non-pituitary tumours.**

The syndrome is usually associated with bilateral adrenocortical hyperplasia and elevated ACTH level in blood and can be suppressed by high doses of dexamethasone.

CLINICAL FEATURES

The symptoms of hypercortisolism are the same regardless of the aetiology and include the following:

Sex Female predominance (3:1), most often in middle adult life. Onset in childhood is suggestive of neoplasm.

Signs and symptoms include

- *Truncal obesity*: Weight gain predominantly in face ***("moon facies")***, neck, shoulders, and abdomen with relatively thin extremities. Many patients develop a characteristic ***"buffalo hump"***, a fat pad on the upper back at the base of the neck.
- *Protein wasting:* With thinning of the skin and development of abdominal ***'Striae'***, easy bruising, muscle wasting and poor wound healing.
- *Hypertension:* Common, owing to cortisol induced sodium and water retention.
- *Abnormal glucose metabolism:* Leading to hyperglycaemia: Impaired glucose tolerance or overt diabetes mellitus.
- *Neuropsychiatric* disturbances.
- *Hirsutism* and *menstrual abnormalities* in females; and *impotence, oligospermia* and *loss of libido* in males.
- *Hyperpigmentation* is common in patients with Cushing's syndrome associated with high ACTH level.
- Decreased ability to limit infection, with **loss of delayed hypersensitivity response,**
- Decreased lymphoid tissue, ***decreased circulating lymphocytes,*** also shows ***eosinopenia.***

LABORATORY INVESTIGATIONS

Laboratory evaluation of a patient with suspected Cushing's syndrome can be done as follows:

- ***To establish the presence of hypercortisolism***
- ***To establish the cause of hypercortisolism, to distinguish between the adrenal, pituitary and ectopic causes of the hypercortisolism.***

A. TO ESTABLISH THE PRESENCE OF HYPERCORTISOLISM

The first step in the investigation must be to establish a diagnosis of presence of hypercortisolism (most crucial step).

In addition to **history** and **clinical features,** certain **"Screening Tests"** will be required.

1. Plasma Cortisol Level and the Adrenal Rhythm

Plasma cortisol level should be estimated in the patient at 8 am and 8 pm to determine the plasma cortisol level whether it is increased above normal level and to determine if the ***normal diurnal variation is present.*** (For normal range and methods—see adrenal function tests).

2. Measurement of 24-hour Urinary Cortisol

Under normal circumstances, less than 1% of the secreted cortisol appears in urine as ***"free"*** cortisol, i.e. the cortisol which is neither bound to protein nor conjugated with glucuronic acid to form glucuronides/or sulfated.

Note

- In general, ***a 24-hour urinary "free" cortisol level less than 100 µg/day excludes the diagnosis of Cushing's syndrome and levels greater than 120 µg/day suggest the diagnosis of Cushing's syndrome and hypercortisolism.***

- The diagnostic accuracy is over 90% when the test is properly performed. ***An elevated excretion rate establishes over production of cortisol.***

Precautions

- Over collection of 24-hour urine collection
- Administration of diuretics/high salt
- Depression and stress.

The above factors ***may cause a false positive*** result.

3. Overnight Low-dose Dexamethasone Suppression Test

This is another reliable "screening test" for the presence of hypercortisolism.

Principle: Dexamethasone, a cortisol analogue, and a strong and potent glucocorticoid suppresses ACTH and cortisol production in normal subjects (inhibition of pituitary-adrenal axis) but not in patient with Cushing's syndrome.

Procedure

- One mg (1.0 mg) of dexamethasone is given orally at 2300 or 2400 hours
- Blood is drawn for determination of plasma cortisol at 0800 hours the next morning.

Interpretation

- ***In normal subjects:*** Plasma cortisol level is suppressed to 3 μg/dl or less after administration of 1 mg of dexamethasone.
- ***Most patients with Cushing's syndrome:*** Will not show adequate suppression and 0800 hour sample will show plasma cortisol level usually greater than 10 μg/dl.

Note

Plasma cortisol level greater than 3 μg/dl may also be seen in various other conditions, viz. in stress, in infections, obesity, alcohol abuse, pregnancy, oral contraceptives use, oestrogen therapy, failure/omission of dexamethasone by patients and under treatment with diphenyl hydantion/or phenobarbitone (these drugs enhance the catabolism of dexamethasone).

These factors are to be taken into consideration, while interpreting the result

Diagnosis of hypercortisolism is highly likely, if

- Plasma cortisol level is higher than normal;
- Loss of diurnal pattern;
- No suppression to low-dose dexamethasone; and
- Urinary "free" cortisol level is greater than 120 μg/dl.

B. TO ESTABLISH THE CAUSE OF HYPERCORTISOLISM

Once a diagnosis of endogenous hypercortisolism is established as per above scheme, then the tests should be performed in conjunction with clinical findings and other special investigations to find out the cause, i.e. where abnormality lies (Table 11.1).

Tests which should be performed to determine the aetiology of overproduction of cortisol are

- Plasma ACTH assay
- High dose dexamethasone suppression test
- Metyrapone test
- CRH stimulation test.

1. *Plasma ACTH Assay*

This test will be able to differentiate between ACTH-independent and ACTH-dependent hypercortisolism.

Principle

- Since cortisol and ACTH interact in a ***"feed-back loop",*** increased plasma cortisol levels will be associated with suppression of ACTH if the syndrome is due to a primary adrenal lesion.
- In contrast, hypercortisolism due to an ACTH producing pituitary adenoma (Cushing's disease) or to "ectopic" production of ACTH would be associated with increased ACTH levels.

Procedure

Plasma ACTH assay is not readily available in most hospital laboratories. It can be measured by RIA method where the radioimmuno assay facilities are available.

Three types **of assays are available:**
- ***Bioassay*** are time consuming and laborious.
- ***Receptor assay*** employ solubilised binding proteins obtained from normal or neoplastic adrenocortical cells. Only biologically active ACTH is measured.
- ***Radioimmuno assays*** most commonly employed where facilities are available. Commercial kits are available for the same.

Interpretation

- ***In normal adults:*** Range is 5 to 60 pg/ml (1.1-13.3 p mol/litre) (morning specimen) 0800-0900 hours.
- ***Plasma ACTH levels are low in adrenocortical tumours***
  - ACTH levels may be normal or increased in Cushing's disease
  - ACTH levels are usually high in ***"ectopic"*** ACTH syndrome. Chromatography of ACTH may demonstrate ***"big" ACTH*** in the "ectopic" ACTH syndrome.

2. High-dose Dexamethasone Suppression Test

- Administration of 2 mg dexamethasone every 6 hours in a normal individual will result in suppression of plasma cortisol and 17-OH corticosteroid excretion. Patients with Cushing's syndrome due to endogenous cortisol production will not suppress with this dosage.
- Administration of high doses of dexamethasone, 8 mg every 6 hours will, however, frequently result in suppression of pituitary Cushing's. In this situation, the set point for suppression of ACTH production by the pituitary tumour seems to be higher than normal, but the "feedback loop" is still intact.
- Patients with adrenal adenoma and carcinoma and "ectopic" ACTH syndrome will not respond to high doses of dexamethasone, since hormone production in these settings has totally "escaped" feedback control.

3. Metyrapone Test

(For detail of the test, refer to Chapter 5, Adrenocortical Function Tests).

Rationale

The test is ***useful in differentiating adrenal tumours from adrenal hyperplasia (pituitary Cushing's).***

Interpretation

- ***In normal persons,*** the administration of this drug results in a decreased production of cortisol, stimulation of ACTH and increase in the metabolic precursors of cortisol. These metabolic precursors are excreted in the urine as 17-OHCS. Hence, a normal response to Metyrapone is an increase in 17-OHCS excretion in urine.
- A similar response is seen in patients with pituitary Cushing's (Cushing's disease) in which adrenal hyperplasia occurs. They are still subject to "feedback" control; even though at a higher level.
- Patients whose cortisol production is completely ***autonomous,*** that is those with adrenal tumours or ***"ectopic"*** ACTH syndrome are already under maximum stimulation and show no response to Metyrapone.

4. CRH Stimulation Test
(Refer to Adrenocortical Function Tests)

- Administration of CRH to patients with Cushing's disease (pituitary adenoma) increases their already elevated ACTH levels. The test produces an exaggerated ACTH or cortisol response or both, in about 90% of patients with Cushing's disease.

Table 11.1: Aetiological diagnosis of hypercortisolism employing biochemical tests

	Plasma cortisol level	*Diurnal rhythm of plasma cortisol*	*Urinary cortisol 17-OHCS*	*Plasma ACTH*	*Response to high dose dexamethasone*	*Metyra pone test*	*ACTH stimulation test*
I. **Normal control gr.**	Normal	8 a.m. value > 8 p.m. rhythm-present	Normal	Normal	Suppressed ↓	Normal	Normal
II. **Iatrogenic**	Variable-depends on steroid used	Not applicable	Variable, depend on steroidused	Decrease ↓	Suppressed ↓	No response	Variable or slightly increased response
III. **Adrenal involvement (primary lesion)**						Usually no response	
• **Adrenal Adenoma**	Increased ↑	No response	Increased ↑	Decreased ↓	Usually no suppression	No response	Decreased ↓
• **Adrenal Carcinoma**	Increased ↑	No response	Increased ↑	Decreased ↓	No suppression	No response	Usually no response
IV. **Pituitary Cushing's (Cushing's disease)**							
Pituitary tumour	Increased ↑	No response	Increased ↑	Normal or increased ↑	Suppression ↓	Normal or Increased response.	Normal or increased response
V. **"Ectopic" ACTH syndrome**	Increased ↑	No response	Increased ↑	• Normal or increased • Chromatography May show **"Big" ACTH (Pre-ACTH)**	No suppression	Decreased ↓ or no response	Normal or slightly increased response

- In contrast, no increase in ACTH is observed when CRH is given to patients with elevated ACTH due to *"ectopic"* ACTH syndrome or to patients with suppressed ACTH due to primary hypercortisolism (adrenal tumours).

This test may thus be useful in distinguishing between causes of hypercortisolism with an elevated plasma ACTH.

4. Other Routine Laboratory Studies

Certain routine biochemical studies will be helpful to demonstrate the effects of hypercortisolism. These tests evaluate the systemic effects of hypercortisolaemia. These are:

- ***Total and differential WBC count*** which demonstrates
  - Lymphopenia
  - Eosinopenia.
- ***Absolute eosinophil count:*** In normal subjects ranges 100 to 300/cumm. In hypercortisolism, the value is usually below 50/c.mm.
- ***Blood sugar estimation:*** shows impaired glucose tolerance:
  - Random postprandial glucose determination may show hyperglycaemia
  - GTT may show hyperglycaemic curve.
- ***Serum electrolytes and CO_2 combining power***
  - *Na^+* may be increased (hypernatraemia)
  - *K^+* may show decreased potassium level (hypokalaemia).
  - May show hypokalaemic alkalosis.
- ***Urinary estimations:*** Quantitative estimation of sodium, potassium and uric acid in 24-hour urine shows:
  - Na^+-diminished ↓
  - K^+ excretion increased (potassium diuresis) ↓
  - Uric acid excretion increased ↓

5. Special Investigations

Certain special investigations may be required for determining the cause in some cases.

1. ***Radiological studies include:***
   - X-ray of skull
   - X-ray of chest
   - X-ray of lumbar spine
   - Intravenous pyelography with nephrotomography for renal stones and detection of adrenal enlargement.
2. If primary involvement of adrenals is suspected like adrenal tumour, adenoma or carcinoma and hyperplasia, the following may be helpful:
   - **Arteriography** for differentiating adrenal hyperplasia and tumour.
   - **CT scanning** of the organs.
   - **Scanning of the adrenal glands** can be done with ^{131}I labelled iodocholesterol which can differentiate hyperplasia, adenoma and carcinoma.
3. ***In suspected pituitary tumour*** following can be helpful:
   - *Pituitary CT scan*
   - *Cerebral arteriography.*
4. ***In suspected case of ectopic ACTH syndrome***
   - **Tomography of lung**
   - **Oncogenic markers.**

Flow chart for investigation of hypercortisolism is given on page 131.

Flow Chart of investigation of hypercortisolism (Cushing's syndrome)

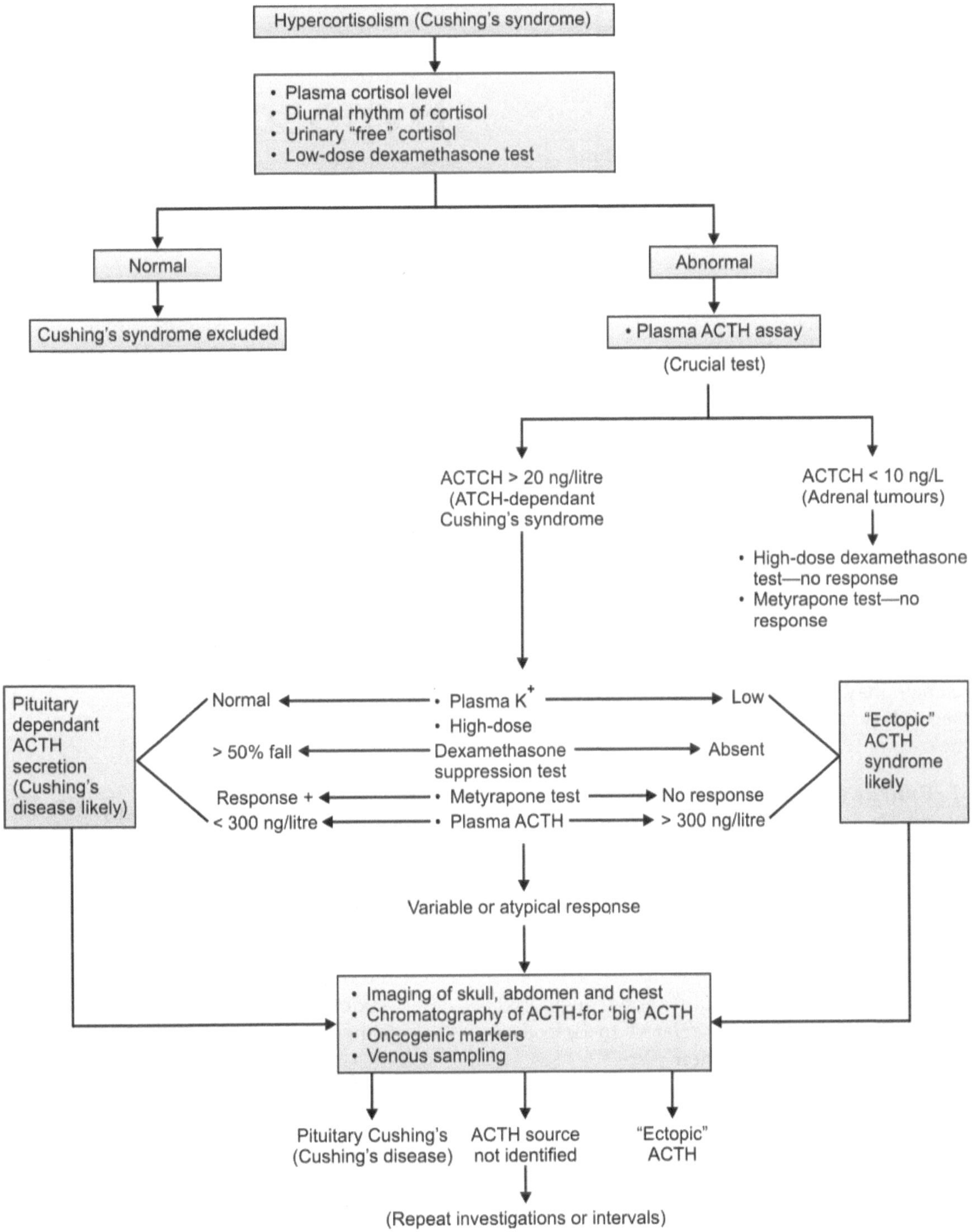

Chapter 12

Hypocortisolism

INTRODUCTION

Plasma cortisol level below normal due to adrenocortical insufficiency is called hypocortisolism.

Decreased production of plasma cortisol may be associated with:

primary adrenocortical disease or may be
secondary to pituitary abnormalities or
tertiary due to hypothalamic lesions resulting in decreased ACTH.

CAUSES

Hypocortisolism due to adrenocortical insufficiency may be of **three types,** i.e. **primary, secondary** and **tertiary.** These are discussed below.

1. Primary (Addison's Disease)

This can be:

- Chronic adrenal insufficiency.
- Acute adrenal insufficiency.

a. *Chronic Adrenal Insufficiency (Idiopathic Adrenal Atrophy)*

Exact cause is not known, but now considered as autoimmune disorder related to defective suppression of T-cell function.

Points in favour

- Association with other autoimmune disorders, viz. Hashimoto's thyroiditis, pernicious anaemia, hyperthyroidism, (thyrotoxicosis), spontaneous adult myxoedema, etc.
- Association with polyglandular autoimmune syndromes—PGA type I and PGA type II

  PGA type I may be associated with mucocutaneous candidiasis.
- Demonstration of presence of antibodies to adrenocortical antigens in more than 75% of cases.

Other causes

- ***Granulomatous diseases, e.g.***
  - Tuberculosis.
  - Sarcoidosis.
  - Histoplasmosis.
- ***Metabolic disorders, e.g.***
  - Amyloidosis.
  - Haemochromatosis.
  - Adrenoleukodystrophy.
  - Adrenomyeloneuropathy, etc.
- ***Neoplastic infiltration***
  - Metastatic cancer.
  - Acquired immune deficiency syndrome.
  - Congenital immune deficiency.
  - Post-bilateral adrenalectomy—surgical removal of the glands
  - Abdominal irradiation.
  - Congenital adrenal hypoplasia.

b. *Acute Adrenal Insufficiency (Addisonian Crisis)*

- ***Vascular haemorrhages:*** Include massive adrenocortical haemorrhage-"***Waterhouse-Friderichsen syndrome***" and non-infectious neonatal adrenocortical haemorrhage.

Waterhouse-Friderichsen Syndrome

It denotes ***acute haemorrhagic necrosis*** secondary to bacteraemia, most frequently with meningococcal infections with meningococcaemia. ***Other organisms involved are:***

- Staphylococci
- Pseudomonads
- Pneumococci
- ***Haemophilus influenzae.***

- ***Rapid withdrawal of steroid therapy:*** It is the most important and common cause clinically. ***"Stress"*** in patients with chronic adrenal insufficiency can precipitate acute episode.
- ***Iatrogenic:*** Anticoagulants and drugs, e.g. aminoglutethamide.
- ***DIC (Disseminated Intravascular Coagulation):*** May be associated with adrenal haemorrhage and excessive utilisation of coagulation factors, producing deficiency.

Note

- At one time tuberculosis was most important cause. But now with specific antitubercular therapy and preventive measures, ***tuberculosis is uncommon.***
- As stated above, most common clinically is the development of adrenocortical insufficiency due to prolonged corticoid therapy and sudden withdrawal. Hence, usual approach to discontinuation of corticosteroid therapy should be to decrease the dose (***taper off***) gradually spread over several days.
- In "primary" disease, it is typically associated with destruction of more than 90% of cortex and all the ***three layers*** are involved, hence, it is accompanied usually by deficiency of mineralocorticoids also.

2. *Secondary*

Due to hypopituitarism.

3. *Tertiary*

Due to hypothalamic disease.

Note

1. Destruction of anterior pituitary or hypothalmus may be caused by:
   - Infarction.
   - Tumours like chromophobe adenoma, craniopharyngioma, meningioma (suprasellar).
   - Granulomatous diseases:
     - Tuberculosis,
     - Sarcoidosis; and
     - Fungal disease.
2. In secondary/tertiary, there is inadequate cortisol production (hypocortisolaemia) and may be due to destructive process at the hypothalamopituitary level resulting in decresed ability to secrete ACTH (secondary) or CRH (tertiary).
3. Mineralocorticoid deficiency is not a problem (c.f. primary), zona glomerulosa remains active, as ACTH plays only a minor role in stimulation of zona glomerulosa.

Clinical Features

Onset

Usually insidious except in acute adrenal insufficiency which is an emergency.

Irrespective of aetiology, in all the types, primary/secondary/or tertiary, the symptoms are:

- Weight loss.
- Easy fatiguability.
- GI symptoms, like anorexia, nausea, vomiting or diarrhoea.
- Asthenia, weekness.
- Lethargy.
- Nervous symptoms, like nervousness and irritability.

Additional Features

The ***differences in primary and secondary adrenal hypofunction*** are as follows.

Primary adrenal hypofunction (Addison's disease)

- Changes in colour of the skin—hyperpigmentation. Due to elevated ACTH and related pituitary peptides.

- Increased numbers of moles and freckles may be present.
- PGA type I may have associated mucocutaneous candidiasis.
- PGA type II may be associated with other autoimmune diseases.

Secondary adrenal hypofunction

- Patients with hypopituitarism may have local symptoms related to underlying cause and some systemic manifestations related to specific tropic hormone deficiencies.
- The patient may have associated:
  - Growth failure
  - Hypogonadism
  - Visual field defects
  - Polydipsia and polyuria, etc.

LABORATORY INVESTIGATION

Laboratory investigations are carried in three steps.

- ***Laboratory investigation of acute adrenal insufficiency—Addisonian crisis.***
- ***Laboratory investigation of chronic adrenal hypofunction.***
- ***To establish hypocortisolism.***
- ***To establish the cause of hypocortisolism.***

1. ACUTE ADRENOCORTICAL INSUFFICIENCY (ADDISONIAN CRISIS)

Acute adrenal insufficiency is a life-threatening medical emergency and the patient must be treated promptly with cortisol replacement and fluids. Time should not be wasted on laboratory investigations, history, clinical features and some biochemical findings will be useful.

Adrenal 'crisis' is characterised by: headache, malaise, restlessness, vomiting, abdominal pain, hyperpyrexia and shock, which may progress to coma and death. Fluid and electrolyte abnormalities associated with primary hypocortisolism complicates the situation and presents a more severe clinical presentation.

Acute adrenal insufficiency can be precipitated, as stated above, under the following situations:

- Following 'stress' in patients with chronic adrenal insufficiency.
- Sudden withdrawal of corticosteroids in steroid-treated patients.
- Following injury to the adrenals by trauma, thrombosis or haemorrhage.
- After bilateral adrenalectomy (surgical).
- Overwhelming sepsis with or without haemorrhagic manifestations.

Biochemical findings in patients with acute adrenal insufficiency include:

- Low serum sodium ↓
- High serum potassium ↑
- Blood sugar low ↓
- Plasma chloride low ↓
- Plasma HCO_3 decreased ↓.

Note

- Low plasma cortisol levels in a setting of vascular collapse ***accompanied with hyperkalaemia, hypoglycaemia and hyponatraemia are diagnostic of acute adrenal insufficiency.***
- In suspected cases of sepsis, a ***blood culture*** will be indicated which can be of help later on.

Once a patient has survived an episode of acute adrenal insufficiency and seen later on or if the diagnosis of chronic adrenal insufficiency is suspected, laboratory evaluation should be:

- ***To establish hypocortisolism***
- ***To establish the cause, i.e. to distinguish primary, secondary, tertiary.***

2. TO ESTABLISH HYPOCORTISOLISM

- ***Plasma Cortisol Level***

Where facilities are available, *plasma cortisol level* should be determined between 8 a.m. and 10 a.m.

- ***In normal:*** The level is 5 to 23 μg/dl.
- ***In primary:*** Plasma cortisol level is decreased 5 μg.dl.

- In ***secondary/tertiary:*** It may be normal (lower range) or usually decreased ↓.
- ***Urinary cortisol level:*** Should be estimated if facilities are available.

3. TO DISTINGUISH PRIMARY AND SECONDARY/TERTIARY

Once hypocortisolism is established, laboratory evaluation to be directed in differentiating primary and secondary/tertiary disease.

Appropriate laboratory tests include the following.

A. ***Plasma ACTH level.***
B. ***"Provocative"/challenging tests:***
   - ACTH stimulation tests.
   - Metyrapone test.
   - CRH stimulation test.

A. Plasma ACTH Level

This is the most important and ***crucial test*** in investigation of hypocortisolism. ***Basal plasma ACTH level***-should be determined between 8 a.m. and 10 a.m.

Interpretation

- ***With primary adrenal disease***: Plasma ACTH levels will be elevated ↑ because the cortisol produced is insufficient to inhibit the ***"feed-back loop".*** (The presence of excess ACTH is suggested clinically by hyperpigmentation)
- If adrenal production of cortisol is decreased because of pituitary disease plasma ACTH level will be low ↓.

B. "PROVOCATIVE"/CHALLENGING TESTS

1. ACTH Stimulation Tests

Several tests are available (for details see Chapter Adrenocortical Function Tests)

- ***Cortrosyn (Tetracosactrin) Test***

It is simple screening test where plasma cortisol level is determined from a blood sample drawn between 8 a.m. and 10 a.m.

Cortrosyn 0.25 mg is given IM and plasma cortisol levels are then determined 30 to 45 minutes after injection.

Interpretation

- ***In normal subjects:*** Plasma cortisol level rises by at least 7 μg/dl in 30 minutes. Usually there is at least a two-fold rise above the control value to 20 μg/dl or above.
- A subnormal response suggests primary adrenocortical failure.

- ***IV ACTH Test***

(See for details and interpretation Chapter Adrenocortical Function Tests)

- ***Multiple-day ACTH Stimulation Test***

Principle: Multiple day ACTH stimulation testing for assessment of adrenal cortex function is required to evaluate adrenal cortisol responsiveness.

Procedure

ACTH gel, 80 U/d, is injected for 3 days. This is followed by a standard 8-hour infusion of ACTH 250 μg of cosyntropin over 8 hours. Urinary "free" cortisol and serum cortisol are measured daily.

Interpretations

- Can be ***useful to distinguish between primary, secondary/tertiary causes of hypocortisolism.*** It is particularly useful when patients have been on corticosteroid therapy.
- ***In primary adrenal insufficiency:*** The damaged adrenal glands do not respond even over several days of ACTH stimulation.
- Patients with secondary/tertiary adrenal insufficiency usually have an inadequate or absent cortisol response, at first, since the adrenal glands have been unstimulated for some time. Eventually, a ***delayed* or *staircase*** response is seen, indicating reactivation of the normal adrenal cortex.

2. *Metyrapone Test*

(For details of the method-see Chapter Adrenocortical Function Tests)

Interpretations

- In patients who show signs of panhypopituitarism or in whom pituitary insufficiency might be expected to develop, the metyrapone test may provide a useful estimate of pituitary reserve.
- Metyrapone blocks ***"11-β-hydroxylase"*** enzyme, the last step in synthesis of cortisol. Decreased amount of cortisol (hypocortisolism) stimulate the pituitary-adrenal axis, resulting in an increased production of cortisol precursors which are excreted in urine as 17 OH-corticoids.

Failure of such an increase to occur after Metyrapone indicates lack of pituitary reserve.

Note

This test must be undertaken with caution because the decrease in cortisol production in a patient with borderline adrenal function may precipitate acute adrenal insufficiency.

3. *CRH Stimulation Test*

(Refer to Chapter Adrenocortical Function Tests)

Interpretations

Theoretically permits differentiation between secondary and tertiary adrenal insufficiency.

- Those with tertiary disease, will show an elevation of plasma ACTH ↑ level, and
- Those with secondary disease will have minimal changes in plasma ACTH concentration.

4. Other Tests

- ***Vasopressin Assay***

Measurements of vasopressin are now available. The determination is best made after a period of water deprivation. Vasopressin acts on the pituitary gland as a corticotropin releasing hormone.

Measurements of plasma cortisol levels following the administration of Vasopressin has been ***used to differentiate between pituitary secondary and hypothalamic disease (tertiary).***

- ***Value of Plasma DHEA-S Determination***

Subnormal basal plasma concentrations of DHEA-S occur in primary/secondary/tertiary foms of adrenal insufficiency. Hence, measurement of basal plasma DHEA-S is of little value in the diagnosis of adrenal insufficiency.

SPECIAL INVESTIGATIONS

Certain special investigations may be required to be carried out for the diagnosis of primary idiopathic adrenocortical insufficiency and for secondary/tertiary hypocortisolism.

1. *For Primary Hypocortisolism*

- Blood sugar estimation.
- Serum electrolytes—Na, K, chlorides.
- CO_2 combining power.
- ***Skin tests:*** For tuberculosis and fungal diseases.
- ***Chest X-ray:*** To exclude pulmonary tuberculosis.
- A KUB film to demonstrate adrenal calcification, which again is suggestive of tuberculosis/or fungal diseases.
- Sputum examination for AFB,
- ***CT scanning:*** Idiopathic primary adrenal insufficiency may be associated with small adrenal glands.
- ***Plasma renin assay:*** In primary idiopathic adrenocortical insufficiency, as all the three layers of the adrenal cortex are involved, may show decreased plasma aldosterone level and ***increased plasma renin.***

Principle: Plasma renin assay (PRA) is defined as the rate of angiotensin I produced from angiotensinogen by renin in a patient's plasma.

Plasma renin activity is expressed in nanograms of angiotensin I produced per millilitre of plasma per hour and is determined by assaying angiotensin I after incubation of plasma at 37°C and then subtracting the amount of preformed angiotensin I in a control aliquot stored at 4°C.

Note

Collection of specimen for renin assay: Blood is drawn in EDTA tube. centrifuge the blood at room temperature to sediment cells, then plasma is frozen at –20°C. Plasma should be transported frozen to the laboratory. EDTA not only acts as an anticoagulant but also inhibits converting enzyme and stops the renin reaction of angiotensin I and inhibits other enzymes that can destroy angiotensin.

Normal value: In adults on normal sodium diet, range is 0.3 to 9.0 ng angiotensin I/ml/hour.

- ***Plasma aldosterone assay:*** Aldosterone levels are markedly decreased.
- ***Demonstration of autoantibodies:***
  - *Antihyroglobulin autoantibodies:* May be present which suggest an autoimmune basis.
  - *Adrenal autoantibodies* when present suggest autoimmune disease.
- ***HLA typing:*** May be indicated, if PGA I or II is suspected.

2. For Secondary/Tertiary Adrenocortical Insufficiency

Secondary adrenocortical insufficiency may be associated with deficiency of other tropic hormones.

(a) ***X-ray of skulls:*** Should be taken to exclude pituitary tumours. If X-rays show pituitary tumours or abnormality of the sella turcica then CT scan of the pituitary gland and arteriography are indicated.

(b) ***Fasting serum growth hormone and prolactin*** determination may be required.

(c) ***Serum TSH by RIA:*** If the TSH is low, TRH infusion with measurement of TSH both before and after the infusion may be carried out to detect pituitary or hypothalamic dysfunction.

- In selected cases, plasma FSH, LH, testosterone and estradiol may have to be determined. If *FSH and LH are low* then LHRF infusion can be carried out.

(d) ***LHRF Infusion Test***

Procedure

- A fasting blood simple is drawn.
- Synthetic LHRF, 100 μg is administered IV
- Blood samples are drawn 20 minutes and 60 minutes after the injection.
- FSH and LH estimated in all the three samples, by RIA methods.

Table 12.1: Biochemical differentiation of hypocortisolism

Tests	*Normal (Control)*	*Hypocortisolism*		
		Primary	*Secondary*	*Tertiary*
I. *Screening Tests*				
• Plasma cortisol (8 am)	5-23 μg/dl	Decreased↓	Normal or decreased↓	Normal or decreased↓
• Plasma ACTH (8 am)	10-85 pg/ml	Increased↑	Normal or decreased↓	Normal or decreased↓
II. *"Provocative"/Challenge Tests*				
1. ***Rapid ACTH stimulation.*** • Peak cortisol.	> 20 μg/dl.	Decreased↓ < 20 μg/dl	Any	Any
2. ***Overnight Metyrapone test***				
• Plasma 11-deoxycortisol	> 7 μg/dl.	Not indicated	< 7 μg/dl.	< 7 μg/dl.
• Plasma ACTH	> 150 pg/ml	Not indicated	< 150 pg/ml	< 150 pg/ml
3. ***CRH stimulation test***				
• Plasma ACTH	Not indicated	Not indicated	Decreased↓ response	Increased↑ response

Interpretation

- *Normally:* A three-fold rise in FSH and LH above the baselines is seen.
- If the 20 minutes or 60 minutes values for both FSH and LH are above normal, the response is regarded as exaggerated.
- When 60 minutes levels are the same as or greater than those found at the 20 minutes interval, the response is considered to be delayed.
- A delayed response in the FSH level is seen in most normal women.

Table 12.1 shows the biochemical differentiation of hypocortisolism—primary, secondary/ tertiary.

Chapter 13

Hyperlipoproteinaemias (Hyperlipidaemias)

INTRODUCTION

Hyperlipidaemia is defined as an excess concentration of lipids in plasma or serum. Lipids are hydrophobic and practically insoluble, hence they are carried in the blood as a soluble complex called *"lipoprotein complex"* Lipids are coated with "polar" substances like phospholipids, cholesterol and cholesterol esters and specific apoproteins characteristic of the particular lipoprotein complex. Therefore, the ***terms hyperlipidaemia and hyperlipoproteinaemia are used synonymously.***

Lipoproteins can be separated by ultracentrifugation and by electrophoresis. However, clinical laboratories usually do not measure the lipoproteins routinely but estimate the lipids, viz., triglyceride (TG), cholesterol, HDL-cholesterol and LDL-cholesterol. Thus, hyperlipidaemia is increase in serum TG, or serum cholesterol or both.

CAUSES

Hyperlipidaemias/hyperlipoproteinaemias are divided mainly into **two groups:**

- *Primary:* these are genetic disorders characterized by distinct clinical syndromes.
- *Secondary:* these are due to underlying disease processes, usually thyroid, liver, renal diseases and malignancies.

I. Primary Hyperlipoproteinaemias

Fredrickson et al (1967)—proposed **five types** based on changes in plasma lipoproteins.

(a) Type-I Familial Lipoprotein Lipase Deficiency (Hyperchylomicronaemia)

It is a rare disorder and is characterized by hyperchylomicronaemia and hypertriglyceridaemia (TG↑). The chylomicrons are grossly increased due to slow clearing of chylomicrons. VLDL (pre-β lipoproteins) may also be increased, and more so in increased carbohydrate intake. There is a decrease in α-lipoproteins (HDL↓) and β lipoproteins (LDL↓).

Inheritance: is autosomal recessive.

Defect:

Deficiency of the enzyme *"lipoprotein lipase"*—a defect in the synthesis of the enzyme or an abnormal mutant enzyme may be the cause. A variant of the disease can be produced by deficiency of apo-C II.

Clinical Features

- Can be seen in children, but may also be found in adults.
- Usual complaint is recurrent episodes of abdominal pain associated with ingestion of dietary fats.
- ***Hepatosplenomegaly*** is common. RE cells of bone marrow, spleen and liver become large and contain droplets of lipids due to phagocytic reaction to excessive lipids in blood.
- ***Eruptive xanthomas*** of the papular type, principally over the extensor surfaces are common.
- ***Lipaemia retinalis*** and ***pancreatitis,*** may be present.

- Lipaemia retinalis when present provides important clue to diagnosis.
- Acute pancreatitis—most serious complication and cause of fatality, may be frequently present.

Note

Serum amylase may be normal *(false)*, probably due to presence of an ***inhibitory factor.*** On dilution of serum with normal saline, increased serum amylase activity consistent with pancreatitis may be obtained.

- Disease is ***fat induced***, patient be effectively treated with low dietary fat. ***Premature cardiovascular disease is not encountered.***

(b) Type-II Familial Hypercholesterolaemia, FHC- (Hyper-lipoproteinaemia)

A common disorder, more common than type-I, has been extensively investigated and is characterized by:

- hyper β-lipoproteinaemia (LDL↑);
- associated with increased total cholesterol ↑;
- VLDL may be raised, hence total TG may be high, but plasma usually remains clear, and
- HDL ↑

Inheritance: is autosomal dominant, frequency is 0.2%.

Defect: There is no enzyme deficiency. ***Metabolic defects are:***

- an increased synthesis of LDL **(β*-lipoproteins*)**; and
- defective catabolism of LDL, deficiency of LDL-receptors in fibroblasts have been demonstrated.

Clinical Features

- Xanthomas tendinous and tuberous have been described.
- Xanthomas may also occur near the eyelids *(xanthelasma).*
- Corneal arcus have been described.

Note

Clinically this type is most important, as it is associated with increased incidence of athero-sclerosis and premature cavdiovascular diseases. This pattern can develop as a result of ***"hypothyroidism" (secondary hyperlipoproteinaemia) and also in nephrotic syndrome.***

Biochemically: two Types of Type-II are described, ***Type-II (a)*** and ***Type-II (b):***

- If ***type-II*** has only hypercholesterolaemia and elevated β-LDL band, it is referred to as Type-II (a).
- If there is ***accompanying increase in pre-β band (VLDL),*** it is called Type-II (b), in which case the ***broad band*** is due to a confluence of β and pre-β bands. In this type, there is increase of both cholesterol and TG in serum.

Cholesterol: TG ratio will always be above > 1.5.

(c) Type-III Familial Dys-β Lipoproteinaemia

- ***"Broad" beta ("floating" beta)*** lipoproteinaemia.
- ***"Remnant" removal disease.***

The disease is less common and is characterized by:

- increase in β lipoproteins (LDL↑);
- increase of cholesterol ↑ and TG in serum↑; and
- Increase in pre-β lipoproteins (VLDL↑), actually rise is in IDL (VLDL "remnant"). This appears as ***"broadbeta-band, ("Floating" betaband);*** β VLDL-on electrophoresis. The density of the lipoproteins accumulating is intermediate to β and Pre-β and the fraction (Sf-12-100) is called "floating" beta.

Inheritance: is autosomal dominant.

Defects:

i. Defect is in "remnant" metabolism i.e., conversion of normal VLDL to β—VLDL (IDL) and its degradation without conversion to LDL.
ii. The precise defect appears to be in remnant metabolism by the liver due to abnormality of apo-E—of the three forms

E_1, E_2 and E_3, only E_2 is present, it does not bind to E-receptor.
- Probably there is also increased synthesis of apo-B.

Clinical Features
- Xanthomas are present. In addition to tuberous and tendinous, there may be planar xanthomas in palms.
- Premature cardiovascular diseases and atherosclerosis are common.
- Foam cells are seen in RE cells of bone marrow, liver and spleen.
- Patients show carbohydrate intolerance.

(d) Type-IV Familial Hypertriglyceridaemia (FHTG)

Synonym: Hyper pre-beta lipoproteinaemia.

The disease is characterized by:
- hyper pre-β lipoproteinaemia (VLDL↑);
- increase in endogenous synthesis of TG↑;
- cholesterol level may be normal, or increased sometimes;
- α- and β-lipoproteins subnormal (decreased HDL↓ and LDL↓); and
- TG: Cholesterol ratio is 5:1 or more.

Inheritance: is autosomal dominant.

Defects:
- Increased endogenous synthesis ↑ of TG.
- Decreased catabolism ↓ of both TG and VLDL; deficiency of a specific *lipoprotein lipase* for elevation of VLDL has been suggested.

Clinical Features
- Xanthomas are not common.
- Usually present in early adulthood (30 Years or more); and is found associated with coronary artery disease and atherosclerosis.
- Abdominal pain with or without pancreatitis, obesity, abnormal GTT.
- May be associated with maturity onset DM, chronic alcoholism, and in women taking progestational hormones.
- Intolerance to sucrose and fructose common.
- Hyperuricaemia may be present.

(e) Type-V Combined Hyperlipidaemias (Hyperchylomicronaemia and Pre-β-lipoproteinaemia)

It is a ***rare disorder*** and a ***combined form of Type-I and Type-IV.*** In this disease, the lipoprotein pattern is complex. Increase in both chylomicrons and pre-β–lipoproteins (VLDL) are seen. Triacylglycerol, cholesterol and phospholipids are also elevated. Concentration of α-lipoproteins (HDL↓) and β-lipoprotein (LDL↓) are decreased.

Inheritance: is autosomal dominant.

Clinical Features:
- The disorder is manifested only in the second or third decade (early adult life).
- Patients are obese and frequently have a family history of diabetes mellitus and obesity.
- Eruptive xanthomas, hepatosplenomegaly, repeated bouts of abdominal pain with abnormal glucose tolerance, ***hyperuricaemia.***
- May have associated pancreatitis.
- Incidence of atherosclerosis is not striking.
- Majority may have ***hyperinsulinaemia.***

Defects

Defects are not known correctly. Type—V of the familial type is of uncertain origin because, unlike Type-I, these patients do not have a significant ***lipoprotein lipase*** deficiency. Diabetes mellitus, nephrotic syndrome and dysproteinaemias may be aetiologic. A further cause suggested is ***overproduction of apo-B*** which influence plasma level of VLDL and LDL.

Table 13.1 shows the differentiating features of ***Five types*** of hyperlipoproteinaemias.

II. Secondary Hyperlipoproteinaemias

Changed lipoprotein patterns may be seen in a number of disease processes and some may

Table 13.1: Hyperlipoproteinaemias—Biochemical Profile

Lipoprotein-pheno type	*Lipoprotein abnormality (Increase)*	*Plasma appearance (after 16 hours at 4°C)*	*Total cholesterol*	*TG*	*LDL cholesterol*	*HDL cholesterol*	*Apolipoproteins*	*Lipoprotein electrophoresis*	*Clinical association*
Type—I	Chylomicrons ↑	• Creamy layer on top • Infranate clear or slightly turbid	Normal to moderate increase	Markedly elevated ↑	Normal	N or Decreased ↓	B_{48} ↑ A-IV ↑ C-II ↑	Intense band of origin	Acute pancreatitis (acute abdomen)
Type—II A	LDL↑	• Clear • Possible increase in yellow-orange tint	• Usually elevated ↑, • Occasionally may be normal	Normal	Elevated ↑	N or Decreased ↓	B_{100} ↑	Increased band in β-region	Markedly increased 'risk' of CAD
Type—II B	LDL ↑ VLDL ↑	Clear to slightly turbid	Elevated ↑ occasionally marginally	Elevated ↑	Elevated ↑	N or Decreased ↓	B_{100} ↑	Increased β and Pre-β band	Increased risk of CAD
Type—III	IDL ↑	• Turbid to opaque • Thin creamy layer-occasionally present	Elevated ↑	Elevated ↑	Normal to Decreased ↓	N or Decreased ↓	E-II ↑ E-III ↓ E-IV ↓	Broad β band	Increased risk of CAD
Type—IV	VLDL ↑	Turbid to opaque	Normal to slightly elevated ↑	Moderate to marked elevation ↑	Normal	N or Decreased ↓	C-II ↑, B-100 ↑	Increased Pre-β band	Increased risk of CAD
Type—V	VLDL ↑ chylomicrons ↑	• Creamy layer (thin), • Infranate turbid to opaque	Slight to moderate elevation	Markedly elevated ↑	Normal	N or Decreased ↓	C-II ↑↓, B-48 ↑, B-100 ↑	Intense band at origin + Increased Pre-β band	Pancreatitis + Increased risk to CAD

resemble Type-II and Type-IV and may be aetiologic factors. The following diseases are important for considerations:

1. *Diabetes Mellitus*

Uncontrolled and untreated diabetes mellitus shows an increase in VLDL↑ and TG (triacylglycerol) ↑. Also there is hypercholesterolaemia (cholesterol ↑). Increased VLDL is due to enhanced endogenous TG synthesis in liver, due to mobilization of FFA from adipose tissue, and due to absolute or relative deficiency of insulin.

2. *Nephrotic Syndrome*

Both LDL and VLDL are increased, on the other hand, α-lipoproteins (HDL↓) is decreased. Serum cholesterol is very high and can be 600 mg/dl or more and TG is also increased (hypertriglyceridaemia).

Defect: Hyperlipidaemia is mainly due to increased hepatic synthesis of lipids and decreased disappearance from blood.

3. *Hypothyroidism*

Cholesterol is increased very much and like nephrotic syndrome in a case of myxoedema it may go up to even 600 mg/dl or more. Characteristically, β-lipoproteins (LDL) is elevated ↑.

4. *Chronic Alcoholism*

Both TG and cholesterol are increased. Lipoprotein profile shows elevated β-lipoproteins (LDL) and VLDL. There is increased synthesis of endogenous hepatic TG. Also there is increased FA synthesis ↑ and cholesterol synthesis ↑.

Biochemically, due to ethanol oxidation, ratio of NADH + H^+: NAD^+↑. Increased NADH + H^+ in the cells make the following biochemical alterations.

1. ***Shift to right*** of the following reaction-

   Dihydroxy-acetone-(P) NAD H α-Glycero-(P).

   Increased ↑ availability of α-glycero-P increases TG synthesis (esterification).

2. ***Shift to left*** of the following reaction.

   Malate NADH H OAA

   Produces relative deficiency of OAA↓ and thus reduces activity of TCA Cycle.

5. *Liver Diseases*

In biliary obstruction, serum cholesterol and β-lipoproteins (LDL) are elevated. α_2-lipoprotein (HDL) is usually decreased.

6. *Pancreatitis*

Both LDL and VLDL are increased. There is mobilization of free fatty acids (FFA) from adipose tissue. ***Lipoprotein lipase*** activity is decreased and there is slow clearance of chylomicrons after a fatty meal. ***Lipoprotein lipase inhibitors have been detected in the blood of patients with acute pancreatitis.***

7. *Multiple Myeloma and Macroglobulinaemia*

Both serum cholesterol ↑ and TG (triacylglycerol) ↑ are increased. Lipoprotein profile shows an increase in LDL↑ and VLDL↑.

Mechanism is not clear. It is suggested that to meet the increased demand for cholesterol by bone marrow plasma cells for their increased synthesis of abnormal β-globulins, the cholesterol synthesis is increased.

8. *Glycogen Storage Diseases GSD_S-Type–1, (von Gierke disease)*

Due to hypoinsulinaemia, there is increased mobilization of FFA from adipose tissue. Endogenous TG synthesis in liver is increased leading to increase VLDL↑. Cholesterol synthesis is also increased and there is increased LDL↑.

LABORATORY INVESTIGATION

Laboratory investigation of hyperlipoproteinaemias can be considered in two steps:

A. *To establish the presence of hyperlipoproteinaemias.*

B. To find out the type and cause of hyperlipoproteinaemias

A. To Establish that Hyperlipoproteinaemia is Present

Following will be useful in establishing hyperlipidaemia.

1. *Appearance of plasma:* Naked eye appearance, followed by **"Refrigeration"** Test.
2. *Complete lipid profile:* Determination of serum cholesterol, triacylgycerol (TG) and HDL cholesterol.

1. *Plasma Appearance*

Plasma appearance (naked eye examination) in a suspected case of hyperlipidaemia is a simple, convenient and inexpensive test that is often overlooked by many clinicians and seldom, if ever, reported by clinical laboratories routinely. **Its value is immense** as the information can be diagnostic, may throw light to aetiology (cause) and provide rough estimate of TG present.

Interpretations

- If the plasma is clear, the TG level is most likely to be either normal or nearly ≤ normal (200 mg/dl).
- When TG level increases to approximately 300 mg/dl, the plasma usually appears hazy, turbid and is not transluscent enough to allow clear reading of newsprints through the tube.
- When plasma TG level exceeds 600 mg/dl, the plasma is usually opaque/milky (lipaemic).
- In patients with hypercholesterolaemia, due only to elevated LDL concentrations, the plasma/serum is usually clear (does not show any turbidity) but may have an orange yellow tint because carotenoids are carried in LDL fraction.

After naked eye examination of the plasma/serum, obtained after at least 12 hours fasting (postabsorptive state), if found turbid and lipaemic then the tube containing the plasma can be placed in a refrigerator at 4°C for 24 hours and again reexamined (see "Refrigeration test" below and its interpretations).

2. Complete Lipid Profile

This includes estimation of total cholesterol, TG (triacylglycerol), VLDL, chylomicrons, HDL and LDL cholesterol.

Routing laboratories estimate the serum total cholesterol and TG.

(a) Estimation of Serum Cholesterol

Serum cholesterol is determined routinely in a clinical laboratory by ***Sackett's method***/or ***Zak's method (colorimetric assay).*** It is better if it is determined by enzymatic method.

Estimation of Cholesterol by Enzymatic Method

Principle: Cholesterol esterase hydrolyzes cholesterol ester to free cholesterol and FA. Free cholesterol is oxidized by the cholesterol oxidase to cholest-4-en-3-one and hydrogen peroxide. Hydrogen peroxide formed reacts with 4-amino antipyrine and phenol in the presence of peroxidase to produce pink coloured quinoneimine dye. The intensity of colour produced is proportional to the cholesterol concentration. A standard of cholesterol solution 200 mg/dl is similarly treated and compared in colorimeter and concentration calculated.

Normal value is 130-250 mg/dl

(b) Estimation of Triacylglycerol (TG)

Principle: Lipoprotein lipase hydrolyzes serum TG to free fatty acids and glycerol. ***Glycerol kinase*** catalyzes the conversion of glycerol in the presence of ATP to glycerol-3-P and ADP. The glycerol-3-P is then oxidized by glycerol-3-P oxidase to yield hydrogen peroxide (H_2O_2). Hydrogen peroxide reacts in the presence of peroxidase with 4-cholorophenol and 4-amino antipyrine to form a coloured complex.

The intensity of the colour is proportional to TG concentration. A standard solution of TG (200 mg/dl) is similarly treated and the colour compared, in a colorimeter and concentration calculated.

Normal value by this method:

- *Men*—60 to 165 mg/dl.
- *Women*—40 to 140 mg/dl.

(c) Estimation of HDL-Cholesterol

Principle: Chylomicrons, very low density lipoproteins (VLDL) and low density lipoproteins (LDL) of serum are precipitated by using buffered polyethylene glycol (PEG-6000). After centrifugation, high density lipoprotein (HDL) are in the supernatent. The cholesterol in the HDL fraction is estimated by the enzymatic method. (See cholesterol estimation above) by addition of cholesterol esterase, cholesterol oxidase, peroxidase, 4-amino antipyrine and phenol. Standard cholesterol used is 50 mg/dl.

Normal values:

- *Males*—35 to 60 mg/dl.
- *Females*—40 to 70 mg/dl.

(d) Estimation of Chylomicrons, VLDL and LDL

These can be estimated by micro-nephelometry.

Note

Concentration of VLDL-cholesterol can be estimated by dividing the TG concentration in mg/dl by 5, provided the TG level is not over 400 mg/dl and the patient does not have Type–III hyperlipoproteinaemia.

(e) Estimation of LDL-Cholesterol

Serum LDL-cholesterol can be calculated by the **"Friedewald formula"**

- *LDL-cholesterol in mg/dl* = Total cholesterol – HDL-cholesterol – TG/5
- *LDL-cholesterol in mmol/l* = Total cholesterol – HDL-cholesterol – TG/22

Note

The formula is not much reliable if the TG concentration is greater than 400 mg/dl (>4.5 m mol/l).

Normal values of complete lipid profile	
Lipid fraction	*Normal values*
• **Total cholesterol**	130– 250 mg/dl
• **Serum HDL cholesterol**	• Males: 35–60 mg/dl • Females: 40–70 mg/dl
• **Serum TG (Triacylglycerol)**	• Males: 60–165 mg/dl • Females: 40–140 mg/dl
• **Serum chylomicrons**	Up to 28 mg/dl (14 hours postabsorptive state)
• **Serum pre-β-lipoproteins (VLDL)**	• Males: up to 240 mg/dl • Females: up to 210 mg/dl
• **Serum β-Lipoproteins (LDL)**	Up to 550 mg/dl
• **Serum LDL-cholesterol**	Up to 190 mg/dl

II. TO ESTABLISH THE TYPE/CAUSE OF HYPERLIPOPROTEINAEMIA

Once it is established that there is hyperlipidaemia, one should proceed to find out the type/cause of the hyperlipoproteinaemia.

1. Refrigeration Test

As pointed out above, many hyperlipidaemias can be at least partially diagnosed at or near the bed side ***by visual inspection of the serum/plasma*** and re-examination 24 hours after keeping in a refrigerator in standing position at 4°C ***("refrigeration test").***

An opaque plasma/serum sample with a thick, creamy layer on top is usually consistent with Type–V pattern. On the other hand, a thick, creamy separate chylomicron layer on top with ***clear*** plasma/serum infranate is usually consistent with Type–I pattern.

A uniformly opaque plasma/serum without any thick layer at top usually denotes a Type–IV pattern.

Different patterns obtained in the five types are shown in Fig. 13.1.

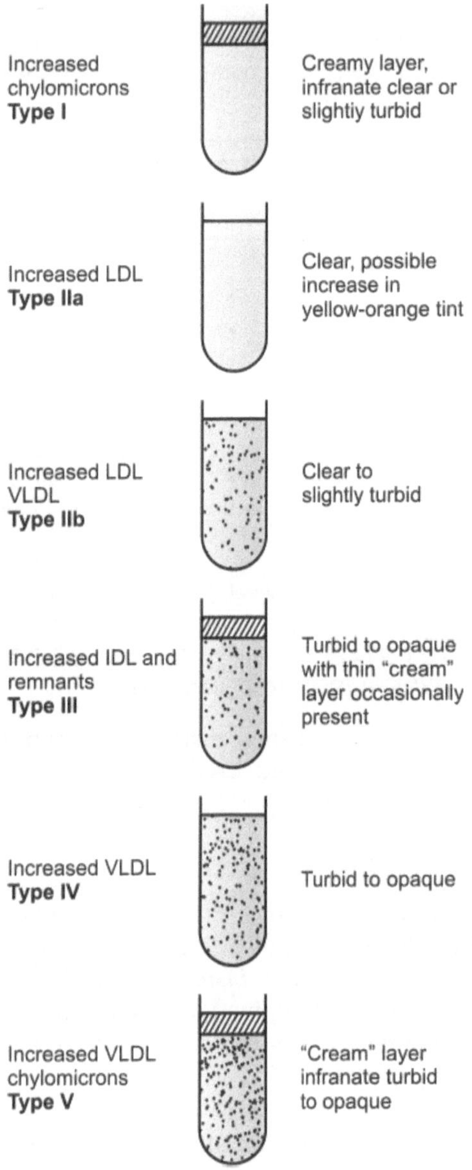

Fig. 13.1: Refrigeration test

Note

- In non-fasting persons, a chylomicron layer may also be found. But it does not constitute an abnormal finding unless the patient fasted for at least 12 to 14 hours before the blood collection.
- If chylomicrons are suspected, but are not clearly discernible, electrophoresis may be of immense help in confirming their presence. Chylomicrons would stay near origin.

2. Lipoprotein Electrophoresis (LPE)

Principle: Lipoporoteins, like other serum proteins, have characteristic migration rates in an electrophoretic field and hence, they can be easily separated in many clinical laboratories by standard electrophoresis method. The electrophoretogram is then ***stained for fats,*** i.e., cholesterol and TG, identified by comparision with a simultaneously run strip that has been stained for proteins.

In such a system

- chylomicrons rich in TG remain at the origin;
- the non chylomicron lipoproteins richest in TG, i.e., VLDL move just in front of β-globulins and are hence called as ***pre-β-lipoproteins;***
- the lipoproteins richest in cholesterol move with β-globulins and hence called as ***β-lipoproteins;*** and
- the lipoproteins richest in PL move with α-globulin and are known as ***α-lipoproteins.***

Media Used

- ***Agarose gel and paper electrophoresis*** produce similar separations of lipoproteins with agarosegel offering increased resolution and occasionally increased separation within classes.
- ***Cellulose-acetate*** may be inadequate to detect chylomicrons that co-migrate with VLDL and it is, therefore, not recommended for routine use.

- ***Paper and Aqarose Gel LPE***

Performed by the same procedures as serum protein electrophoresis, **except** for:

- sample size;
- duration of run; and
- staining procedures.

Paper electrophoresis is carried out for 16 hours at 120 V with albumin—containing barbital buffer. Albumin is added to the buffer to improve separation and definition of the lipoprotein bands.

The paperstrips are stained in an alcoholic solution of Oil Red 0, rinsed and air-dried before qualitative visual inspection.

Agarose gel electrophoresis is performed for about 90 minutes with a barbital buffer and is followed by fixing, drying and staining with Fat Red 7 B or Sudan Black B.

Value of LPE in Hyperlipoproteinaemias

- Value of lipoprotein electrophoresis as part of routine lipid/lipoprotein profile remains debatable. Clinical and analytical experts now discourage use of lipoprotein electrophoresis (LPE) in primary/initial assessment.
- They recommend instead, quantitative assays of TG, total cholesterol and HDL-cholesterol, calculation of VLDL-cholesterol and LDL-cholesterol and naked eye inspection of plasma/serum followed by "standing test" ("refrigeration" test) which are more informative.
- If any abnormal findings, it should be followed-up with ultracentrifuge separation to establish the Phenotype,
- Though above scheme is ideal, but facility of ultracentrifuge is not available as a routine in hospital laboratories.
- As lipoprotein electrophoresis is easy to perform and the facility is available in all routine hospital laboratories, LPE remains valuable test as a supplemental, qualitative adjunct.
- LPE does help in typing of the hyperlipoproteinaemias. It can specially be useful in characterization of Type-III hyperlipoproteinaemia ***(broad or "floating" β-disease), in a abetalipoproteinaemia and in Tangier's disease.***
- LPE also continues to be important for assessing post heparin lipolytic activity.
- It is useful in detecting a sample, which may have been collected without fasting (12 to 14 hours) and non-post absorptive state. ***A small chylomicron band at the origin alerts a physician to retest the patient after proper preparation.***
- LPE is also ***useful for detection of LP-X an abnormal lipoprotein that is "marker" in obstructive jaundice*** (Refer to Laboratory investigation of jaundice).

For Lipoprotein pattern seen in LPE (refer to Fig 13.2).

- **Type-I** — shows heavy chylomicron band, faint β-lipoprotein and pre-β-bands.
- **Type-II (a)** — shows heavy β-lipoprotein band.
- **Type-II (b)** — shows heavy β-lipoprotein and pre-β-lipoprotein bands.
- **Type-III** — shows ***"broad" β-band***
- **Type-IV** — shows heavy pre-β-lipoprotein band.
- **Type-V** — shows heavy chylomicron and pre-β-lipoprotein bands.

3. Ultracentrifugation

Lipoproteins can be characterized not only by their electrophoretic mobility but also by their ***density on ultracentrifugation***. If ultracentrifuge is available, this will be ideal for phenotyping. The largest and least dense particles are the chylomicrons with a density from 0.9 to 0.96 g/ml.

Next comes the pre-β-lipoproteins (very low density lipoproteins, VLDL) and have a density from 0.96 to 1.006 g/ml.

The low density lipoproteins (LDL), the β-lipoproteins in the ultracentrifugal separation have a density of 1.006 to 1.063 g/ml.

Finally, the high density lipoproteins (HDL) having a high density of 1.063 to 1.20 g/ml settles at the bottom and it corresponds to α-lipoproteins by LPE.

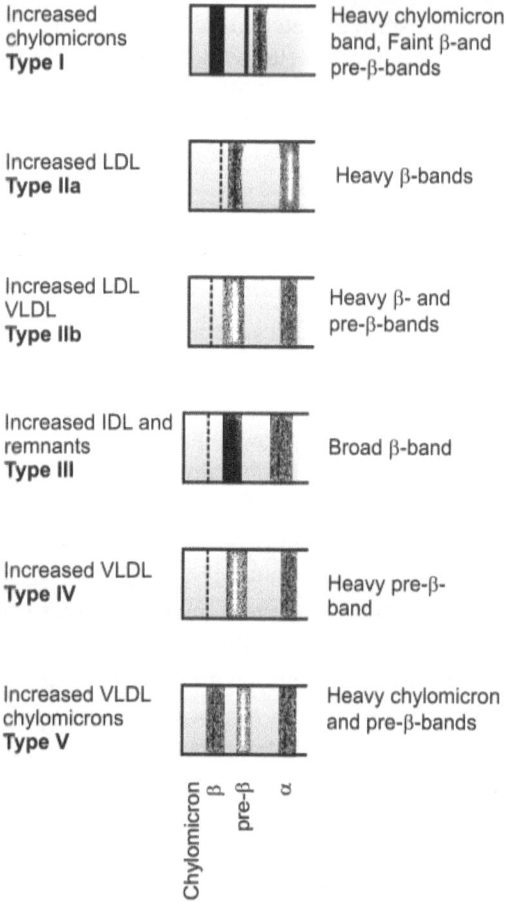

Fig. 13.2: Lipoprotein electrophoresis pattern

4. Measurement of Apolipoproteins (Apo-proteins)

Measurement of apo-lipoproteins (apo-proteins) is rapidly gaining in popularity as specific antisera and various purified apo-lipoproteins have become more widely available and being, used in immunochemical assays that are more ***sensitive, specific*** and ***reproducible.***

A number of established immunochemical techniques are now available for apolipoprotein assays, viz.:

- Radioimmunodiffusion assay (RIDA)
- Electroimmunoassay (EIA) in agar or agarose-gel,
- Enzyme-linked immuno assay (ELISA).
- Fluorescence immunoassay (FIA) and radio immunoassay (RIA).

Out of these ELISA, and RIA methods are most commonly used. ELISA has been used for measurement of apo-A-I, A-II, E, B, apo-C-II and apo-C-III.

RIA, if facilities available, is the most traditional approach to apolipoprotein measurement. It has been used for most of apolipoproteins, viz., apo-A-I, A-II, B, apo-CII, apo-C-III, apo-E and apo-D.

5. *Measurement of Lipoprotein Lipase*

Lipoprotein lipase can be released from capillary endothelium of tissues after administration of IV heparin (100 units per kg). The enzyme is released in the circulation, allowing its measurement in plasma/serum. This is of immense value in investigation of Type-I hyperlipoproteinaemia.

Heparin-released lipoprotein lipase can be assessed by following two methods:

a. *Lipoprotein Electrophoresis (LPE)*

First Lipoprotein electrophoresis is carried out on plasma collected ***before*** heparin injection and then on the sample collected 15 minutes after heparin injection.

Interpretation

In persons with normal ***lipoprotein lipase*** activity, the heparin-induced lipolysis of chylomicrons leads to release of FFA which then bind to other LP_S. This results in ***smeared*** Pre-β, β and α-bands.

b. *RIA Method*

In a more recently developed assay, lipoprotein lipase is measured directly by RIA, using specific antisera.

Chapter 14

Jaundice

INTRODUCTION

Jaundice is a clinical syndrome in which there is yellow colouration of conjunctivae, mucous membranes and skin due to increased bilirubin level in blood and body fluid. Normal bilirubin level in blood is in the range of 0.2 to 0.6 mg/dl and does not exceed 1.0 mg/dl. ***Jaundice is clinically visible when serum bilirubin exceeds 2.4 mg/dl.***

CAUSES AND CLASSIFICATION OF JAUNDICE

I. Rolleston and McNee (1929) as modified by Mclagan (1964)

They classified jaundice in *three groups.*

1. Haemolytic or Prehepatic Jaundice

In this there is increased breakdown of Hb, so that liver cells are unable to conjugate all the increased bilirubin formed.

CAUSES

(For details see haemolytic anaemia). There are **two main groups:**

Intrinsic

Abnormalities within red blood cells, viz.
- Haemoglobinopathies and abnormal Hbs,
- Hereditary spherocytosis,
- G-6-PD deficiency and other enzyme deficiencies,
- Favism, etc.

Extrinsic

Factors external to red blood cells, e.g.
- Incompatible blood transfusion.
- Haemolytic disease of the newborn (HDN).
- Autoimmune haemolytic anaemia (AIHA)
- Malaria, infections, etc.

2. Hepatocellular or Hepatic Jaundice

In this, there is disease of the parenchymal cells of liver. This may be divided into *three groups,* though there may be overlapping.
- Conditions, such as viral hepatitis and toxic jaundice, in which there is extensive damage to hepatic cells and associated with intrahepatic cholestasis.
- Conditions in which there is defective conjugation. There may be a reduction in the number of functioning liver cells, e.g. chronic hepatitis, ore

  Or, there may be a specific defect in the conjugation process, e.g.
  - Gilbert's syndrome.
  - Crigler-Najjar syndrome Type I and Type II.
- "Cholestatic" jaundice occurs due to administration of drugs/steroids, e.g.
  - Chlorpromazine;
  - Steroids.

3. Obstructive or Posthepatic Jaundice

In this there is obstruction to flow of bile in the extrahepatic ducts, e.g.
- Gallstones.

- Enlarged lymph nodes pressing the bile duct.
- Carcinoma of head of the pancreas.

II. Rich's Classification

According to this classification jaundice is divided into **two main groups.**

1. Retention Jaundice

In this there is impaired removal of bilirubin from the blood, or excessive amount of bilirubin is produced and not cleared fully by liver cells. This group includes haemolytic jaundice and those conditions characterized by impaired conjugation of bilirubin.

2. Regurgitation Jaundice

In this there is excess of conjugated bilirubin and this group includes obstructive jaundice and those conditions in which there is considerable degree of intrahepatic obstruction (cholestasis).

Note

In clinical practice, the most common causes of jaundice are:

- Viral hepatitis
- Haemolysis
- Iatrogenic (Drugs)
- Bile duct calculi
- Carcinoma of head of pancreas
- Carcinoma metastatic to the liver.

III. Physiological Classification of Jaundice

A classification of jaundice ***based on the site of altered bilirubin metabolism*** is given below:

1. Unconjugated Hyperbilirubinaemia

a. ***Increased production of unconjugated bilirubin from haeme***
   - Haemolysis
     - Hereditary
     - Acquired.
   - Ineffective erythropoiesis.
   - Rapid turnover of increased red blood cells mass (in the neonate).

b. ***Decreased delivery of unconjugated bilirubin (in plasma) to the hepatocyte***
   - Right sided congestive heart failure.
   - Portocaval shunt.

c. ***Decreased uptake of unconjugated bilirubin across hepatocyte membrane***
   - Competitive inhibition, drugs, others?
   - Gilbert's syndrome.
   - Sepsis.

d. ***Decreased storage of unconjugated bilirubin in cytosol (decreased Y and Z proteins)***
   - Competitive inhibition.
   - Fever.

e. ***Decreased conjugation in hepatic cells***
   - ***Hereditary***
     Crigler-Najjar syndrome
     —Type I (complete enzyme deficiency)
     —Type II (partial enzyme deficiency).
   - Hepatocellular dysfunction.
   - Gilbert's syndrome?
   - Inhibition (drugs).
   - Neonatal jaundice (physiological).

2. Conjugated Hyperbilirubinaemia (Cholestasis)

a. ***Decreased secretion of conjugated bilirubin into bile canaliculi***
   - Dubin–Johnson syndrome
   - Rotor syndrome
   - Hepatocellular disease
     - Hepatitis
     - Cholestasis (intrahepatic).
   - Drugs (oestradiol).

b. ***Decreased drainage***
   i. Extrahepatic obstruction
      - Calculi,
      - Carcinoma,
      - Enlarged lymphnodes
      - Stricture
      - Biliary atresia
   ii. Intrahepatic obstruction
      - Primary biliary cirrhosis,
      - Granulomas,
      - Tumours,
      - Drugs (steroids, chlorpromazine).

LABORATORY INVESTIGATION

- ***To establish the presence of jaundice***
- ***To assess the severity of the jaundice and its cause***

I. TO ESTABLISH THE PRESENCE OF JAUNDICE

1. *Clinical Examination*

If the bilirubin level is more than 2.4 mg/dl the jaundice is clinically visible and can be ascertained from examination of conjunctivae of eyes and mucous membranes/skin.

2. *Estimation of Serum Bilirubin*

Serum bilirubin gives a measure of the intensity of jaundice. An elevated serum bilirubin indicates either the presence of hepatobiliary disease, over production of bilirubin or both.
In sub-clinical jaundice, where the jaundice cannot be ascertained clinically, demonstration of small increases in serum bilirubin 1.0 to 3.0 mg/dl is of great diagnostic value. Higher values are usually seen in obstructive jaundice than in haemolytic type.

Elevations over 35 mg/dl generally indicates presence of renal insufficiency in addition to hepatobiliary disease. Uncomplicated haemolysis seldom causes a total serum bilirubin of more than 5 mg/dl unless hepatobiliary disease is also present.

II. TO ESTABLISH THE SEVERITY OF JAUNDICE, TYPE AND CAUSE

Proper history and physical examination gives good information and points to causative factor.

a. *History*

- Insidious onset of jaundice in a young patient associated with loss of appetite, nausea and vomiting, malaise and fever points to viral hepatitis.
- A family history of jaundice raises the suspicion of inherited disorders like Gilbert's disease, haemolytic disorders, Crigler-Najjar syndrome, etc.
- History of chronic ingestion of alcohol for long time will point to alcoholic liver disease-cirrhosis liver.
- Onset of jaundice in middle aged elderly patient, specially woman with obesity, associated with episodes of right hypochondial pain is suggestive of cholelithiasis.
- A history of administration of drugs specially ***steroids, chlorpromazine,*** etc. or ***anaesthetic*** agents prior to onset of jaundice is a pointer to drug-induced liver diseases with cholestasis.
- If jaundice is preceded by chronic weight loss and weakness, it is suggestive of malignancy—liver cell carcinoma/carcinoma of head pancreas.

b. *Clinical Examination of the Patient*

Certain physical findings, typical of certain diseases will be helpful in diagnosis.

- Presence of ascites, enlarged spleen and dilated umbilical veins suggestive of ***portal hypertension.***
- Presence of xanthomas will be a pointer to ***primary bilary cirrhosis.***
- Palpable gallbladder, non-tender associated with weight loss and weakness is suggestive of ***carcinoma of head of pancreas.***
- Presence of gray pigmentation points to ***haemochromatosis.***
- Presence of spider naevi, palmer erythema, gynaecomastia suggestive of ***cirrhosis liver.***

c. *Laboratory Tests*

These will be helpful to determine severity of jaundice and its type—whether obstructive or hepatocellular.

1. VD Bergh test and determination of conjugated and unconjugated bilirubin. (For details—refer to chapter on Liver Function tests in Textbook of Medical Biochemistry).

2. Enzyme studies

- Serum aminotransferases (AS-T and AL-T).
- Serum alkaline phosphatase (ALP).
- Serum leucine aminopeptidase (LAP).

- Serum gamma-glutamyl transpeptidase (GGT)
- Serum 5' nucleotidase.

3. ***Determination of prothrombin time (PT)***
4. ***Floculation tests***

1. VD Bergh Test and Differential Bilirubin

• *VD Bergh Reaction*

Depends on the type of bilirubin present, whether conjugated or unconjugated.

- ***Haemolytic jaundice*** there is an increase in unconjugated bilirubin and indirect VD Bergh reaction is obtained, occasionally it may be a delayed direct reaction. (For investigation: refer to Laboratory investigation of haemolytic anaemia.)
- ***In obstructive jaundice*** conjugated bilirubin is increased and an immediate direct positive VD Bergh reaction seen.
- ***In hepatocellular jaundice*** either type of bilirubin or both may be present. In viral hepatitis, direct reaction is the rule as it is accompanied with certain amount of intrahepatic cholestasis.

An immediate direct VD Bergh reaction points to obstructive jaundice which may be intrahepatic or extrahepatic and thus has limited value.

• *Serum Bilirubin*

It gives a measure of intensity of jaundice—higher values are found in obstructive jaundice.

2. Enzyme Studies

(a) S-GOT and S-GPT

Serum aspartate transminase (AST also called S-GOT) and serum alanine transaminase (ALT also called S-GPT) are most commonly done enzymes in laboratory.

Normal range:

- Aspartate transaminase (SGOT) 4 to 17 IU/L (7 to 35 units/ml).
- Alanine transaminase (S-GPT): 3 to 15 IU/L (6 to 32 units/ml).

Both the enzymes are found in most tissues, but the relative amounts vary. ***S-GOT*** is found in following organs in order of decreasing concentration: heart, liver, skeletal muscle, kidney, pancreas. ***S-GPT,*** although much more widely distributed is predominantly confined to liver and is, therefore, ***more specific for liver diseases.*** Increases in both transminases occur in liver diseases, with S-GPT much greater than S-GOT.

These two enzyme tests are ***sensitive indicator of hepatocellular necrosis.*** In general, levels greater than 10 to 15 times the upper limit of normal indicate acute hepatocellular injury as seen in the viral hepatitis, drug and toxin induced hepatitis (other than alcohol), ischaemic liver disease or transient cholangitis. Very high values of S-GPT are seen in viral hepatitis/and toxic hepatitis in thousand IU/L in severe cases.

Lesser elevations are non-specific and may be seen with any other form of liver injury, including cholestasis or infiltrative liver diseases.

In obstructive jaundice, increase occur but does not usually exceed 200 to 250 IU/L.

(b) Serum Alkaline Phosphatase (ALP)

This enzyme is derived from liver in normal health. It is also produced by bone, small intestine, kidney and placenta. ***Placental ALP is heat-stable.***

In normal subjects: serum ALP varies from 3 to 13 KA units/dl (23-92 IU/L).

Main clinical value of ALP is its sensitivity in detecting early intrahepatic or extrahepatic bile duct obstruction. It has been used in ***differentiating obstructive jaundice from non-obstructive.***

Dividing line suggested is 35 KA units/dl. A value higher than 35 KA units/dl is highly sug-

gestive of extrahepatic obstruction (often before jaundice appears). Normal ALP value excludes obstruction. Higher values also point to presence of "infiltrative" diseases like TB, sarcoidosis, amyloidosis, or to ***"space-occupying"*** lesions like abscess, hepatoma, metastatic cancer.

Value of Combination of S-GPT and Serum ALP

- In obstructive jaundice and cholestatic jaundice usual finding is high serum ALP and low S-GPT activity.
- In hepatocellular jaundice without intrahepatic cholestasis, S-GPT is usually very high with normal or slightly raised, serum ALP.

Note

Serum ALP is also increased in bone diseases, hence it is somewhat non-specific in liver diseases. Two other enzymes which are more specific and not affected by bone diseases are serum gamma-glutamyl transpeptidase (GGT) and serum 5-nucleotidase.

(c) Serum Leucine Aminopeptidase (LAP)

Normal serum LAP activity ranges from 15 to 56 m-Iu.

- In obstructive jaundice marked increase in serum LAP activity is seen, similar to serum alkaline phosphatase (ALP).

  Increase has been more in malignant obstruction as compared to benign obstruction. In benign obstruction, serum LAP activity ranges from 75 to 185 m-Iu, whereas in malignant obstruction higher ranges seen up to 350 m-Iu or more.

  Serum LAP activity has got added advantage over serum ALP in that it is not increased in osseous involvement. Increase in serum LAP activity is seen in viral hepatitis and cirrhosis liver but rise in much less.

(d) Serum Gamma-glutamyl Transpeptidase (S-GGT)

Also called as serum γ-glutamyl transferase (γ-GT).

Normal range is 10-47 Iu/L.

The enzyme is microsomal. The activity of this enzyme has been found to increase in most of the hepatobiliary diseases. The main clinical value of this enzyme determination is its specificity for liver diseases. In patients with elevated serum ALP due to bone diseases or pregnancy, the serum GGT levels are usually normal. Thus, an elevated serum GGT (γ-GT) implies that an elevated serum ALP is of hepatic origin.

Note

- Elevated level of serum GGT may be due to enzyme induction by certain drugs such as phenobarbitone, warfarin, phenytoin sodium and alcohol.
- ***Recently the importance of this enzyme in alcohol abuse has been stressed.*** Sudden increase in serum GGT in chronic alcoholics suggests recent bout of drinking alcohol.

(e) Serum 5'—nucleotidase

Normal range: is 2 to 17 Iu/L. Similar to serum GGT, this enzyme is also raised in hepatobiliary diseases along with serum ALP in a parallel manner and it has ***the added advantage that the enzyme is more specific in hepatic diseases and is not affected in bone diseases and pregnancy.***

3. Determination of Prothrombin Time

Prothrombin time (PT) is the time required for clotting to take place in citrated plasma to which optimum amounts of thromboplastin and Ca^{2+} have been added.

Prothrombin time reflects the activities of fibrinogen, prothrombin and factors V, VII, and X.

It is dependent on hepatic synthesis of these factors and conversion to active factors for which vitamin K is required. In liver, ***"pre-prothrombin"*** which is inactive is converted to active prothrombin in presence of vitamin K which produces carboxylation of glutamic acid residues. Hence, proper intestinal absorption of vitamin K is necessary.

Malabsorption of vitamin K occurs with impaired lipid absorption, as is commonly found with ***bile salt deficiency secondary to prolonged cholestasis.***

PT is helpful in assessing the extent of liver cells damage and also in assessing the prognosis.

- ***Normal prothrombin time:*** Normal levels of prothrombin in control subjects gives a PT of approximately 14 second (range 10-16 sec).

  Results are always expressed as patient's PT in seconds compared to normal control.
- PT is increased ↑ from 22 seconds to as much as 150 seconds in liver cells damage. PT is also increased in obstructive jaundice due to absence of bile salts, due to defective absorption of vitamin K.

Thus, PT is increased in both obstructive jaundice as well as in hepatocellular diseases due to damage to liver cells. Hence, PT as such cannot be used to differentiate these two types of jaundice.

But, if vitamin K is administered ***parenterally,*** the PT returns rapidly to normal in obstructive jaundice but not in hepatocellular jaundice, ***thus, obstructive jaundice can be differentiated.***

Note

- PT is helpful in assessing the extent of liver cells damage and the prognosis.
- Little diagnostic significance should be given to a prolonged PT, unless it is measured again at least 24 hours after parenteral injection of vitamin K.
- Hypoprothrombinaemia related to bile salt deficiency will be corrected and come back to normal, whereas that secondary to hepatocellular disease will not show improvement.

3. Flocculation Tests

Large number of flocculation tests have been used in jaundice and in assessing liver function. Common ones done but now because outdated in laboratory are:

- ***Thymol turbidity and flocculation test.***
- ***Zinc sulphate turbidity and flocculation test.*** *(Refer to Chapter 2—Liver Function Tests)*
- ***Jirgl's Flocculation Test***

This test is not performed routinely. **Jirgl (1957)** first described a new serum flocculation test, called Jirgl's flocculation test for differentiating obstructive from hepatocellular jaundice. He observed that the sera of patients with obstructive jaundice become turbid and formed a thick precipitate on addition of Folin-Ciocalteau phenol reagent. He observed a positive reaction in 44 out of 46 patients with extrahepatic obstructive jaundice. Since then, number of reports have appeared and strong positivity was reported varying from 87.7 to 93.3% in extrahepatic obstructive jaundice.

Procedure

- In a clean test tube, 0.8 ml of serum and 2 ml of 0.1 N KOH are taken, mixed and allowed to stand at room temperature for 45 minutes.
- Then 2 ml of 20% sulphosalicylic acid is added and the mixture shaken thoroughly.
- Tube is then left for 10 minutes at room temperature and then filtered.
- Of the filtrate, 2.5 ml is taken in another clean centrifuge tube, mixed with 0.5 ml tungsten reagent (5% phosphotungstic acid in 2 N HCl), and allowed to stand for 10 minutes at room temperature, then centrifuged for 15 minutes.
- Discard the supernatant, the inside of the tube is wiped dry and the sediment is re-dissolved in 3.25 ml of 10% sodium carbonate and 0.25 ml of Folin-Ciocalteau reagent (diluted 1 in 3 with distilled water) is added.

Results and Interpretation

- The flocculation is read immediately and also after 12 hours, the result is read against a dark background using a strong incident light. The result is graded as follows:

Negative	= Tube contents clear
+	= Slight turbidity
++	= Definite flocculation
+++	= Heavy precipitate

- *In extrehepatic obstructive jaundice:* more than 93% cases show ++ to +++ positivity.
- In less than 15% of viral hepatitis slight turbidity (+) is obtained.
- A control group and cirrhosis liver cases show negative result.

Mechanism of Flocculation

Underlying mechanism is not clear. It has been suggested that the flocculation is dependent on a factor present in bile which is retained in the serum in obstructive jaundice cases.

Remarks

It has been stressed that a positive Jirgl's flocculation test (++ to +++) in a case of clinical jaundice with negative thymol turbidity/flocculation and serum ALP greater than 50 KA units/dl will be almost diagnostic for extrehepatic obstructive jaundice.

Other Laboratory Tests

1. Biochemical Tests

(a) Serum Proteins—Total and Differential and A:G Ratio

- ***Serum albumin concentration like PT*** is a good indicator of hepatic functional reserve, but because of its half-life (20 to 26 days) changes are slow in reflecting liver damage. Jaundice can occur in cirrhosis liver and in this condition serum albumin reduced↓, globulin shows increase↑ and A : G ratio is reversed. It is characteristic of cirrhosis liver.
- ***α-globulins tend to be low*** in hepatocellular diseases.
- ***An absent α_1*** Globulin suggests a homozygous α_1-antitrypsin deficiency.
- ***γ globulin concentration tends to increase*** with most forms of chronic liver diseases. Marked increase, in serum level of γ-globulin greater than 3.0 gm/dl is suggestive of chronic active hepatitis.

(b) Immunoglobulins (Igs) Assay

- ***In acute viral hepatitis*** initial increase is found in IgM, which comes down to normal in 2 to 3 months. (IgG and IgA are normal.)
- ***In chronic hepatitis*** major increase is found in IgG (IgA and IgM are normal).
- ***In primary biliary cirrhosis*** there is marked increase in IgM, greater than in acute viral hepatitis. IgG and IgA are normal.

(c) Serum Cholesterol

As a rule, obstructive jaundice shows an increase in serum cholesterol level and such increase parallels with increase in serum bilirubin. Very high values of serum cholesterol is found in biliary atresia and xanthomatous biliary cirrhosis.

(d) Lipoprotein Electrophoresis (LPE)

Detection of "LP-X" an abnormal lipoprotein which is a "marker" in obstructive jaundice. This abnormal serum LP called Lipoprotein-X (LP-X) can be identified by its peculiar electrophoretic behaviour. On most support media except agar gels, ***LP-X migrates with the β-lipoproteins.*** In agar gels, in which endosmosis is strong, LP-X migrates cathodically behind the origin. "LP-X" is characterized by a low protein content and relatively large amounts of phospholipids and cholesterol and ***is found only in sera of patients with obstructive jaundice.***

(e) BSP Excretion Test

Dubin-Johnson syndrome an autosomal recessive disorder characterized by conjugated hyperbilirubinaemia and jaundice in childhood and in adult life.

A BSP test when performed in a suspected case of Dubin-Johnson syndrome shows ***a secondary rise*** in plasma concentration due to reflux of the conjugated BSP ***(pathognomonic of the disease).***

(f) Urinalysis

- ***Bilirubin:***
  - Bilirubin is found in the urine of obstructive jaundice cases and in choles-

tatic jaundice, as conjugated bilirubin can pass through the glomerular filter.
- Bilirubin is not present in urine in most cases of haemolytic jaundice, as it is accompanied with unconjugated hyperbilirubinaemia.
- ***Bilirubinuria in obstructive jaundice and cholestesis is always accompanied with direct VD Bergh reaction.***

- *Urobilinogen:*
  - Normally there is trace of urobilinogen in urine, average 0.64 mg, maximum normal 4 mg in 24 hours urine. No urobilinogen is detected in urine in obstructive jaundice, in complete obstruction whereas in haemolytic jaundice urobilinogen is increased in urine.

Note
- ***Bilirubinuria accompanied with positive VD Bergh reaction, absence of urobilinogen in urine strongly suggests obstructive jaundice.***
- ***Absence of bilirubinuria, accompanied with indirect VD Bergh test and increased urobilinogen in urine is strongly suggestive of haemolytic jaundice.***

(g) Bile Pigments in Faeces

Bilirubin is not normally present in faeces since intestinal bacterial flora reduce it to urobilinogen.

Faecal urobilinogen

- Normal quantity of urobilinogen excreted in the faeces per day is from 50 to 250 mg. The amount of faecal urobilinogen will depend primarily on the amount of bilirubin entering the intestine.
- Faecal urobilinogen is increased in haemolytic jaundice, in which dark-coloured faeces is passed.
- ***In obstructive jaundice,*** as there is obstruction to flow of bile, faecal urobilinogen is decreased or absent and ***clay-coloured faeces*** is passed. ***A complete absence of faecal urobilinogen is strongly suggestive of malignant obstruction in case of presence of jaundice.***

2. Serological Tests

- *Hepatitis Antigens and Antibodies*

a. In hepatitis A (HAV)

- ***IgM hepatitis antibody (IgMHAAb)*** appears early and present in the serum at the onset of symptoms and disappears in a few months (2 to 3 months) during convalescence.
- ***IgG hepatitis A antibody (IgGHAAb):*** This antibody appears in convalescence; it increases as IgM declines and persist for years, perhaps for life, conferring immunity.

b. Hepatitis B (HBV)

- Hepatitis B surface antigen (HBA): HBsAg appears first and is a serologic ***'marker'*** of active HBV infection, appearing before the onset of symptoms, ***reaches its peak during 'overt' disease*** and declining over 3 to 6 months.
- ***Hepatitis B surface antibody (HBsAb):*** This antibody becomes detectable in the serum at a variable time after disappearance of the antigen and usually persists for life.
- ***HbeAg, HBV-DNA and DNA polymerase:*** They appear in serum soon after HBsAg and before the onset of acute disease. ***All of them are 'serologic markers', indicating active viral replication.***

Note

These decline usually within a few weeks, but ***persistence of serum HBeAg indicates that viral replication is continuing*** and persistence of infectivity indicates progression to chronic disease.

c. Hepatitis B core antibody (HBcAb)

- IgM anti-HBc is usually the first antibody to appear, followed shortly by anti-HBe, indicating that acute infection has reached the peak and is on the decline.
- IgG anti-HBc slowly replaces the IgM over months. ***HBcAb is present during "Window Period", between disappearance of HBsAg and appearance of HBsAb.***

- IgM hepatitis Bc core antibody titres can be determined. High serum titres usually are present early in the course of hepatitis B (HBV) infection and disappears within 3 to 4 months.

Note

In the laboratory evaluation of the patient with acute viral hepatitis, determination of IgM-HAAb, HBsAg, and HBcAb allow one to diagnose whether HAV (Hepatitis A) or HBV (Hepatitis B) is present. ***If all are negative, provisional diagnosis of non A, non B (NANB) hepatitis may be made.***

d. Antimitochondrial Antibody

Significant raised titres of antimitochondrial antibody is seen in ***primary biliary cirrhosis***. Positivity is observed in more than 85% of cases.

Note

- It is ***not specific*** for primary biliary cirrhosis, as elevated titres are occasionally observed in chronic active hepatitis.
- Though it is not specific for primary biliary cirrhosis, absence of the antibody goes against a diagnosis of the disease ***(negative finding is useful).***

SPECIAL INVESTIGATIONS

Certain specialized investigations when undertaken may be informative and help to find out the aetiology.

1. *Radiological*

- ***Plain X-ray of right hypochondrium and oral cholecystography:*** are useful to detect presence of gallstones, if any, and evaluate gallbladder function.
- ***Biliary scan:*** a radionucleotide biliary scan (HIDA scan) will be of immense help in evaluating the patient with suspected acute cholecystitis. Visualization of the bile ducts and not the gallbladder on acute and delayed films may suggest cystic duct obstruction.
- ***Liver scan:*** an isotopic liver scan may be useful in detecting ***"space occupying lesions";*** specially when biochemically high serum ALP is present.

- ***Gastrointestinal Series***

An upper GI series may reveal enlargement of head of pancreas suggesting carcinoma head of pancreas, with extrahepatic obstruction.

2. *Liver Biopsy*

A percutaneous liver biopsy and histopathological examination of biopsy material may be of, immense use in diagnosing the cause of jaundice and assessing the liver pathology.

3. *Oncogenic Markers*

Refer chapter on "Oncogenic Markers"

- Serum AFP (alphafetoprotein)—in liver cell carcinoma.
- CA19: carcinoma of pancreas.

4. *Ultrasound and CT Scanning*

These may be specially useful in detecting:
  - space occupying lesions in liver;
  - bile duct enlargement; and
  - pancreatic tumours.

5. *Percutaneous Transhepatic Cholangiography and Endoscopic Retrograde Cholangiopancreatography*

These techniques may provide more detailed information regarding the cause of extrahepatic obstruction. Pancreatic duct can also be examined usually. These are sophisticated techniques and local expertise is necessary.

Biochemical Differentiation of Jaundice

(Refer to Table No. 2.2 in Part 1, Chapter on Liver Function Tests)

A proposed flow chart for investigation of a case of jaundice is given in page 158.

Flow Chart for laboratory investigation of a case of jaundice

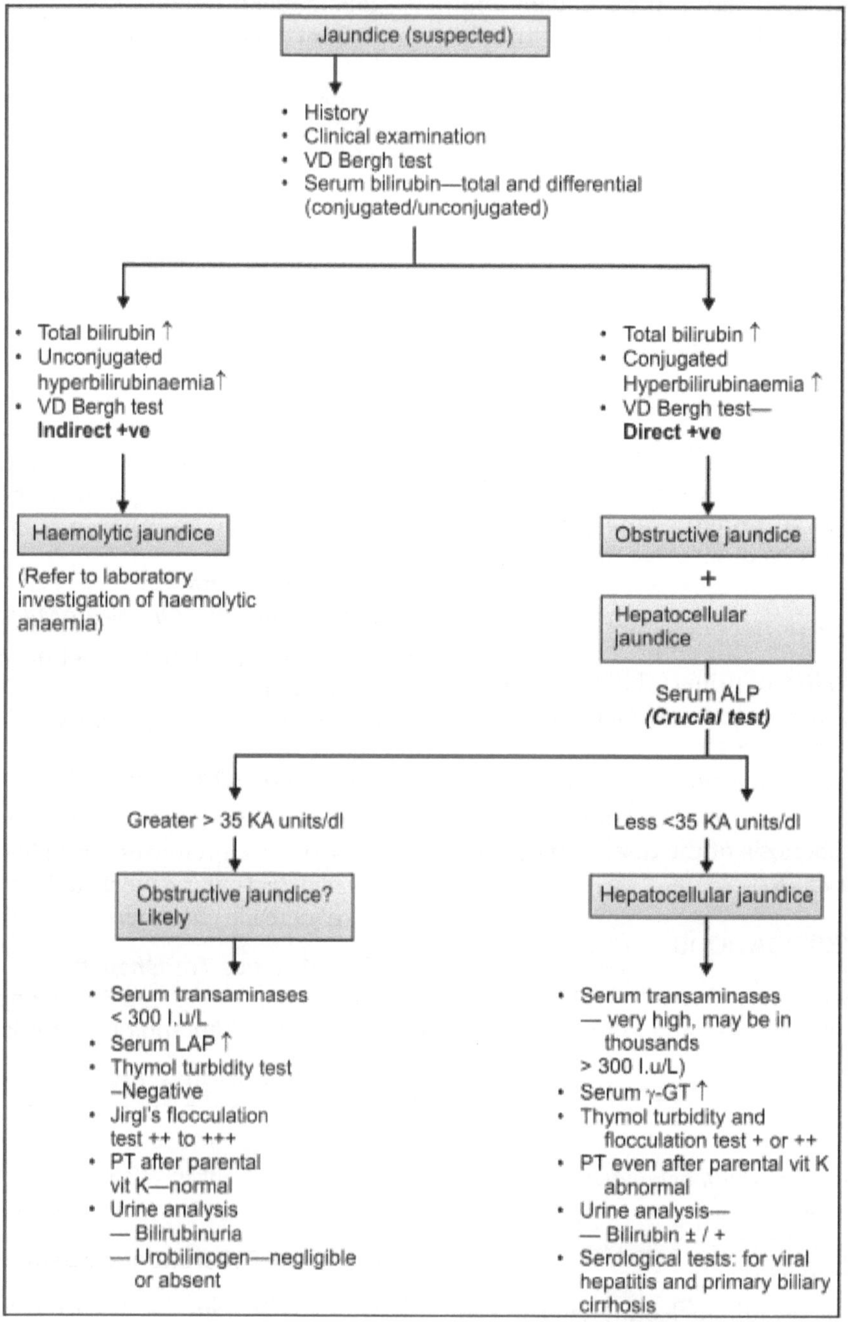

Chapter 15

Neonatal Jaundice

INTRODUCTION

Jaundice in the neonatal period has a different approach from that seen in the adults. Most newborn infants, immediately after birth may show an unconjugated hyperbilirubinaemia and jaundice which may be a transient phenomenon. This results from delayed development of the enzyme, ***"glucuronyl transferase"*** which conjugates bilirubin to form water soluble bilirubin diglucuronide.

Factors which enhances this effect like:

- prematurity;
- certain drugs; and
- factors in maternal serum or milk will aggravate the problem.

Haemolytic disease also affects neonates due to Rh/ABO incompatibility. Hence, an increase in lipid-soluble unconjugated bilirubin is of frequent occurrence and carries with it the ***"risk" of fatal "kernicterus" (bilirubin encephalopathy),*** which is not seen in adults. ***The risk becomes greater if the amount of bilirubin bound to serum albumin is decreased.*** The neonates are particularly prone to viral and other infections which do not cause jaundice in an adult. Congenital abnormalities like jaundice associated with biliary atresias and congenital toxoplasmosis can produce jaundice and become manifest soon after birth. Certain metabolic abnormalities such as enzyme deficiency like ***glucose-6-phosphate dehydrogenase (G-6-PD)*** may also produce jaundice in this period. Hence, the aetiology of jaundice in neonates is slightly different as compared to jaundice in adult.

CAUSES

The important conditions which may be responsible for neonatal jaundice be classified as follows:

- ***Physiological and prematurity jaundice***
- ***Haemolytic disease of the newborn*** (HDN)-ABO/Rh incompatibility.
- ***Jaundice due to certain maternal factors and drugs***
  - Serum enzyme inhibition (Lucey-Driscoll syndrome).
  - Factor present in maternal milk.
  - Drugs.
- ***Enzyme deficiency***
  - G-6-PD deficiency.
  - Galactosaemia.
  - Hereditary fructose intolerance.
  - Crigler-Najjar syndrome Type I.
- ***Hepatitis***

a. Giant cell hepatitis.

b. Other hepatitis due to various viral infections.
   - Cytomegalovirus infection.
   - Congenital rubella syndrome.
   - Herpes simplex.
   - Group B coxsackievirus.
   - Adenoviruses.

- ***Pyogenic infections—umbilical sepsis***
- ***Congenital disorders***
  - Congenital syphilis
  - Congenital toxoplasmosis
  - Congenital biliary atresias.
- ***Other causes*** (See below)

1. Physiological and Prematurity Jaundice

In normal newborn babies, jaundice can appear immediately after birth, reaching peak levels within 2 to 5 days and disappears in two weeks time. Prematurity can aggravate; and is liable to have Kernicterus. It is ***unconjugated hyperbilirubinaemia.***

Causes

- It may be due to haemolysis of surplus foetal red blood cells.
- Relative deficiency of the enzyme ***"glucuronyl transferase"***—more so in premature babies.
- Probably defective hepatic excretion plays part.

2. Haemolytic Disease of the Newborn (HDN) (Erythroblastosis Foetalis)

Pathogenesis

Antigens of foetal red cells entering into maternal circulation may provoke the development of maternal antibodies which on passing into the foetal circulation produce haemolysis of the foetal red blood cells.

Causes

- Commonest incompatibility is in the Rhesus blood factors. ***Rh incompatibility which is common, occurs in a D positive foetus with mother being D negative.***
- HDN also occurs by ABO incompatibility or other blood group antigens. ABO incompatibility between maternal plasma and foetal red blood cells may result in HDN. It is significant that most cases of ABO haemolytic disease occur in infants of Gr A or Gr B with Gr O mothers. ***Some authorities feel that ABO incompatibility is more common*** than previously assumed, accounting for as much as 2/3 of all HDN cases.

Note

- It is believed that ABO incompatibility is not detected/missed as:
  - Due to frequent inability to demonstrate antibodies in the infant (except for elevated bilirubin).
  - Due to direct Coombs' test being negative or weekly positive.
- ***Essential differences between HDN of Rh incompatibility to that of ABO incompatibility are shown in Table 15.1.***
- Characteristically, the first born baby escapes the disease, unless the mother's blood has been sensitized by a previous transfusion of Rh D positive blood. A normal first pregnancy sensitizes the mother's blood sufficiently to provoke haemolytic disease in subsequent infants.

Clinical Features

The clinical forms of HDN vary in severity but the underlying pathological lesions are similar. According to severity, ***three types*** are recognised.

- ***Hydrops foetalis:*** The most severe form of HDN, presents with congenital oedema of the foetus terminating in still birth or death due to cardiac failure within few hours of birth.
- ***Icterus gravis neonatorum:*** The amniotic fluid is yellow at delivery and within 12 hours the baby is deeply jaundiced. Jaundice is deeper in premature infants in which there is hepatic immaturity. There may be haemorrhages/petechiae in skin and splenomegaly may be present.

  Biochemically, unconjugated hyperbilirubinaemia and urine contains bilirubin and urobilin.
- ***Anaemia gravis:*** this is the mildest clinical variant characterized by:
  - Haemolytic anaemia
  - Splenomegaly
  - Reticulocytosis
  - Mild jaundice.

Note

- Both prematurity jaundice and haemolytic disease of the newborn (HDN) can have a frequent and fatal complication called **"kernicterus"** *(bilirubin encephalopathy)*, if not treated early.
- Kernicterus can also occur in other forms of neonatal jaundice especially hepatitis.
- Certain drugs, viz. salicylates and sulphonamides and certain organic anions, e.g. FFA, haematin can displace unconjugated bilirubin from binding site of albumin and likely to produce kernicterus at reduced concentration of plasma bilirubin specially in a premature infant.

3. Jaundice due to Certain Maternal Factors/and Drugs

- ***Serum Enzyme Inhibition (Lucey-Driscoll Syndrome)***

A rare form of transient familial, neonatal ***unconjugated hyperbilirubinaemia*** occurring during the first 48 hours of life. An inhibitor present in both maternal and infant's serum is responsible; exact nature not identified.

Factor Present in Maternal Milk

A form of prolonged unconjugated neonatal hyperbilirubinaemia has been found in breast-fed babies. The condition lasts from 2 weeks to more than 2 months after delivery.

Cause

Maternal milk may contain an abnormal steroid ***"pregnanane-3 (α)-20(β)-diol"***. The steroid factor competitively inhibits the enzyme ***glucuronyl transferase.*** It is not certain whether the maternal defect is inherited or acquired.

Note

- 5% of mothers of normal infants, secrete milk containing this factor which inhibits ***glucuronyl transferase*** by more than 20%, but concentration of the inhibitor is less than that found in jaundiced infants.
- Stopping breast-feeding decreases hyperbilirubinaemia and jaundice, but resumption of feeding increases the jaundice again.

- ***Drugs (latrogenic) V/s Neonatal Liver***

Drugs can produce jaundice:

- By increasing the serum unconjugated bilirubin level by haemolysis.
- Interfering with its combination with albumin.
- Acting as a competitive inhibitor of the enzyme ***glucuronyl transferase.***

Examples

- ***Novobiocin*** is a competitive inhibitor of ***glucuronyl transferase enzyme.***
- ***Sulphonamides and salicylates:*** competes for the binding site on albumin for unconjugated bilirubin and displaces the bilirubin from albumin.
- ***Any oxidant drugs:*** causing haemolysis may produce jaundice specially if there is underlying tendency such as ***glucose-6-phosphate dehydrogenase (G-6-PD) deficiency.***
- ***Vitamin K:*** watersoluble synthetic vitamin K analogues may produce jaundice, but the effect is not seen when given IV. The toxic effects of synthetic vitamin K preparations to produce hyperbilirubinaemia may be due to increased haemolysis or to a direct hepatoxic effect.

4. Enzyme Deficiency

- ***G-6-PD Deficiency***

Infants having a deficiency of the enzyme ***glucose-6-phosphate dehydrogenase (G-6-PD)*** in their erythrocytes may develop jaundice with unconjugated hyperbilirubinaemia.

The precipitating agent is an oxidant drug like phenacetin, salicylates, sulphones, sulphonamides transmitted in the mother's milk.

It is a common cause of neonatal jaundice in Mediterranean zone, far East and Nigeria.

- ***Galactosaemia***

(For details—refer to laboratory investigation of hypoglycaemia).

The disease starts *in utero* and the infant presents with feeding difficulties, with vomiting/diarrhoea, malnutrition and often accompanied with *jaundice.*

- ***Hereditary Fructose Intolerance***

(For details—refer to laboratory investigation of hypoglycaemia).

The condition is marked by jaundice, ascites, albuminuria and aminoaciduria. Hypoglycaemia follows fructose administration.

5. Hepatitis

- ***Giant Cell Hepatitis***

Clinical presentation is variable. Sometimes there is ***still birth*** or infant may die soon after or before jaundice has had time to develop. More usually a ***fluctuant type*** of jaundice appears during the first two weeks of life. Often the baby fails to thrive and expires within a few days or weeks. A ***genetic factor*** may be involved, an autosomal recessive mode of inheritance has been suggested. Viral etiology is controversial.

Biochemically

- Serum transminases are increased ↑ more than 800 I.u/l; and
- There may be hypoprothrombinaemia.

- ***Other Hepatitis due to Various Viral Infections***

- *Cytomegalovirus infection:* The virus may be transferred from an asymptomatic mother transplacentally. It causes jaundice, hepatosplenomegaly and purpura.

  Jaundice may be prolonged for months and usually it is ***conjugated hyperbilirubinaemia.***

Note

It is not a frequent cause of neonatal hepatitis.

- ***Congenital rubella syndrome:*** Produces hepatitis which is marked by jaundice, commencing within first 1 to 2 days and may be associated with hepatosplenomegaly.

  Jaundice is ***conjugated hyperbilirubinaemia*** but haemolytic process may complicate the rubella syndrome. This disease, ***contracted in the first trimester of pregnancy may cause focal malformations.*** The infection may persist through the neonatal period and continue into later life. The hepatitis may resolve completely with restitution of a normal liver structure.

- ***Herpes simplex infection:*** The liver may be involved in the course of a fulminating viraemia, contracted at birth from herpes simplex infection of the maternal birth canal. Jaundice may be a manifestation, due to viral involvement of the liver which shows white nodules.
- ***Coxsackie B virus infection:*** These viruses may cause neonatal hepatitis and can produce jaundice. It is not a usual cause (rare).
- ***Adenoviruses:*** These may disseminate in babies with decreased resistance due to thymic alymphoplasia and agammaglobulinaemia. Not a common cause of neonatal jaundice.

6. Pyogenic Infections: Umbilical Sepsis

Jaundice appears suddenly in a baby who does not look so ill initially. Hepatomegaly may not be present and splenomegaly is never great. Earlier, it used to be a common cause of neonatal jaundice but decreased with the advent of broad-spectrum antibiotics. Increase in Gram-negative infections, particularly *E. coli* in nurseries has led to increase in jaundice due to this cause.

Origins may be:

- Umbilical sepsis.
- Pneumonia.
- Otitis media.
- Gastroenteritis.
- Exchange blood transfusion.

Diagnosis sometimes become difficult as focal signs are minimal or absent.

7. Congenital Disorders

- ***Congenital Syphilis***

This condition is now very rare. Visceral involvement is late in acquired syphilis but common in foetal infection. Large numbers of treponemata may be found in the liver, which leads to fine ***pericellular cirrhosis*** with a marked connective tissue reaction. ***Jaundice is usual.***

- ***Congenital Toxoplasmosis***

The infection by this protozoon is transmitted to the foetus from an inapparent maternal infection.

Jaundice may develop in such cases within a few hours of birth and it may be associated with *hepatomegaly, encephalomyelitis, hydrocephalus, microcephaly, choroidoretinitis* and *intracerebral calcification.* The jaundice may be difficult to relate to the extent of hepatic damage and haemolysis may be a contributory factor.

- ***Biliary Atresias***

These are defined as the inability to excrete bile associated with malformations of biliary tree. The abnormality may be in any part of the biliary tract from the ductules to the common bile duct. Biliary atresias produce ***cholestatic jaundice: conjugated hyperbilirubinaemia. Jaundice*** starts soon after birth, the baby becomes icteric by the first week and the icterus continues unremittingly and the baby may be deeply jaundiced with following features:

- Pruritus is severe usually.
- Bleeding tendency due to vitamin K deficiency.
- Ascites is a late and terminal feature.

Biochemically

- **Urine** is dark coloured;
- **Stools**—pale;
- **Serum transaminases** increased ↑ considerably;
- Serum cholesterol may rise to very high level—leading to xanthomatosis; and
- Baby may have prolonged ***steatorrhoea*** leading to osteomalacia ***(biliary rickets).***

8. Other Causes

- ***Extravascular Blood***

Cephalhaematomatas, cerebral or pulmonary haemorrhage or any occult bleeding may lead to an elevated serum bilirubin from breakdown of extravascular red cells and can cause jaundice.

- ***Polycythaemia***

- Twin-twin transfusion.
- Maternal—foetal transfusion.
- Anything that produces an elevated Hb level,
- Or an increase in red cell mass.

All above conditions can increase the bilirubin load to liver producing hyperbilirubinaemia and jaundice.

- ***Increased Enterohepatic Circulation***

This may occur with any form of intestinal obstruction or delay in bowel transit time, allowing more time for bilirubin deconjugation and reabsorption. Thus, jaundice may occur in infants with:

- Small bowel obstruction.
- Pyloric stenosis.

- ***Congenital Hypothyroidism***

The infants may develop prolonged unconjugated hyperbilirubinaemia and jaundice.

Cause is the absence of haemolysis. It is suggested that hepatic uptake and conjugation or both are affected.

LABORATORY INVESTIGATIONS

These can be discussed under two heads:

- ***To establish that jaundice is present and to determine the type whether it is unconjugated or conjugated hyperbilirubinaemia.***
- ***To determine the cause of the jaundice.***

I. TO ESTABLISH THAT JAUNDICE IS PRESENT AND ITS TYPE

For this to achieve, the following will be useful:

- ***Proper clinical examination of the baby,*** evidence of clinical jaundice to be looked for in conjunctivae of eyes, mucous membranes.

- ***Total serum bilirubin and differential bilirubin,*** both conjugated and unconjugated bilirubin to be determined.
- ***van den Bergh's reaction:*** a direct positive test will indicate conjugated hyperbilirubinaemia and an indirect one, unconjugated hyperbilirubinaemia.

The clinical examination supported by total and differential bilirubin and van den Bergh's test will establish the presence of jaundice and its type.

- ***Urine analysis*** for presence of bilirubinuria and urobilinogen should be carried out.

II. TESTS TO ESTABLISH THE CAUSE

Before any laboratory investigation is started, a proper history and clinical examination of both mother and the infant should be carried out which will be of immense help in coming to aetiology.

1. History and Clinical Examination

- ***Family History***

Parent or sibling with history of jaundice or anaemia, suggests hereditary haemolytic anaemia, such as hereditary spherocytosis. Previous siblings with neonatal jaundice, suggests HDN with ABO/Rh incompatibility or breast milk jaundice.

- ***Maternal History***
  - History of liver disease in siblings or disorders such as galactosaemia, Crigler-Najjar syndrome, etc, to be elicited.
  - History of diabetes mellitus: increased incidence of jaundice observed in diabetic mothers.
  - History of any drugs by mother, e.g. sulphonamides, salicylates, or antimalarials, etc. oxidant drugs can produce haemolysis in G-6-PD deficiency.
  - Unexplained illness/fever in mother during pregnancy associated with lymphadenopathy and rash suggests congenital infections like cytomegalovirus, rubella, herpes simplex, toxoplasmosis, congenital syphilis, etc.

- ***History of Labour and Delivery***

History of labour and delivery earlier to the current pregnancy is important. Increased incidence of hyperbilirubinaemia and jaundice seen in following:

- Vacuum extraction—cephalomata.
- Asphyxiated infants (Apgar score).
- Delayed cord clamping.
- Oxytocin—induced labour.

- ***History of the Infant***
  - ***Vomiting:*** suspect sepsis, pyloric stenosis, galactosaemia.
  - ***Cephalohaematoma:*** entrapped haemorrhage associated with haematoma
  - ***Microcephaly (small head):*** suggest intrauterine infection.
  - ***Macrocephaly (large head):*** suggests diabetic mother.
  - ***Caloric intake:*** inadequate calorie intake results in delay in development of *glucuronyl transferase* and delay in conjugation.
  - ***"Small" babe (small or gestational age):*** infants frequently polycythaemic and jaundiced, intrauterine infection should be considered.

- ***Clinical Examination of the Infant***
  - ***Marked pallor*** suggestive of haemolytic anaemia.
  - ***Enlargement of liver and spleen*** suggests haemolytic anaemia, or congenital intrauterine infections.
  - ***Petechiae*** suspect congenital infection, hepatitis, severe sepsis or severe HDN.
  - ***Umbilical cord stump and its appearance*** inflammation and sepsis of umbilical stump to be looked for. *Omphalitis and sepsis may cause jaundice.*

– ***Examination of optic fundus (ophthalmoscopy)*** presence of chorioretinitis suggests congenital infection as cause of jaundice.

LABORATORY TESTS

After ascertaining presence of jaundice and after performing total and differential bilirubin and VD Bergh tests for further evaluation the following investigations are to be carried out.

I. In Unconjugated Hyperbilirubinaemia

- ***Coombs' Test***

This is the ***most crucial test.*** If unconjugated hyperbilirubinaemia is present and VD Bergh test is indirect positive, the most crucial test to perform is Coombs' test.

a. ***If direct Coombs' is +ve:*** HDN should be suspected—isoimmunization of Rh, ABO or minor blood group. Diagnosis of HDN depends on both clinical and laboratory findings.

- ***Blood grouping*** of mother and infant to be re-checked.
- Demonstration of presence of an antibody in mother's serum to a blood factor present in infant's cells but not in the mother.
- Titration of antibodies present in mother's serum (Refer Table 15.1).

Note

- Serologic diagnosis of ABO haemolytic disease is more difficult to make than that of Rh. The direct Coombs' test is frequently negative or only weakly positive, hence, it is missed.
- An antiglobulin serum which has a high level of anti-non-γ-globulin reactivity will often be able to detect coating of infant's cells with maternal antibody.
- ***Witebsky test:*** **Witebsky** has shown that red cells sensitized with Rh antibody agglutinate by the slide technique more strongly in a mixture of 1 part of normal adult serum with 2 parts of 30% bovine albumin than in serum alone, while cells sensitized with

Table 15.1: Essential differences—clinical and laboratory in case of HDN due to Rh and ABO incompatibility

	HDN due to Rh incompatibility	*HDN due to ABO incompatibility*
(a) In infant		
• *Jaundice*	Moderate (++ to severe +++)	Mild to moderate (+ to ++)
• *Hb*	Low	Frequently normal or higher side
• *Anaemia*	Moderate to severe	Slight to moderate
• *Osmotic fragility of RBCells*	Normal	Increased↑
• *Spherocytes*	Absent	Present
• *Reticulocyte count*	Mild to moderate increase	Marked increase ↑
• *Nucleated red cells increase*	Moderate to marked	Marked
• *Direct Coombs' test*	Positive	*Weakly positive or sometimes negative
• *Eluate of infant's cells*	Contains Rh antibodies	Contains anti-A or anti-B
• *Indirect Coomb's with cord (infant's) serum*	Positive with cells of appropriate Rh type	Positive with A_1 or B Cells
• *Incidence*	About 1 in 300 deliveries	May be greater
• *Occurrence in first born*	Unlikely	Likely
(b) In Mother		
• *Haemolysis*	No anti-Rh haemolysins	Anti-A and/or anti-B haemolysins present
• *Indirect Coombs' with mother's serum*	Positive with cells of appropriate Rh type	Positive with A_1 or B cells after neutralization of isoagglutinins

immune anti-A or anti-B agglutinate more strongly than in the mixture.

- *Munk-Andersen test:* **Munk-Andersen** has developed a conglutination test, using dextran, capable of detecting immune antibody coated infant's cells as well as free immune antibodies in infant's serum.

b. *If Coombs' test is -ve:* then perform Haematocrit.

1. *If haematocrit value is high* consider:
   - Twin-twin transfusion.
   - Materno-foetal transfusion.
   - Delayed cord clamping.
   - Small babe for date.
2. *If haematocrit value is normal or low* the following tests are required to be carried out:
   - Red cell morphology (Peripheral smear),
   - Reticulocyte count.
3. *If the above tests, i.e., red cell morphology and reticulocyte count are normal:* the causes are to be looked for:
   - Extravascular blood,
   - Increased enterohepatic circulation
   - Metabolic and endocrine conditions, viz.
     - Crigler-Najjar Type 1;
     - Galactosaemia; and
     - Hypothyroidism.
   - Drugs and hormones.
   - Infants of diabetic mother.
   - Inadequate calorie intake.

For Galactosaemia

The following investigations will be helpful in a suspected case:

- *To demonstrate the presence of free galactose in the blood and urine of the suspected patient,* paper and thin layer chromatography (TLC) of the blood/urine after deproteinisation can be done using either pyridine: isoamyl alcohol: water in ratio of 10 : 10 : 7 or isopropanol: water in ratio of 4 : 1. After running the chromatogram, galactose can be stained with aniline hydrogen oxalate or aniline phthalate as spraying agents. On heating to 120 to 150°C for 10 minutes brown spots are seen. This is to be compared with standard of galactose run along with.
- *Enzyme assays in RB Cells:*
  - galactos-1-p uridyl transferase,
  - galactokinase: marked decreased activity or absence of enzyme activity; and
  - G-6-PD activity may also be lowered in RB Cells.
- *Other investigations:*
  - blood sugar: low (hypoglycaemia);
  - galactose tolerance is impaired;
  - ophthalmoscopy: may demonstrate the presence of cataract; and
  - hepatic function tests may be abnormal, if cirrhosis liver is present.

4. *If the red cells morphology and reticulocyte count are abnormal* it indicates:
   - Specific morphological abnormalities:
     - Hereditary spherocytosis; and
     - Elliptocytosis
   - Non-specific abnormalities:
     - ABO incompatability: spherocytes are seen;
     - enzyme deficiencies: viz. G-6-PD and PK deficiency;
     - α-thalassaemia: Hb-H and Hb-Bart's; and
     - DIC.

All the above are ***associated with haemolytic anaemia.*** (Refer to Chapter on laboratory investigations of haemolytic anaemia for above disorders.)

5. In general, routine blood examinations like Hb, ESR, RBC count, peripheral smear, total and differential WBC count, platelet count and reticulocyte count provides information, suggesting the nature of the disease as follows:

- **Hb:** Low Hb suggests haemolytic disease or large entrapped haemorhage, Hb > 22 gm/dl is associated with increased incidence of jaundice.
- **Red cells morphology (peripheral smear):** Presence of spherocytes suggest ABO incompatibility or hereditary spherocytosis, red cells fragmentation (schistocytes) are seen in DIC.
- **Platelet count:** Low platelet count (thrombocytopenia) suggests infection.
- **Reticulocyte count:** Elevation suggests haemolytic disease.
- **WBC count:** Leucocytosis or band forms greater than 200/cmm suggests infection.
- **ESR:** values in excess of 5 during the first 48 hours indicate infection or ABO incompatibility.

IV. In Conjugated Hyperbilirubinaemia

If total bilirubin is increased and the increase is in conjugated bilirubin and VD Bergh test is direct positive, the following should be suspected, according to priorities.

- ***Sepsis:*** umbilical cord.
- ***Intrauterine infections:***
  - Cytomegalovirus infection.
  - Rubella syndrome.
  - Herpes simplex and other viral infections.
  - Congenital syphilis.
- ***Biliary atresias.***
- ***Giant cell hepatitis.***

In addition to history and clinical examination, certain laboratory tests will help in making the diagnosis.

- **Sepsis**
  - Primary focus to be looked into.
  - Total WBC count: leucocytosis usually >12000/c.mm with increase in band forms.
  - Blood culture: aerobic/anaerobic, antibiotic sensitivity test (AST).
  - Urine examination: RE and deposit, urine culture and antibiotic sensitivity test.
  - Umbilical stump:
    - smear examination if frank pus is there; and
    - culture of a swab taken from umbilical stump.

- ***Giant Cell Hepatitis***
  - Serum transminases high ↑.
  - PT ↓ (hypoprothrombinaemia).
  - ***Liver biopsy*** is diagnostic. In liver biopsy, histopathology shows:
    - normal zonal architecture is lost;
    - most prominent and characteristic feature is ***large multinucleated giant cells*** containing 30 to 40 nuclei in a cytoplasmic mass; and
    - evidence of ***cholestasis, focal necrosis, haemosiderosis*** is a constant feature.

- ***Cytomegalovirus Infection***
  - Isolation of virus: the responsible virus can be isolated from liver biopsy, blood and urine.
  - Urinary deposits may show cytoplasmic inclusions in epithelial cells.
  - Demonstration of IgM antibodies in blood.
  - Liver biopsy examination: histopathologically, it is identical to giant cell hepatitis. Intranuclear inclusions may or may not be present.

- ***Congenital Rubella Syndrome***
  - Isolation of the virus: virus can be isolated and identified from the liver biopsy.
  - Antibodies can be demonstrated in serum.
  - Serum transaminases are elevated ↑, slight to moderate.
  - ***Liver biopsy:*** histopathologically,
    - a focal hepatocellular necrosis;

- portal fibrosis;
- erythroid haemopoietic tissue is relatively increased;
- bile in swollen Kupffer cells and ductules; and
- a typical giant cell hepatitis may be present.

- ***Congenital Syphilis***

Serological tests, like VDRL in both mother and the baby are to be performed.

- ***Congenital Toxoplasmosis***

  - Microscopical examination of aspirates and fluids for *Toxoplasma.*
  - Total and differential WBC count: relative lymphocytosis with atypical mononuclear cells may be seen.
  - ***Sabin-Fieldman dye test:*** is sensitive but because it requires the use of live *Toxoplasma,* it is not as widely used as the other serological tests.
  - ***Serological tests:*** other recent serological tests include:
    - an indirect fluorescent antibody test (IFAT);
    - an indirect haemagglutination test (HAI);
    - recently, enzyme-linked immuno-absorbent assays (ELISA) introduced; and
    - ***test for IgM antibodies:*** demonstration of IgM antibodies in the serum of the infant is important and diagnostic. If such antibodies are present, they must have been formed by the infant in response to an active infection because IgM antibodies cannot cross the placenta.
  - ***X-ray skull:*** may show evidence of ***intracerebral calcifications.***
  - ***Liver biopsy:*** histopathology shows—
    - infiltration of portal zones with mononuclear cells;
    - extramedullary haematopoiesis with increased stainable Fe is conspicuous; and histiocytes containing *Toxoplasma* may be present.

Table 15.2 depicts the essential differentiating features of jaundice due to transplacental infection and HDN (erythroblastosis foetalis)—clinical.

- ***Biliary Atresias***

  - Jaundice is ***cholestatic type,*** severe in nature and prolonged.
  - Conjugated hyperbilirubinemia.
  - ***Urine:*** dark coloured, bilirubinuria +.
  - ***Stool:*** pale and clay coloured, urobilinogen absent
  - Serum transaminases increased ↑ but usually do not exceed 300 units.
  - Serum cholesterol usually markedly elevated.
  - Serum calcium may be low ↓ (hypocalcaemia).
  - ***Liver biopsy:*** shows characteristic features:
    - ducts may be absent or replaced by fibrous strands;
    - cholestatic jaundice with a variable number of giant cells—in that way resemble other neonatal hepatitis and makes the diagnosis difficult; and
    - Site and extent of atresia is variable.

VALUE OF LIVER FUNCTION TESTS IN NEONATAL JAUNDICE (IN INFANTS)

- The usual adult tests do not give consistent results in neonates.
- Bilirubinuria is found in jaundiced infants.
- Urobilinogen is also present in haemolytic jaundice and neonatal hepatitis; its occasional presence in total biliary atresia is unexplained.
- Faecal stercobilinogen (urobilinogen) may be useful in the distinction between hepatocellular and obstructive jaundice in the neonatal period.
- Total and differential serum bilirubin and VD Bergh test are useful in assessing the

Table 15.2: Differential diagnosis of neonatal jaundice—clinical/laboratory tests—in transplacental infections and HDN (erythroblastosis foetalis)

Findings	*Congenital syphilis*	*Toxoplasmosis*	*Cytomegalic inclusion disease*	*Rubella syndrome*	*HDN (erythroblastosis foetalis*
• *Jaundice*	++ to +++	+++	+++	+	+++
• *Anaemia*	Marked +++	++	++	–	Very severe
• *Hepatomegaly*	Marked +++	++	Marked +++	++	++
• *Splenomegaly*	Marked +++	+++	+++	++	+++
• *Thrombocytopenia*	++	+	+++	+++	+
• *Purpura*	++	+	+++	+++	+
• *Skin rash*	+	+	Nil	?	Nil
• *Chorioretinitis*	+	+++	+	+	Nil
• *Generalized oedema*	++	+	+	?	+
• *Intracranial calcifications*	Nil	+	+++	?	Nil
• *Special features*	• MC lesions • Periosteitis • Snuffles • Positive serology (VDRL +ve)	• Microcephaly • Hydrocephaly • Lymphadenopathy • Demonstration of the organism • Positive dye test • IgM antibody	• Pneumonia • Cytomegalic inclusions in renal epithelial cells in urinary deposit • Isolation of virus • Demonstration of IgM antibody	• Cataract • Glaucoma • Deafness • Heart defects • Microcephaly • Hydrocephaly • Bone lesions • Isolation of rubella virus • IgM antibody	• Coombs' test +ve • Evidence of blood group incompatibility between mother and infant • Increased titre of immune antibody in mother

severity of jaundice and type, whether increase is in conjugated or unconjugated bilirubin.

- Total serum bilirubin level serves as a useful guide to the development of kernicterus.

  Serial levels are useful in the assessment of prolonged jaundice. The level rises slowly and continuously in atresia of the bile ducts, whereas it reaches a rapid peak and gradually falls with recovery in haemolytic disease of the newborn (HDN). Total serum bilirubin level fluctuates in neonatal hepatitis.
- Bromsulphalein (BSP) is retained in the newborn, not through deficiency of cojugation but through deficiency in hepatic excretion.
- Serum cholesterol determinations are unhelpful, although extremely high levels may be recorded in biliary atresias.
- Serum alkaline phosphatase level (ALP) is normally somewhat higher than in the adult, but it is of no diagnostic importance in neonatal jaundice.
- Serum GOT/GPT levels, probably reach 120 units/dl in normal neonates. High levels over 800 or more units suggests hepatitis.

Refer flow chart 15.1 for laboratory investigation of neonatal jaundice.

Flow Chart 15.1: Laboratory investigation of neonatal jaundice

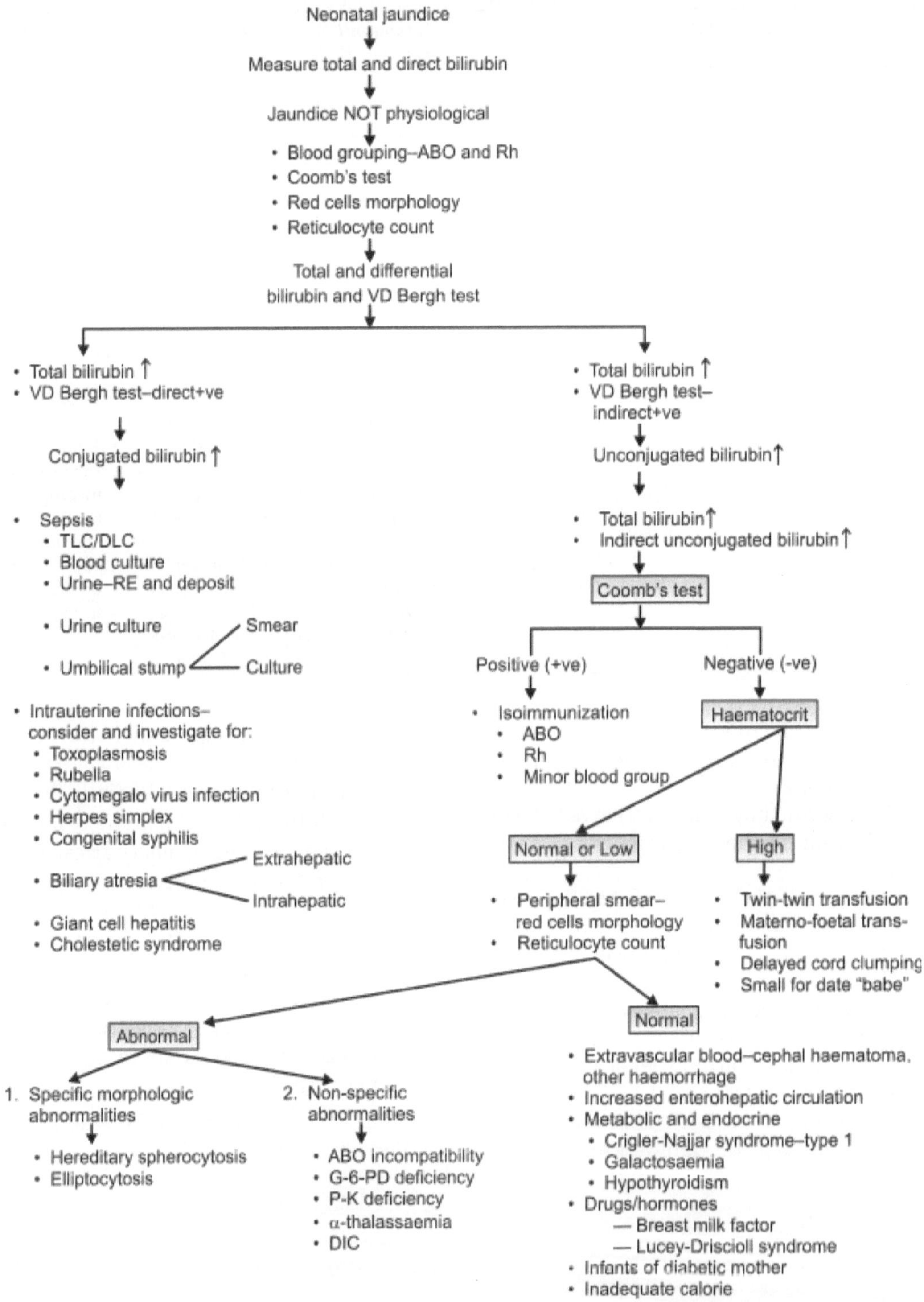

Chapter 16

Hyperthyroidism*

INTRODUCTION

The term hyperthyroidism denotes the biochemical, physiological and clinical findings associated with hyperactivity of thyroid gland. The condition is characterized by generalized enhancement of metabolic rate and oxygen consumption with or without weight loss. Common manifestations of the disease comprise nervousness, emotional lability, insomnia, frequent bowel movements, heat intolerance, excessive sweating and increased weight loss. Dyspnoea and palpitations along with oligomenorrhoea and amenorrhoea in premenopausal women also tend to occur.

THYROTOXICOSIS

TYPES AND CAUSES

The term thyrotoxicosis signifies the clinical condition when tissues are exposed and respond to excess thyroid hormones. The aetiology of the condition might be primary hyperfunction of thyroid gland or any other abnormality leading to increased plasma thyroid hormone levels. Therefore, thyrotoxicosis is not a specific disease but a clinical condition which can originate from a variety of problems (Table 16.1) and may or may not be associated with hyperthyroidism. The sustained overproduction of thyroid hormones by the gland itself may be due to excessive secretion of TSH which, in turn, might originate from a pituitary tumour or associated with resistance of pituitary to the raised levels of thyroid hormones. Sometimes, the source of thyroid hormones can be extrathyroidal also, e.g., functioning metastatic carcinoma of thyroid and thyrotoxicosis factitia (Hamburger's toxicosis) that results from accidental ingestion of meat containing animal thyroid tissue.

Table 16.1: Types and causes of thyrotoxicosis

- *With hyperthyroidism*
  - I. Hyperthyrotropism (increased TSH)
    - Pituitary tumour
    - Pituitary resistance to thyroid hormones
  - II. Abnormal stimulation
    - Graves' disease
    - Trophoblastic tumour
  - III. Functionally autonomous tissue
    - Adenoma
    - Multinodular goitre
- *Without hyperthyroidism*
  - Thyrotoxic factitia
  - Functioning carcinoma
  - Struma ovarii
  - Transient thyrotoxicosis with thyroiditis

Autoimmunity also plays a significant role in the causation of thyrotoxic state. In the most common form of hyperthyroidism, i.e., Graves' disease, the culprit is specific antibodies

*Contributed by Professor R Chawla, MSc, DMRIT, PhD, Professor of Biochemistry , Faculty of Medicine, Addis-Ababa University, Ethiopia, ex-Professor of Biochemistry, Christian Medical College, Ludhiana (Punjab)

against the TSH receptors, which provide homeostatically unregulated stimulation of the gland, known as ***long acting thyroid*** stimulator (LATS). Thyrotoxic state also appears, albeit transiently, in Hashimoto's thyroiditis because of the leakage of preformed thyroid hormones from the gland due to inflammatory injury.

Note

The distinction between hyperthyroidism and thyrotoxicosis is, thus, very much essential and must be considered not only for diagnosis but also in selecting the treatment protocol. Although, the diseases that cause thyrotoxicosis make their own contribution to the overall clinical picture, the manifestations of the thyrotoxic state are largely the same.

Multinodular toxic goitre (MNG) is frequently associated with hyperthyroid state and autonomy of the nodules is an underlying phenomenon. Most often than not, it is a consequence of a long standing simple goitre and therefore, multinodular goitre is a disease of the elderly.

Sometimes ***hyperthyroidism*** is also observed in case of trophoblastic tumours, e.g., choriocarcinoma and hydatidiform mole.

The Jodbasedow phenomenon is another unusual type of thyrotoxicosis and is induced by exposure to large doses of iodine particularly in areas of endemic iodine deficiency. Similar situation can develop in patients with non-toxic nodular goitre on receiving large doses of iodine.

LABORATORY INVESTIGATIONS

The diagnosis of hyperthyroidism is far less enigmatic than hypothyroidism and most often than not the clinician is able to make a diagnosis on the basis of clinical presentation and the laboratory investigations play a supportive role only. The evaluation of thyroid status under these circumstances also serves as baseline for monitoring of the therapy and progression of the disease. The various thyroid function tests available for evaluation and diagnosis of hyperthyroidism are described under the heads of *in vivo* and *in vitro* investigations.

I. "*In Vivo*" Thyroid Function Tests

Although the *in vitro* estimation of the thyroid hormones and related tests have virtually eclipsed the *in vivo* tests of thyroid function, they still find their application in specific conditions as discussed below.

1. Radioiodine Thyroid Uptake (RTU)

(Refer to Chapter on thyroid function tests)

Interpretation

- Since percentage uptake of the administered radioiodine is proportional to activity of the follicular cells, the increased uptake or early peaking normally are seen in all disorders producing hyperthyroidism. Two hours as well as 24 hours uptake are increased.
- Rarely, in Graves' disease the 2-hours uptake is elevated and 24-hours-uptake is normal due to very high turnover. Such high turnover is always associated with obvious clinical hyperthyroidism. In such a situation, another 8-hours observation is recommended and an ***8-hour-uptake rather than 24-hour-uptake is diagnostic of hyperthyroidism with a very high turnover (Fig. 16.1).***

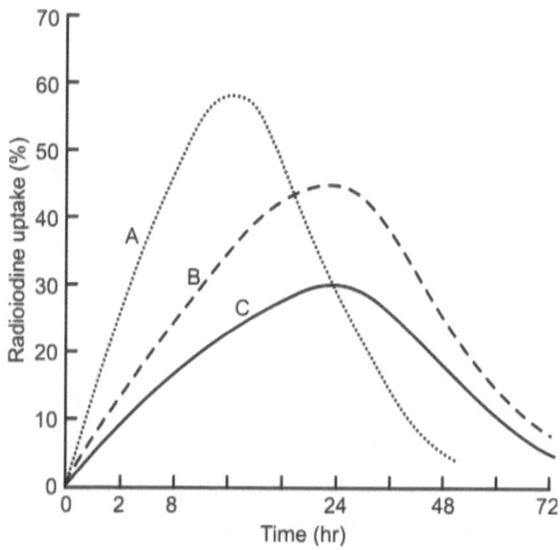

Fig. 16.1: Typical radioiodine uptake curves under various conditions (A) hyperthyroidism; (B) Euthyroid; (C) Thyrotoxicosis without hyperthyroidism

- Thyrotoxicosis not associated with hyperthyroidism, is characterized by subnormal values of RTU. Subacute thyroiditis and chronic thyroiditis with spontaneously resolving thyrotoxicosis are the most common examples in this category.
- In thyrotoxicosis factitia and thyrotoxicosis due to ectopic thyroid tissue, the thyroid gland is suppressed. Therefore, RTU is low and most of the administered radioiodine is excreted in urine.
- In places with endemic goitre, due to chronic iodine deficiency, elevated iodine uptake is common and could interfere with the diagnosis. Earlier, the plasma radioiodine levels were investigated in these situations to distinguish hyperthyroidism from iodine deficiency. In the former case, plasma levels of radioiodine were significantly higher than the later. But these days, plasma radioiodine is seldom measured due to the availability of estimations of thyroid hormones in circulation.

Note
- **Several foods and drugs** are known to interfere with the thyroid uptake studies and are known to depress the uptake values. Ingestion of food rich in iodine such as seafood and medications including amoebicides and antitussives keep the iodine uptake depressed for even up to 30 days.
- **Iodine contrast materials** may decrease uptake, from a few weeks (in cases of excretory urography) to several months and even years in cases of contrast myelography and bronchography.
- **Exogenous T_3 and T_4 hormones** decrease TSH secretion and hence depress iodine uptake.
- The **drugs** like propylthiouracil block thyroid hormone synthesis, but not trapping step, therefore, actually increasing the uptake.
- Prolonged ingestion of ***goitrogenic foods*** as turnips and cabbage liberate thiocyanates, which competitively suppress the iodine uptake.

2. T_3 Suppression Test

Principle
- **Werner** (1955) recognized the application of this test in confirming hyperthyroidism. The premise for the test is that increased levels of circulating T_3 inhibit the secretion of TSH. As the TSH levels fall, thyroid uptake diminishes.

Method
T_3 (25 μg) is administered orally for seven days and radioiodine uptake is measured before and after the therapy.

Interpretations

- Normally, the uptake falls by more than 60% of the baseline value due to decreased levels of TSH.
- The principal application of the test lies ***in differentiating borderline hypethyroidism from euthyroid state.*** In the former, the thyroid uptake does not decrease because of autonomous nature of the disease.

3. Thyroid Scintigraphy

Thyroid imaging can be achieved with a number of techniques including ultrasound and computed tomography, but the most popular and useful modality is scintigraphy with ^{131}I or ^{99m}Tc-pertechnitate.

Indications
The major indications of thyroid scanning are:
- Palpable nodule(s) in the neck.
- Assessment of substernal mass.
- Postoperative search for functioning metastasis.
- Suspicion of occult malignancy but it has also been used for the evaluation of goitre.
- Progress of thyroiditis. Evaluation of the effects of thyroid stimulating and suppressive therapy.

Method

The first radioiodine (^{131}I) thyroid scans were obtained with the help of collimated Geiger-Muller tubes which were followed by rectilinear scanners. Currently, thyroid scans are obtained with gamma camera or SPECT units after oral or i.v. administration of radioiodine (^{131}I) or technetium (^{99m}Tc) pertechnitate. Another technique available for the purpose is fluorescent scanning, which measures the K X-ray given off when iodine atoms are excited by an incident photon beam. The instruments based on fluorescence have been developed and are available commercially but are not very popular.

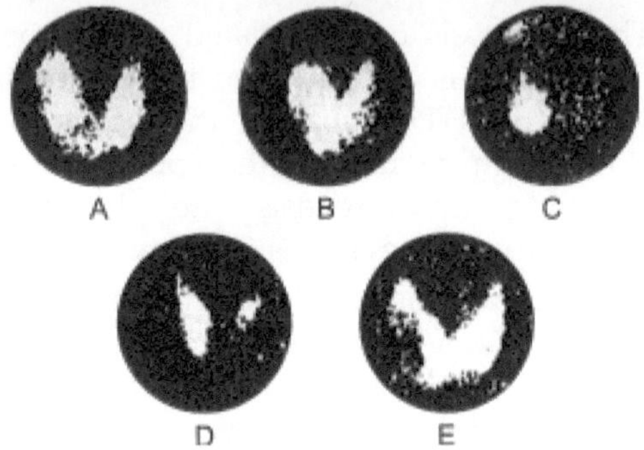

Figs 16.2A to E: Thyroid scintigraphy using ^{99m}Tc pertechnitate (A) Graves' disease, (B) Multinodular goiter, (C) Solitary functioning nodule, (D) Thyroid carcinoma involving left lobe, (E) Colloid cyst

Interpretations

- Thyroid scintigraphy provides the information regarding morphology of the gland, e.g., size and position of the gland, congenital absence of one lobe, sublingual thyroid or substernal extension, etc.
- Also provides the regional information like functioning or non-functioning nodule(s). The functioning nodules concentrate the radioiodine to much higher extent than normal thyroid tissue and therefore appear brighter on the scan called **"hot spots"** whereas non-functioning nodules appear as **"cold nodules"** because they are unable to concentrate radioactive iodine or pertechnitate.
- Hyperfunctioning nodules may be multiple or single and are very prominent on the scan because they suppress the surrounding normal thyroid tissue. In Graves' disease, characterized by diffuse hypertrophy, the gland is usually large and more uniform in size (Fig. 16.2) and on scan appears very bright with well defined margins but nodularity associated with Graves' disease has also been reported. On the other hand in multinodular goitre, a number of **"hot spots"** are observed interspersed with minimal normal tissue which is poorly visualized due to suppression by the raised thyroid hormone levels.
- ***The cold spots on a thyroid scan have for long been associated with malignancy.*** The incidence of malignancy in cold-nodules (20%) is far higher than that in hot-nodules (2%). A number of cold areas interspersed with patches of normal tissue might indicate multiple non-functioning nodules. The clinical findings like number, feel and fixation of the nodules are very important in interpreting a cold nodule on a thyroid scan. Nodules that involve an entire gland are most likely to be caused by subacute thyroiditis. Similarly, large soft nodules with smooth borders are most often benign cysts. Further, the nodules associated with hyperthyroidism are most often benign.

Note

The thyroid gland is, sometimes, not visualized in an iodine scan due to:

- increased iodine pool;
- acute thyroiditis;
- chronic thyroiditis;
- suppressive or antithyroid medication;
- surgical or radioiodine ablation; and
- congenital absence of one or both lobes.

II. *"In Vitro"* Tests for Thyroid Function

In vivo tests have predominated for a long time, but with the advancement of laboratory techniques, the ***in vivo*** tests are becoming more or less redundant in the diagnosis of hyperthyroidism, particularly where it is not accompanied by nodular goitre in which case radioiodine thyroid scan may be very helpful. As in case of hypothyroidism, a wide range of *in vitro* tests are now available in the hands of clinician. Further, the clinical picture in case of hyperthyroidism is much more clear than that in hypothyroidism and many a times the laboratory investigations just serve as baseline for evaluation of therapy rather than necessary diagnostic aids.

The earliest methods developed for the estimation of serum levels of thyroid hormones were protein bound iodine (PBI) and butanol extractable iodide (BEI), both of which were painfully laborious and involved extraction of iodine associated with the serum proteins. These assays served the clinicians for a number of decades before being replaced by two ingenuous assays, i.e., T_3 uptake and competitive protein binding assays; the later then paved the way for the radio and enzyme immunoassays.

1. T_3 Red Cells Uptake Test

Principle

The T_3 red cell uptake test was developed by ***Hamolsky et al*** (1959) and was the first attempt to measure the circulating thyroid hormones and their interaction with the plasma proteins. The test was based on competition between serum thyroid hormone binding proteins and washed red cells to bind labelled T_3. The test involves incubation of test serum with radiolabelled T_3 along with washed RBC. The greater the plasma T_4 concentration is, fewer the unoccupied binding sites on the transport proteins, hence, larger proportion of the added labelled T_3 will be free to be adsorbed on the RBCs. The principle is described in Fig. 17.2 (Chapter 17 on hypothyroidism). The RBCs in the test were later replaced with a different resins by different manufacturers and a number of commercial kits known as T_3-resin uptake kits became available. These days the resins have themselves been replaced by the use of specific anti-T_3 antibodies, many times coated on the surface of the polypropylene tubes.

Interpretations

The T_3 uptake test finds its application in the indirect estimation of free T_4 known as ***free thyroxine index*** *((FTI)* and is particularly useful in conditions where alterations in the total T_3 and T_4 levels are suspected to be due to changes in the levels of binding proteins especially TBG. Various conditions influencing TBG concentrations are described in Table 17.2 (Chapter 17 on hypothyroidism). The test continues to serve the thyroid clinicians even after four decades of its inception.

2. Competitive Protein Binding (CPB) Assays

Murphy et al (1966) introduced a technique called as **saturation analysis.** This replaced the earlier cumbersome and less reliable estimates of circulating hormones, e.g., protein bound iodine (PBI) or butanol extractable iodide (BEI) and T_4 by column. In this test serum T_4 was extracted by alcohol, which was then incubated with TBG saturated with labelled T_4. The labelled T_4 displaced from TBG was then scavenged with the help of a resin. The test results could differentiate hyperthyroidism but were not as good for hypothyroidism in which case considerable overlap was observed between hypothyroid and euthyroid ranges. The major drawback of the assay again was the interference by the serum proteins albeit in the opposite dir-ection to that in T_3 uptake.

3. Radioimmunoassays of Thyroid Hormones

Principle

The radioimmunoassay (RIA) technique was introduced in 1959 by **Berson and Yalow** when they developed an assay system for insulin. Their technique was adapted for the estimation of thyroid hormones by **Gharib et al. (1970) and Chopra et al. (1971).** The RIA tests are based on the competition between the hormone in serum with exogenously added labelled hormone for the limited number of binding sites on the antibodies against that hormone. The assays for circulating thyroid hormones involve the release of hormones from the binding proteins which is generally achieved with the help of 8-anilino-1-naphthalene-sulphonic acid (ANS).

Advantages

Advantages of RIAs involve their extreme sensitivity and simplicity of the procedure which are now available in different formats including IRMA.

Procedure

- ***Immunometric assays (IRMA):*** employ multiple sets of highly specific monoclonal antibodies; one of which is labelled with radioiodine and hence, differ from conventional RIAs in their use of labelled antibodies rather than labelled antigens.
- ***Enzyme-linked immunosorbent assay (ELISA) techniques:*** These were developed primarily to avoid the radioisotopes and the associated restrictions/hazards. There are various types of ELISA tests available in different formats including the most recent microwells, for the estimation of thyroid hormones. These assays are almost as sensitive as RIA and have become more popular due to no requirement of technical personnel and less expensive infrastructure.
- ***Chemiluminescence immunoassays (CIA) and fluorescence immunoassays (FIA),*** both of which are again based on the principle of RIA or IRMA but use luminescent or fluorescent chemicals as labels are the next addition to the list of immunoassays.

Table 16.2: Various conditions associated with hyperthyroxinemia

Clinical condition	T_4	T_3
• *Increased T_3/T_4 Binding:*		
A. Increased TBG	H	H
B. Increased TBPA	H	N or H
C. FDH*	H	N or H
D. Anti-T_4 antibodies	H	N
E. Anti-T_3 antibodies	N	H
• *Pituitary and peripheral resistance*	H	H
• *Non-thyroidal illness (NTI)*	L	L
• *Acute psychiatric illness*	H	N or H
• *Hyperemesis gravidarum*	H	N
• *Drugs:*		
A. Radiographic contrast agents	H	L
B. Propranolol	H	L
C. Amiodarone	H	L
D. Heparin	H	N
E. Levothyroxine therapy	H	N

• FDH: Familial dysalbuminic hyperthyroxinaemia, TBG: Thyroxine binding globulin, TBPA: Thyroxine binding prealbumin, H: High, N: Normal, L: Low

(a) Serum Total T_3 and T_4 Assays

Interpretations

- Serum T_3 and T_4 levels are the most common laboratory investigations of hyperthyroidism because both of them are elevated in most of the hyperthyroidism cases. The serum thyroxine RIA can detect hyperthyroidism with a sensitivity as high as 90%, whereas tri-iodothyronine has been found to be raised in about 70% of the cases. Sometimes, normal T_4 values have been found along with raised T_3 levels in so-called T_3-thyrotoxicosis.
- Increased serum T_4 levels can occur from a variety of other causes also (Table 16.2). The most common among these is the ***increased serum binding proteins.*** The patients with ***acute hepatitis*** may have increased serum T_4 levels secondary to increases in TBG. ***In hospitalized patients isolated hyperthyroxinaemia in euthyroid patients is almost as common as true hyperthyroidism.***
- ***Non-thyroidal illnesses (NTI)*** mostly present with low levels of T_3 and T_4, but rarely increased T_4 concentration has also been observed.
- ***In familial dysalbuminaemic hyperthyroxinaemia,*** inherited as autosomal trait, the plasma concentration of an albumin variant, with an unusally high affinity for T_4, is increased. As a result, ***the serum T_4 is markedly elevated although clinically, the patient is essentially euthyroid.*** In such a

situation even T_3 uptake does not reflect the increase in the intensity of T_4 binding (because affinity rather than capacity of T_4 binding is raised) and hence free T_4 index (FT_4I) is raised, often leading to mistaken diagnosis of thyrotoxicosis. Estimation of free T_4 by radioimmunoassay are mostly normal and hence, can help in the diagnosis; but rarely, high free T_4 levels may also be observed in familial dysalbuminaemic hyperthyroxinaemia.

- Spuriously increased levels of thyroid hormones (T_3 or T_4) are also found in patients who have developed ***antibodies against*** T_3 ***or*** T_4. The condition can be demonstrated by incubating the patient's serum with radiolabelled T_4 and measuring the radioactivity in the immune complexes precipitated with polyethylene glycol (PEG). The increased activity over a parallel run control, would indicate the presence of antibodies to T_4.
- ***Serum*** T_3 ***estimation has been found to be a poor indicator for diagnosing hyperthyroidism,*** particularly in hospital settings where presence of NTI lowers an otherwise elevated T_3 level to bring it within normal limit; whereas the T_4 level is affected in very severe disease only.
- T_3 hyperthyroidism occurs in about 4% of the hyperthyroidism patients, but in areas of iodine deficiency, the incidence might be much higher. In ***endemic iodine deficiency patients,*** the T_3 concentration is usually higher than T_4 levels and the TSH levels are raised, although the patients are clinically euthyroid.

(b) Serum Free Thyroxine Assay

With the increases in thyroxine binding proteins the corresponding increase in serum T_3 and/or T_4 occur that are not reflected in clinical state. ***In these situations, the free*** T_4 ***(or even free*** T_3***) is more closely correlated with the patient's clinical status.*** The assays for the estimation of free hormones in the presence of bound ones have been elusive or cumbersome and hence indirect assays like free T_4 Index (FT_4I) have found much popularity under these conditions (explained above). The RIA as well as EIA are now available which can measure the free thyroid hormones with reasonable reliability. ***Free*** T_4 ***assays are in general more reliable than free*** T_3 ***assays and correlate better with the clinical findings.***

Interpretations

- Typically, in hyperthyroidism, whether primary or secondary in origin, the ***free*** T_3 ***and*** T_4 ***levels are found to be increased.*** These elevations correlate very well with the clinical condition and are not affected by the changes in the binding proteins. Although it has been claimed that the free T_4 levels are within normal limits in non-thyroidal illness (NTI), there are reports that contradict this claim. In general, it is agreed that free T_4 values represent thyroidal status very well even in hospitalized patients. FT_4I has also been found to be helpful in NTI patients but is low in critically ill patients.

Note

Certain drugs are known to interfere with free T_4 estimations, e.g., serum total T_4 as well free T_4 levels in patients on *phenytoin* are about 15 to 30% lower than in normal subjects. Similar findings are also observed with *carbamazepine* treatment. ***Heparin also interferes with free*** T_4 ***estimations, hence, use of heparinized blood should be avoided for free*** T_4 ***assays.***

- In ***familial dysalbuminaemic hyperthyroxinaemia*** total T_3 and T_4 as well as FT_4I might be elevated although the patient is essentially euthyroid. Free T_4 assays mostly yield normal values in these patients.

In view of the above, it appears that the free hormone assays are much more useful in the diagnosis of thyroid diseases, in all clinical conditions, than the total T_3/T_4 estimations and with the technical improvements in the assay procedures, are becoming more and more popular with the clinicians. In the coming years, the free hormone estimations may totally replace the total hormone assays.

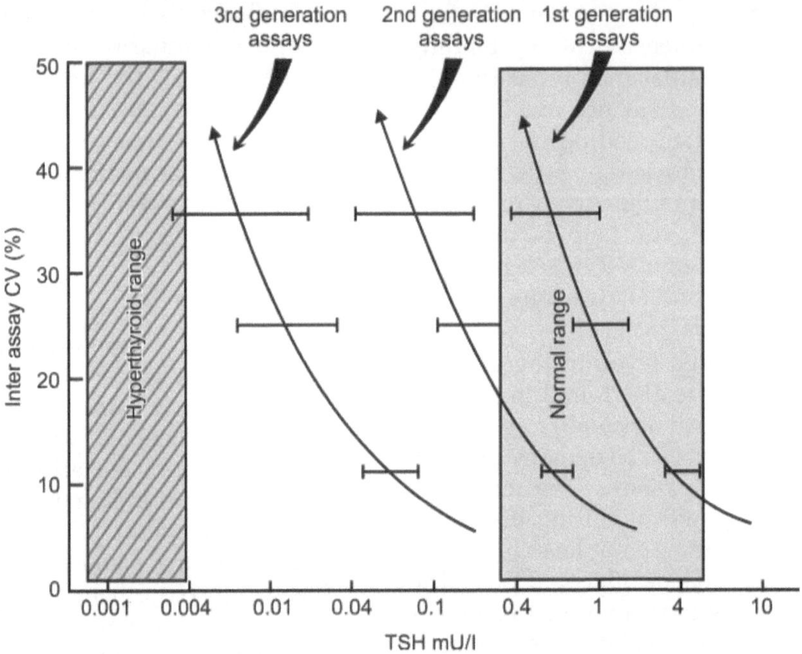

Fig. 16.3: Development of the TSH assays

C. Serum Thyrotropin Assay

Principle and Methodologies:

Thyrotropin (TSH) estimation has shown tremendous developmental strides over the last two decades. The earliest TSH assays suffered lack of both sensitivity as well as specificity. Therefore, falsely elevated TSH levels, due to cross reaction with HCG or FSH and LH, were observed in conditions like pregnancy or postmenopausal states. Further, the sensitivity of these assays was higher than the lower limit of normal range and, hence, could not be used for the diagnosis of hyperthyroidism. ***These problems have been solved by the use of highly specific monoclonal antibodies*** and ***by immunoradiometric assay (IRMA).*** The latest TSH assays, popularly called ***"sensitive TSH assays"*** or ***"third generation TSH assays"*** have sensitivity extending much below the lower limit of normal range (Fig. 16.3) and are claimed to have absolute specificity to TSH only. These assays have opened the use of TSH estimations to the till now forbidden hyperthyroid state also.

Interpretations

- Various reports are available emphasizing the application of TSH estimations in hyperthyroidism. A new strategy is now developing under which ***major emphasis is on using TSH as the single primary screening test for all the thyroid disorders including hyperthyroidism.*** The sensitivity of third generation TSH assays for detecting hyperthyroidism has been reported to be as high as 90 to 98% by various workers.
- The very low or absent TSH in a third generation assay is almost diagnostic of an excess of thyroid hormone levels. Further, the low TSH levels in these assays are almost certain signs that the patient will have a suppressed response to TRH, thus obviating the need, in most patients, of performing a TRH stimulation test.

Note

- The test still has to be used with a great degree of caution because falsely suppressed TSH levels might be observed in a number of clinical conditions. The ability of TSH measurement to appropriately assess the thyroid status is, by definition, ***dependent on the functional and structural integrity of hypothalamic-pituitary axis.***

- Rarely, tumours or other lesions of pituitary or hypothalamus may affect TSH feed-back response leading to inappropriate release of TSH.
- Most commonly, disparities between TSH and free T_4 levels are related to systemic illnesses, major psychiatric disturbances, acute dopamine or glucocorticoid therapy and pharmacological use of some hormones which may transiently inhibit pituitary TSH secretion. Therefore, in such conditions TSH measurement alone might not be enough to provide us with a clear decision.
- In hospitalized euthyroid patients (NTI) again the low TSH levels might be observed, although the level of depression is much above than that found in hyperthyroidism.
- ***TSH estimations can also serve as an excellent tool for monitoring the response to antithyroid therapy for hyperthyroidism.*** But during the first few months of therapy, the TSH measurements are of little significance because the hypothalamic-pituitary system takes a long time to stabilize against the new thyroid hormone status. The persistence of low TSH for prolonged periods reflect a prolonged recovery from profound TSH suppression or a persistent state of subclinical hyperthyroidism.

d. TRH Stimulation Test

The test monitors the integrity and status of hypothalamus-pituitary axis and is still ***one of the most reliable tests for diagnosing borderline hyperthyroidism.***

Procedure

TRH (500 µg Thypinone) is injected IV and the serum TSH levels are measured before and after 30 and 120 minutes of injection.

Interpretation

- ***In euthyroid cases,*** the TSH levels increase within 30 minutes but ***in hyperthyroidism*** the response to TRH stimulation is either not observed or is very diminished. It must be noted that poor TRH response is also observed in case of treated Graves' disease because circulating TSH is already increased (Table 16.3).

Table 16.3: TRH stimulation test—thyroid and pituitary disorders

	Pre-TRH TSH	*Post-TRH TSH*
• Normal	<5 µU/ml	Approx. 25 µU/ml at 30 minutes
• Graves' disease	↓	↓
• Nodular goitre	↓	↓
• Pituitary hyperthyroidism	↑	No response

III. Special Tests for Hyperthyroidism

1. Serum Thyroxine Binding Globulin (TBG) Assay

Estimation of TBG is possible by radioimmunoassay and by electrophoresis and can be helpful in the patients with suspected changes in binding capacity of serum proteins. ***The ambiguous results of T_3, T_4 and TSH measurements, incompatible with the clinical findings can be sorted out by estimating the TBG levels.***

2. TBG: T_4 Ratio

Another parameter, i.e., ***ratio of TBG : T_4*** has also been used in patients with binding protein abnormalities. Some workers have advocated that TBG : T_4 ratio better compensates for TBG alterations than even the free thyroxine. But since the TBG estimation by RIA is relatively newer test and is not included in the routine thyroid function protocol, further reports are awaited to prove its utility.

3. Serum Antithyroid Antibodies

Normal thyroglobulin circulates systemically in very low amounts and may induce a "low zone" T-lymphocyte tolerance with weak synthesis of antithyroglobulin antibodies. This antibody levels increase gradually with age. Sometimes due to exposure to chemicals or infection, an immune response against one or more components of thyroid gland may be induced. In clinical conditions, these antibodies are present in most of the thyroiditis and follicular carcinoma patients, 70 to 90% of Graves' disease and about half of the thyrotoxicosis cases. The antibodies in these autoimmune states do not seem to have a primary pathogenic role, but once formed may cause further tissue damage.

Classically, autoantibodies to thyroid antigens have been measured by precipitation reactions, haemagglutination and by immunofluorescence. However, these tests are subjective and lack high sensitivity. ELISA and RIA methods are these days available for all kinds of antibodies separately.

Other 'antitissue' autoimmune states like pernicious anaemia, myasthenia gravis, systemic lupus erythematosus and rheumatoid arthritis may also have the antithyroid antibodies, but mostly titre in these diseases is not as high as in thyroiditis and Graves' disease. (Refer to Chapter on thyroid function test for details).

4. Serum Thyroglobulin Assay

Thyroglobulin (Tg) normally circulates in blood in very low quantities, but in case of tissue damage as in thyroiditis or Graves' disease Tg is released into plasma in greater amounts and hence the Tg levels in blood are raised. In well differentiated follicular carcinoma cases, the thyroglobulin is systhesized in large amounts due to increase in cellular mass and the levels of Tg are elevated. In serum; the elevated levels of thyroglobulin can be demonstrated by RIA or ELISA.

Measurement of Tg is also useful to confirm thyrotoxicosis factitia. Levels are elevated in Graves' disease and thyroiditis but are subnormal in thyrotoxicosis factitia is due to suppression by the exogenous hormones.

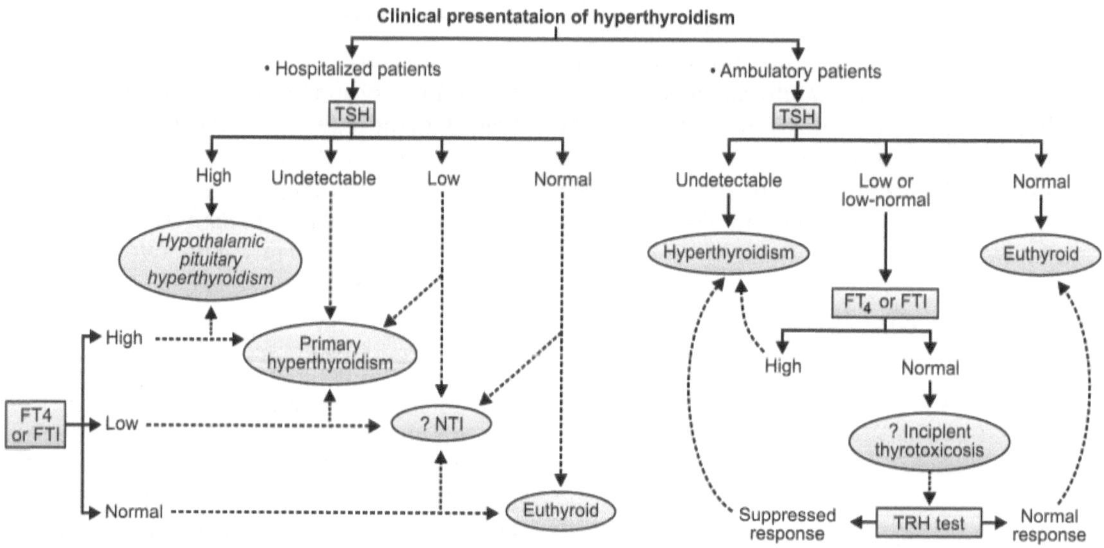

Fig. 16.4: Test profile for hyperthyroid patients utilising 3rd generation TSH assays (TSH and FT4 estimation are recommended for hospitalized patients, whereas TSH alone is required for primary screening of ambulatory patients.)

5. Long Acting Thyroid Stimulator (LATS)

The basic factor responsible for Graves' disease is the perpetual stimulation by an immunoglobulin or family of immunoglobulins directed against the TSH receptors. Two opposing type of antibodies (stimulatory and inhibitory) have been implicated and the disturbance of the homeostasis has been proposed to be the precipitant for autoimmune state leading to Graves' disease. The levels of these antibodies, i.e., stimulatory (LATS) as well as inhibitory (thyroid inhibitory immunoglobulin, TII) can be estimated by RIA and ELISA techniques and can be very helpful in establishing the diagnosis. In patients with unilateral or bilateral ophthalmopathy not associated with thyrotoxicosis, the demonstration of significantly high titres of LATS suggests that the cause is Graves' disease.

GUIDELINES FOR THE DIAGNOSIS OF HYPERTHYROIDISM

The flow chart given on page 180 (Fig. 16.4) represents the general guidelines for the diagnosis of hyperthyroidism in view of the latest developments in laboratory technology. The additional tests may be required to support or augment the diagnosis in specific conditions as discussed above.

Chapter 17

Hypothyroidism*

INTRODUCTION

The normal function of thyroid gland is directed to the secretion of L-thyroxine (T_4) and 3, 5, 3'-triiodo-L-thyronine (T_3), the hormones that influence a number of metabolic processes, Hypothyroidism, characterised by decreased caloric expenditure or a hypometabolic state can result from any of a variety of abnormalities that lead to insufficient synthesis of thyroid hormones. If hypothyroidism is present since birth and results in developmental abnormalities, it is termed as ***cretinism***. In the adult form, accumulation of hydrophilic mucopolysaccharides in the ground substance of dermis and other tissues results in thickening of facial features and skin and the condition is termed as ***myxoedema***.

Over the last few decades a number of thyroid function tests have been developed, some based on the use of radioisotopes and others without them. Each one of these tests has its own advantages and hence application, but none of these is without disadvantages. Therefore, the clinician has to interpret the results critically in the light of the clinical situation. Before we discuss the application of each of these tests, we must look into aetiology of hypothyroidism.

CLASSIFICATION

A classification of hypothyroidism is presented in Table 17.1. It has been observed that about 95% of the hypothyroidism cases are thyroid in origin with suprathyroid variety accounting for only 5% of the patients. The ***most common cause of primary hypothyroidism appears to be autoimmunity*** and is associated with circulating antithyroid antibodies and sometimes might have originated from the action of antibodies that block the TSH receptors. Hashimoto's

Table 17.1: Classification of the causes of hypothyroidism

Primary to thyroid	*Suprathyroid*
I. *Non-goitrous*	I. *Pituitary*
• Congenital	• Panhypopituitarism
• Primary idiopathic	• TSH deficiency
• Post-ablative (Radioiodine, Surgery)	
II. *Goitrous*	II. *Hypothalamic*
• Hereditary biosynthetic defect	• Congenital defects
• Iodine deficiency	• Encephalitis
• Chronic thyroiditis (Hashimoto's)	• Infiltrative (Sarcoidosis)
• Maternally transmitted	• Neoplastic
• Drug induced	

Contributed by Professor R Chawla, MSc, DMRIT, PhD, Professor of Biochemistry , Faculty of Medicine, Addis-Ababa University, Ethiopia, ex-Professor of Biochemistry, Christian Medical College, Ludhiana (Punjab)

thyroiditis is characterised by defective organification of iodine along with or due to the presence of antithyroid antibodies. ***Another common cause of hypothyroidism is radioiodine or surgical ablation of the gland in the treatment of thyrotoxicosis.***

- Inability to synthesise adequate amount of thyroid hormones results in hypersecretion of TSH and hence goitre. This compensatory response may or may not be sufficient to achieve euthyroid state. Therefore, ***the most common finding in hypothyroidism is increased TSH levels in serum.***
- ***In suprathyroid hypothyroidism,*** the thyroid is intrinsically normal but is deprived of stimulation by TSH. Deprivation of TSH may be due to postpartum necrosis or a tumour of pituitary. Hypothalamic hypothyroidism is rare.

LABORATORY INVESTIGATIONS

The earliest laboratory investigations of thyroid function were based on metabolic impact of thyroid hormones. ***Measurements of oxygen consumption in the basal state (Basal metabolic rate, BMR), once mainstay in the diagnosis of thyroid disorders, are only of historical interest today.*** Several blood tests may be abnormal in patients with thyroid disease, but lack of specificity limits their utility. For example, serum ***concentration* of *creatinine phosphokinase*** and less frequently, ***lactate dehydrogenase*** and ***aspartate aminotransferase*** are increased in hypothyroidism. Increases in cholesterol levels are common in hypothyroidism of thyroid origin.

Laboratory investigations can be discussed under the following heads:

I. ***In vivo tests for thyroid function***
II. ***In vitro tests for thyroid function.***

I. *In Vivo* Tests For Thyroid Function

The radioactive iodine studies provide excellent way of assessing the thyroid function and have been extensively used for a long time. Among all the tests designed to assess thyroid function, only those which involve *in vivo* administration of radioactive iodine, test glandular function 'per se'. The radioactive iodine concentration by the thyroid tissue can either be quantitated as in uptake studies to test hypo-or hyper-functioning gland or imaged (thyroid scanning) to give us regional distribution of iodine in the gland.

- ***Radioiodine Thyroid Uptake***

The thyroid uptake is the percentage of an administered radiopharmaceutical (^{131}I or ^{123}I or ^{99m}Tc) incorporated by the thyroid gland in a defined period of time. The radiopharmaceutical is given ***orally*** or ***intravenously*** and its concentration by thyroid gland is monitored with the help of a detector probe placed in front of the neck. If radioiodine is administered orally, the measured uptake increases progressively, reaching a plateau between 18 and 24 hours after intake (Fig. 17.1). Generally, two observations, i.e. at 2 hours and 24 hours are adequate.

Interpretations

- ***The slow and subnormal uptake is observed in hypothyroidism.*** The two-hour uptake is occasionally useful, especially in diagnosing thyroiditis in which trapping function is normal or increased and organification is impaired. This condition results in normal

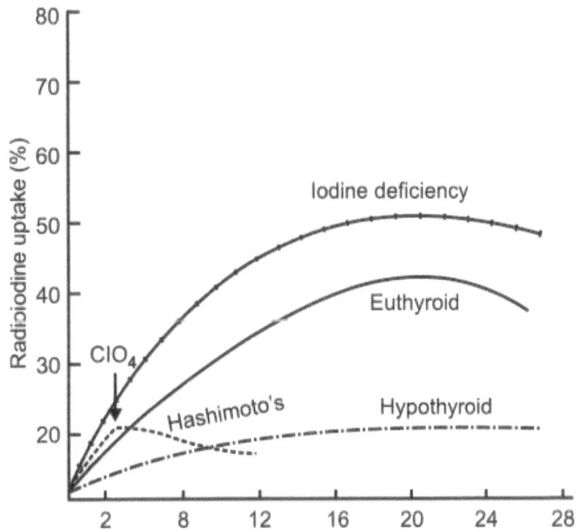

Fig. 17.1: Thyroid uptake curves in hypothyroidism and Hashimoto's disease

or elevated 2-hour uptake and low 24-hour uptake.

- *In iodine deficiency goitre* (fully or partially compensated), the 2-hour radioiodine uptake is supranormal due to iodine-starved tissue, the 24 hours uptake is generally normal or marginally elevated.

• Modifications of Thyroid Uptake Studies

1. Absolute Iodine Uptake and Plasma/Urinary Levels

The absolute iodine uptake measures the quantity of iodine extracted by the thyroid per unit time. The test is seldom used because the method involves measurements of plasma and urinary radioactivity along with stable urinary iodine levels. Its utility has been particularly emphasised in the study of endemic goitre but is of historical importance only.

2. Perchlorate Washout Test

Principle:

The test is based on the fact that ClO_4 is trapped by thyroid tissue and can displace unorganified iodine. In organification defects, such as ***peroxidase deficiency***, unorganified iodine is discharged from the gland.

Procedure

The patient is administered with 20 μCi ^{131}I orally and 2-hour uptake is measured. The patient is then given $KClO_4$ and the thyroid radioactivity is measured every 15 minutes for 90 minutes.

Interpretation

If a significant organification defect exists, the thyroid activity falls at least 15% below the 2-hour level. The ***test is positive in congenital goitres and Hashimoto's thyroiditis.***

• TSH Stimulation Test

Principle:

The test measures the thyroid gland's ability to respond to stimulation by its natural stimulant, i.e. TSH. Since TSH affects almost all the steps in hormonogenesis by the thyroid tissue, the effects of exogenous TSH can be evaluated at almost any level.

Procedure

The test is performed by first obtaining a baseline 24-hour radioiodine uptake. The patient is then given 10 units of bovine TSH intramuscularly for three days followed by repeat uptake study next day.

Interpretations

- More than 50% increase in iodine uptake is normally observed.
- ***The test has been used to differentiate between primary and secondary hypothyroidism.***
- In secondary hypothyroidism, since the endogenous synthesis of TSH is defective, the thyroid responds well to exogenous TSH.
- In primary disease, the glandular function is subnormal accompanied by increased levels of TSH, the thyroid tissue does not show any change in radioiodine uptake upon TSH administration.

Note

With the development of sensitive radioimmunoassay methods for measuring TSH levels, TRH stimulation test has largely replaced TSH stimulated iodine uptake test. In countries where TRH preparations are not available, TSH stimulation can still be used very effectively.

• Thyroid Scanning (Scintigraphy)

Principle:

Thyroid gland can be scanned with the help of ultrasonography, computed tomography and magnetic resonance imaging to get information like thyroid mass, presence of any cyst or solid tumour, etc. But the information provided by the radioiodine ^{131}I or ^{99m}Tc scintigraphy is much more comprehensive. The scanning is done with the help of gamma camera after administering 10-25 μCi of ^{131}I or 2 mCi of ^{99m}Tc pertechnitate.

Interpretations

• The radioisotope scanning can be useful to know the • extent of the goitre, • to detect any thyroid mass like thyroglossal duct or sternal extensions, etc. and • in case of multinodular goitre where thyroiditis is included in the differential diagnosis.

• ***In thyroiditis,*** the gland may be completely non-visualised, may have a faint outline of an enlarged gland or, more commonly, may show patchy irregularity consisting of cold areas interspersed with areas of hyperplasia.

II. *"In Vitro"* Tests for Thyroid Function

Over the last three decades, a number of ***in vitro*** thyroid function tests have been developed, some based on the use of radioisotopes and others without them. Each one of these tests has its own advantages and hence application, but none of these is without disadvantages. Therefore, the clinician has to interpret the results critically in the light of the clinical situation.

The ***earliest methods*** developed for the estimation of serum levels of thyroid hormones were ***protein bound iodine (PBI)*** and ***butanol extractable iodide (BEI),*** both of which were painfully laborious and involved extraction of iodine associated with the serum proteins. These assays served the clinicians for a long period of time before being replaced by two ingenuous assays, i.e. T_3 uptake and competitive protein binding assays; the later then paved the way for the most significant methodological advancement in analytical sciences, i.e. radioimmunoassays.

• *Radioimmunoassays of Thyroid Hormones*

Principle and Methodologies:

The radioimmunoassay (RIA) technique was introduced in 1959 by **Berson** and **Yalow** and was adapted for the estimation of thyroid hormones by ***Gharib et al (1970)*** and ***Chopra et al (1971).*** The RIA tests are based on the competition between the hormone in the serum with exogenously added labelled hormone for the limited number of binding sites on the antibodies against that hormone. The assays involve the release of hormones from the binding proteins which is generally achieved with the help of 8-anilino-l-naphthalene sulphonic acid (ANS). Advantages of RIAs involve their extreme sensitivity and simplicity of the procedure.

Note

- The recent advancements in RIAs have been the introduction of ***immunometric assays (IRMA)*** which ***employ highly specific monoclonal antibodies*** and the use of labelled antibodies rather than labelled antigens as in conventional assays. These assays have shown a tremendous improvement in sensitivity over RIAs particularly in case of TSH measurement (third generation ultrasensitive assays).
- ***The enzyme-linked immunosorbent assay (ELISA) techniques*** were developed primarily to avoid the radioisotopes and the associated restrictions/hazards. There are various types of ELISA tests available in different formats including the most recent microwells. These assays are almost as sensitive as RIAs and have become more popular due to non requirement of technical personnel and less expensive infrastructure.

• *Serum Triiodothyronine (T_3) and Thyroxine (T_4) Assays*

The serum estimation of T_3 and T_4 levels by RIA, ELISA or recently by chemiluminescence and fluorescence assays are the most popular indices of thyroid function evaluation. ***The T_4 assays are more reliable*** because of relatively constant levels of T_4 in a patient and also due to lesser variability of estimates of T_4 assays as compared to T_3. Further, there is considerable overlap between the hypothyroid and normal ranges for T_3.

Interpretations

- About 20 to 30% hypothyroid patients might show normal T_3 levels.

- Low T_3 values might be observed only in severe cases, i.e. patients having T_4 levels at less than 2.5 μg/dl.
- In addition, ***T_3 is reduced in a number of non-thyroid illnesses (NTI)***, particularly, in myocardial infarction where the decrease in T_3 is very rapid, declining to about 50% of the reference value within three to four days.
- It has also been reported that T_3 levels fall progressively with advancing age.
- ***A decrease in serum T_4 levels is almost uniformly observed in all types of hypothyroidism*** but the levels of T_3 may not be decreased to that extent. This lesser reduction in T_3 may be due to compensatory hypersecretion of TSH which skews the ratio in favour of T_3 either at the synthesis step or by activating the peripheral deiodinases leading to more efficient conversion of T_4 to T_3.
- ***In endemic goitre*** the levels of T_3 and T_4 are grossly normal although near upper limit values are more common.

- ***Serum Thyrotropin (TSH) Assay***

Interpretations

- ***Serum TSH assay is the single most useful measurement in hypothyroidism.*** The thyrotropin levels are raised in goitrous as well as non-goitrous varieties of primary hypothyroidism and is usually normal or low in pituitary or hypothalamic hypothyroidism.
- Some ***euthyroid patients*** show laboratory evidence of hypothyroid state much before it manifests clinically ***(subclinical hypothyroidism).*** Initially, only TSH levels are found to be raised along with normal (near the lower margin of normal range) T_3 and T_4. As the disease advances T_4 levels fall below the normal range but T_3 still might be normal due to hypersecretion of TSH as explained above.
- ***Subclinical hypothyroidism is most often encountered in Hashimoto's disease.***
- ***In the patients treated with ^{131}I or surgery,*** the supranormal levels of TSH with or without low T_4 might be indicative of the developing hypothyroidism. Therefore, these patients along with other high risk patients like neonates of hypothyroid mothers should be routinely screened for TSH and T_4 levels.

- ***T_3 Red Cells Uptake Test (RT_3u)***

Principle:

The T_3 red cell uptake test was developed by ***Hamolsky et al (1959)*** and was the first attempt to measure the circulating thyroid hormones and their interaction with the plasma proteins. The test was based on the competition between serum thyroid hormone binding proteins and washed red cells to bind labelled T_3 and involved incubation of test serum with radio-labelled T_3 along with washed RBC. The greater the plasma T_4 concentration is, fewer the unoccupied binding sites on the transport proteins, hence larger proportion of the added labelled T_3 will be free to be adsorbed on the RBCs. The principle and interpretation of the test is described in Figure 17.2.

Note

The RBCs in the test were later replaced with different **resins** by different manufacturers and a number of commercial kits known as T_3-resin uptake kits became available. ***Recently, the resins have been replaced by the use of specific anti-T_3 antibodies mostly coated on the tubes.***

Interpretations

- The test finds its application in the ***indirect estimation of free hormones known as free thyroxine index (FT_4I) and free T_3 index (FT_3I)*** and is particularly useful in conditions where alterations in the total T_3 and T_4 levels are suspected to be due to changes in the levels of binding proteins especially TBG (Table 17.2). FT_4I and FT_3I are the product of total T_4 or T_3 concentrations with T_3 uptake. The two indices are proportional to free T_4 and free T_3 levels.
- The patients with decreased TBG may show subnormal T_3 and T_4 levels but FTI is normal or increased (Fig. 17.2).

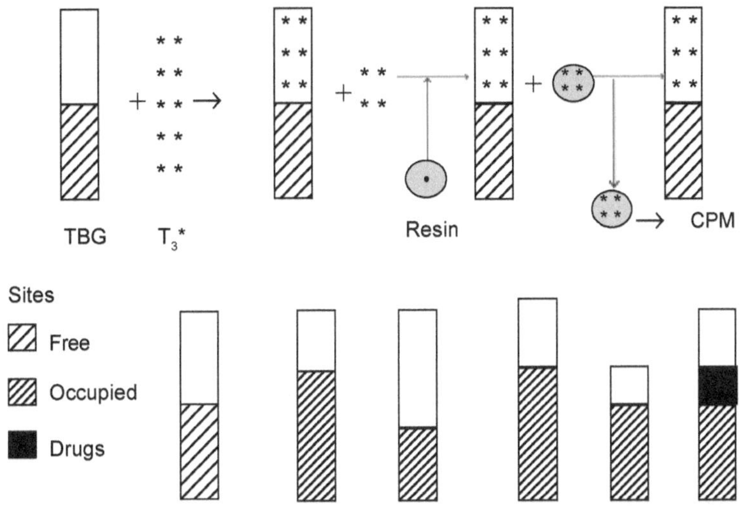

	Normal	Hyper-	Hypo-	↑ TBG	↓ TBG	Drugs
Binding capacity	N	↓	↑	↑	↓	↓
T_3 uptake	N	↑	↓	↓	↑	↑
T3 or T_4	N	↑	↓	↑	↓	↓
TSH	N	↓	↑	N	N	N
Free T_4	N	↑	↓	N	N	N
FT_4I	N	↑	↓	N	N	N

Fig. 17.2: Principle and interpretation of T_3 uptake

Table 17.2: Conditions associated with altered TBG concentrations

Increased TBG	*Decreased TBG*
• Pregnancy	• Androgens
• Oral contraceptives	• Glucocorticoids
• Oestrogen	• Chronic liver disease
• Infectious and chronic hepatitis	• Active acromegaly
• New born state	• Nephrosis
• Acute intermittent porphyria	• Severe systemic illness
• Tamoxifen	
• Biliary cirrhosis	

- ***In severely ill patients (non-thyroidal illness, NTI or sick euthyroid syndrome, SES),*** the intensity of binding of thyroid hormones to plasma proteins is decreased (greater decrease for T_4 than T_3). As a result RT_3U is increased concomitant to the decrease in total T_4 levels. The FT_4I in such cases is normal or increased.
- SES is also associated with lesser production of T_3 hence total T_3 is low in such cases. ***Estimation of reverse T_3 (rT_3) are helpful in this situation because rT_3 is increased in SES*** in proportion to the severity of the disease (Fig. 17.3) owing primarily to retardation in its degradation. Low T_3, T_4 and TSH values in SES may be confused with pituitary hypothyroidism. ***Thus, rT_3 could be a useful parameter in such a condition. Serum rT_3 is decreased in hypothyroidism thus finding of***

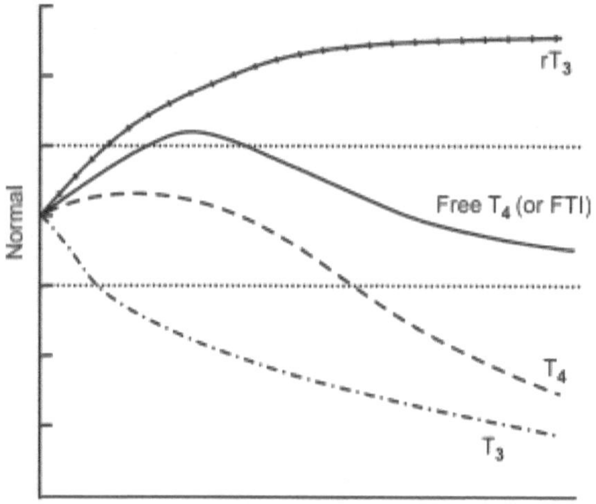

Fig. 17.3: Effect of non-thyroidal illness on thyroid parameters

elevated levels of rT_3 along with low total T_3 and/or T_4 is indicative of non-thyroid illness (NTI or SES).

- ***Free Thyroid Hormones Assay***

The free T_4 levels are the second most reliable test in hypothyroidism after TSH. In fact free T_4 levels closely correlate with the clinical status in all the conditions where total T_4 levels might be misleading. The test has not found its deserved role in the diagnosis of hypothyroidism because of technical reasons. The free T_4 has been estimated by equilibrium dialysis and two step RIA procedures involving extraction of unbound thyroxine; both of these techniques have been too tedious, technically demanding and prone to the technical errors. Further, the cost of these tests have been prohibitory. The recent advances leading to increased sensitivity of RIA and EIA methods have now made the estimation of free T_4 and free T_3 much more reliable as well as cost effective.

Interpretations

- In all kinds of primary as well as suprathyroid hypothyroidism, the free T_4 levels are below the normal range.
- Whereas, in case of euthyroidism with or without protein abnormalities, the free T_4 is always below normal limit of normal range.
- In patients with non-thyroid illness, the FT_4I might be subnormal because T_3 uptake values are low due to reduced binding of T_4 with TBG in NTI, but free T_4 is found to be normal in such circumstances.
- The free T_3 values mostly correlate well with the clinical hypothyroidism, but are inferior to free T_4 estimation.

- ***Serum Thyroxine Binding Globulin (TBG) Assay***

Estimation of TBG is possible by radioimmunoassay and by electrophoresis and can be helpful in the patients with suspected changes in binding capacity of serum proteins. The ambiguous results of T_3, T_4 and TSH measurements, incompatible with the clinical findings can be sorted out by the TBG levels.

TBG: T_4 Ratio

Another parameter, i.e. ratio of TBG : T_4 also ***has been used for the diagnosis of hypothyroidism*** in patients with binding protein abnormalities. Some workers have advocated that TBG : T_4 ratio better compensates for TBG alterations than even the free thyroxine. But since the TBG estimation by RIA is relatively newer test and is not included in the routine thyroid function protocol, more reports are awaited to prove its utility.

- ***Antithyroid Antibodies***

Normal thyroglobulin circulates systemically in very low amounts and may induce a "low zone" T-lymphocyte tolerance with weak synthesis of antithyroglobulin antibodies. This antibody levels increase gradually with age. ***Sometimes due to exposure to chemicals or infection, an immune response against one or more components of thyroid gland may be induced. Hashimoto's thyroiditis*** is an autoimmune inflammatory condition characterised by gland enlargement due to lymphocytic infiltration and is associated with induction of a number of antithyroid antibodies. High titres of antithyroid peroxidase and/or antimicrosomal antibodies are seen in most patients with Hashimoto's thyroiditis and many of the thyroprivic hypothyroidism cases. The antibodies in most of thyroid autoimmune states do not seem to have a primary pathogenic role, but once formed may cause further tissue damage.

The detection of antithyroid antibodies have been done with ***immunofluorescence staining*** and with ***tanned red cells haemagglutination test.*** Former can detect antithyroperoxidase, antithyroid microrsomal as well as antithyroglobulin antibodies, whereas the later is more specific for antithyroglobulin antibodies. ELISA and RIA methods are available for all kinds of antibodies separately these days. Table 17.3 shows the prevalence of antithyroid antibodies in different clinical conditions.

Other antitissue autoimmune states like pernicious anaemia, myasthenia gravis, systemic lupus erythematosus and rheumatoid arthritis may also have the antithyroid antibodies, but mostly titre in these diseases is not as high as in thyroiditis and Graves' disease (Refer to the Chapter on Thyroid function tests for details).

- ***TRH Stimulation Test***

The test monitors the integrity and status of hypothalamus-pituitary axis. TRH (500 μg Thypinone) is injectedd IV, and the serum TSH levels are measured before and after 30 and 120 minutes of injection.

The test is primarily useful for differentiating borderline hyperthyroidism from euthyroidism, also finds its application in establishing the cause of hypothyroidism (Table 17.4) and in the diagnosis of the rare hypothalamic hypothyroidism.

Table 17.4: TSH secretion before and after TRH stimulation in thyroid and pituitary disorders

TSH values by RIA/IRMA	*Pre-TRH*	*Post-TRH*
• **Normal**	<5 μU/ml	Approx. 25 μU/ml at 30 minutes
• **Primary hypothyroidism**	↑↑	↑↑
• **Pituitary hypothyroidism**	↑ or N	↑
• **Hypothalamic hypothyroidism**	↑ or N	Delayed (peak at 60-180 min)
• **Decreased thyroid reserve**	↑	↑

A. Monitoring the Hormone Replacement Therapy

Laboratory measurements also serve as useful guides in the treatment of hypothyroidism with exogenous hormones (levothyroxine sodium). The goal of replacement therapy should be to normalise not only the clinical symptoms but also the FT_4 and TSH levels in hypothyroid patients. Therefore, estimation of serum FT_4 (or FT_4I) and TSH levels in these patients is obligatory. The availability of ultrasensitive TSH (IRMA) assays, which are able to differentiate between normal and suppressed levels of TSH, now enable the clinicians to select a dose of levothyroxine that maintains TSH above

Table 17.3: Prevalence of thyroglobulin and antithyroid antibodies

Clinical condition	*Thyroglobulin*	*Microsomal antibodies*	*Anti-Tg (Ca-2)*
• **Hashimoto's**	75-95	70-90	40-70
• **Idiopathic myxoedema**	75	65	40
• **Non-toxic goitre**	20-30	20	-
• **Ca-thyroid**	40	15	10
• **Graves' disease**	40	50	5-10
• **Pernicious anaemia**	25	10	-
• **Normal**	10	10	-
• **Normal (>70 Yr)**	20	20	-

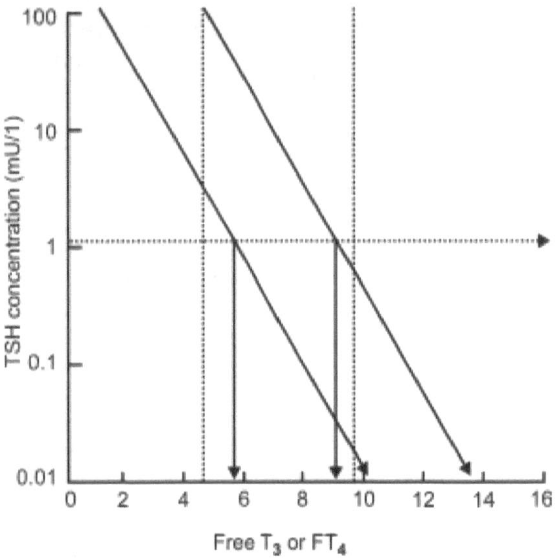

Fig. 17.4: Log-linear relationship between TSH and FT_4 A & B: set points of two patients to achieve midnormal TSH levels

the lower limit of normal range hence preventing the risk of overdosage. This is further emphasized that the dose adjustment must be done on individual basis rather than a universal per kg body weight dose of levothyroxine. The patients do differ in regard to their 'set-point' of FT_4-TSH relationship (Fig. 17.4), i.e. a level of FT_4 which may be sufficient to bring the TSH to midnormal value in one patient (with high-FT_4-TSH set-point) might push another patient (having a low set-point) into hyperthyroid state.

However, it may be stressed that the TSH levels should be measured only after the patient has reached a near euthyroid status based on clinical assessment and serum FT_4 levels. A minimum of 8 weeks should be allowed after the last thyroid hormone dosage adjustment before retesting serum TSH levels in order to ensure that a new steady state has been achieved. Once the FT_4 as well as TSH levels have been normalized, annual or semiannual estimations of TSH are satisfactory for subsequent monitoring as long as the dosage is kept unchaged and patient compliance is maintained.

In case of pituitary or hypothalamic hypothyroidism, since TSH secretion is impaired, restoration of serum FT_4 to normal range along with alleviation of clinical symptoms is the only criteria available for selecting the appropriate dosage of levothyroxine.

B. Guidelines for the Laboratory Management of Hypothyroidism

The preceding discussion of thyroid function testing has been designed with the object of giving the reader an overview of the general principles and applications of various tests available. ***It is generally believed that the 'gold standard' for hypothyroidism testing is TSH levels and second line of testing would be free T_4 or free thyroxine index (FT_4I).*** This has proved to be true to a greater extent, but one must keep in mind the clinical circumstances and the objective of the tests, i.e., the 'clinical question' before ordering the test profile (Table 17.5).

Table 17.5: Suggested test profile for hypothyroidism

Clinical question	*FT_4(FTI)*	*S-TSH*	*Miscellaneous*
• ***Population Screening***			
Ambulatory—well	O	R	-
Hospitalised—sick (SES)	R	R	-
Neonatal Screening*	R	R	TBG (in case of low T_4)
• ***Exclude Hypothyroidism***			
Suspect Disease:	O	R	
Primary hypothyroidism	O	R	Thyroid autoantibodies
Hypothalamic-pituitary disease	R	R	TRH stimulation test
• ***Associated with Protein Abnormalities***	R	R	TBG
Replacement Therapy			
Acute dose adjustment	R	O	
Fine tune/monitoring	O	R	

R—recommended; O—optional; •—might be required.
* Neonates should be screened only after 2-5 days of birth.

Chapter 18

Malabsorption Syndrome

INTRODUCTION

It is a syndrome chiefly characterized by chronic diarrhoea, wasting and weight loss resulting from defects in digestion and/or malabsorption of one or more of the nutrients like lipids, carbohydrates, proteins, vitamins, minerals and water. Malassimilation of nutrients may occur with diseases of small intestine or pancreas. Even stomach may be involved in that the failure of secretion of intrinsic factor can lead to defect in absorption of vitamin B_{12}.

In our country, the necessity of proper understanding of the syndrome cannot be overemphasized, as the condition is widespread. Proper investigation and management of the condition result in marked improvement of the patient.

CAUSES/CLASSIFICATION

1. Defects in Gastric Function

Failure in secretion of intrinsic factor (IF) by stomach. This leads to defective absorption of vitamin B_{12}. Postgastrectomy malabsorption can involve several factors/nutrients.

2. Defective Digestion

a. Defective Luminal Digestion

It involves digestion of major nutrients in the lumen of duodenum and upper part of jejunum. This is due to following conditions.

- ***Defective bile salt secretion*** observed in,
  - Cirrhosis liver.
  - Extrahepatic biliary obstruction.
  - Deconjugation of bile salts.

  In these, emulsification of fat is impaired leading to malabsorption of lipids and lipid-soluble vitamins like vitamin A, D, E and K.
- ***Deficient secretion of pancreatic enzymes*** *seen in:*
  - Chronic pancreatitis
  - Pancreatic calculi
  - Fibrocystic disease of the pancreas
  - Carcinoma of pancreas
  - Inherited trypsinogen deficiency (rare disorder).
- ***Inhibition of pancreatic enzymes*** occurs in Zollinger-Ellison syndrome due to excessive acid secretion in stomach leading to disturbed small intestinal pH (more acidic).

b. Defective Brush Border Digestion

- ***Disaccharidase deficiency:*** affects the maldigestion of the disaccharides leading to malabsorption of disaccharides.
- ***Secondary deficiency of enzyme synthesis:*** seen in protein energy malnutrition (PEM), viz. Kwashiorkor.
- ***Severe deficiency of dietary protein intake:*** can lead to decreased synthesis of enzymes in brush border and also pancreatic enzymes.

3. Defective Intestinal Absorption (Malabsorption)

Most common and important causes are described as follows:

a. Acquired

- *Lesions of intestinal mucosa:*
  - Gluten-induced enteropathy or coeliac disease in children and adults (idiopathic steatorrhoea).
  - Tropical sprue (cause unknown).
- *Infiltrative lesions of small intestinal mucosa and/or lymphglands*
  - Leukaemic infiltrations
  - Lymphoma and lymphosarcoma
  - Hodgkin's disease
  - Small intestinal tuberculosis
  - Sarcoidosis
  - Amyloidosis
  - Scleroderma.
- *Inflammatory lesions of terminal ileum or Crohn's disease:* interfere severely with absorption of vitamin B_{12}.
  Also there is reabsorption of bile salts leading to maldigestion and malabsorption of fats and fat soluble vitamins.
- **Surgical resection of small intestine**
  - Massive resection
  - Gastroileostomy
  - Gastrojejunocolic fistulae.

Note

Effects depend on site and extent of resection. If extensive resection, absorption of all nutrients can suffer. If only jejunum is involved it is compensated by ileal absorption. If terminal ileum is involved, it affects vitamin B_{12} absorption permanently.

- *Iatrogenic* i.e. various drugs viz. neomycin, cholestyramine, colchicine, triparanol, phenidione, mefenamic acid, etc. can interfere with absorption.
- *Effects of radiation*
  - Damages to intestinal mucosa.
  - Overdose can produce nausea, vomiting and interferes with absorption.
- *Endocrine disorders:* may result in disordered absorption, viz:
  - Addison's disease
  - Diabetes mellitus
  - Hypothyroidism
  - Carcinoid tumour etc.
- *Bacterial contamination and bacterial overgrowth in small intestine:* can occur in stagnant areas, e.g.
  - Diverticulosis of jejunum
  - Affarent "Loop syndrome"
  - Strictures, fistulae and anastomosis.
- *Lesions of vessels:*
  - Arterial disorders: mesenteric arterial occlusion
  - Venous congestion:
    - congestive heart failure
    - constrictive pericarditis
- **Abnormalities of lymphatics**:
  - Whipple's disease
  - Intestinal lymphangiectasis
- **Parasitic infestations of the gut:**
  - Giardiasis.
  - Ankylostomiasis
  - Strongyloidosis
  - Dibothriocephalus latus.

b. Congenital Defects of Intestinal Mucosa

- *Glucose transport defect:* interferes with glucose absorption
- *Amino acid transport defect:* interferes with absorption of amino acids.
- *Abetalipoproteinaemia:* interferes with absorption of fats and fat soluble vitamins.

LABORATORY INVESTIGATION

The following should be the aims/objectives of investigation:

- *To confirm or exclude the clinical diagnosis*
- *To find out the nature of malabsorption syndrome-defect is digestive (pancreatic) or only absorption (small intestine).*

- ***To establish the degree and extent of malabsorption.***
- ***To identify the cause of malabsorption.***

Large number of tests are available; being used mainly to demonstrate the malabsorption of lipids, carbohydrates, proteins, vitamins and minerals. Lipid digestion and absorption being complex, is often the first to be disturbed, and malabsorption of fats results in increase in faecal fat called as ***"steatorrhoea"***, which is present in generalized malabsorption and in many cases involving a more limited disturbance.

Before the various laboratory tests are discussed it is necessary to have a proper history and clinical examination of the patient which throw light on the nature of malabsorption and the cause.

A. HISTORY AND CLINICAL FEATURES

- ***Alteration in Bowel Habits***

In majority of cases, frequency of stool is increased 3 to 8 per day. Frequency of stool is usually greater in small bowel diseases (3-8/day), as compared to pancreatic disorders (2-3/day).

In ***giardiasis***, patients have an urgent desire to defecate after meals and complain of colicky pain just before defecation. In pancreatic diarrhoea, it is aggravated with fatty foods.

In ***tropical sprue***, bowel habits increase on taking milk, spices.

- ***Abdominal Pain***

In *intestinal tuberculosis, Crohn's disease* or stricture of bowel there is severe colicky pain in umbilical region.

In ***tropical sprue***, mild, colicky pain occurs after taking milk, diets rich in spices.

In patients with ***pancreatic carcinoma/chronic pancreatitis*** there may be dull aching pain in back.

In gluten-induced enteropathy, pain in abdomen is usually absent.

- ***Weight Loss***

Marked and progressive weight loss, in spite of adequate food intake, is suggestive of malabsorption syndrome.

- ***Nutritional Deficiency***

Anaemia (due to deficiency of Fe, vitamin B_{12}, folic acid), glossitis, and cheilosis due to vitamin B_2 (riboflavin) deficiency.

The above are seen usually in small bowel diseases and they are uncommon in patients with pancreatic diseases.

- ***Abdominal Distention***

In ***small bowel diseases***, patients usually complain of fullness and heaviness of abdomen after 1 to 2 hours of taking food.

In tropical sprue, distended coils of small bowels may be seen.

In Crohn's disease, a palpable lump in abdomen may be felt.

Intestinal tuberculosis may be associated with ascites and generalized tenderness of abdomen or palpable lump.

- ***Pigmentation***

In patients with ***small bowel diseases***, pigmentation over dorsum of fingers has been described along with vitamin B_{12} deficiency.

- ***Nervous System Involvement***

Presence of peripheral neuritis and posterior and lateral column sclerosis (subacute combined degeneration of cord) indicates vitamin B_{12} deficiency due to an ileal lesion.

- ***Bone Disease***

Presence of evidences (radiological) for osteomalacia and/or osteoporosis, with low serum calcium and tetany indicates malabsorption of vitamin D, which can occur in post gastrectomy and idiopathic steatorrhoea and also in obstructive jaundice.

Malabsorption of vitamin D leads to deficient formation of "calcitriol" (1,25-di (OH)-D_3) resulting in impaired calcium absorption and hypocalcaemia.

B. LABORATORY TESTS

After proper clinical evaluation, certain laboratory tests are required to find out the malabsorption of the nutrients concerned. Large number of tests are available which are described under the following heads.

1. TESTS TO DETECT MALABSORPTION OF FATS

a. "Screening" Tests

- ***Examination of Faeces***

NE examination provides valuable information whether steatorrhoea is present or not. ***Typical steatorrhoeic stool is bulky, pale, greasy, malodorous*** and ***frothy. The stools float readily*** in water and difficult to flush.

Note

1. *Pale colour* is due to increased fat content and frothy nature is due to bacterial fermentation of unabsorbed carbohydrates.
2. *Stools float* due to increased fat content and due to increased gas content.
3. *In pancreatic steatorrhoea,* the stools have highest fat concentration and it is more severe.
4. *In biliary steatorrhoea,* due to extrahepatic obstruction and absence of bile salts, there is increased fat content but due to absence of bile and thus urobilin, stools are *"clay-coloured"*.

- *Microscopic examination* reveals the presence of ***fatty crystal*** and ***globules:*** stool is mixed with 2 to 3 drops of 95% ethyl alcohol on a slide and 2 to 3 drops of Sudan III added and mixed. The slide is seen under microscope after putting a cover slip.

Interpretation

- Neutral fat appears as yellow or reddish refractile globules and fatty acid crystals stain a pale orange colour.
- In steatorrhoea, more than 3 to 5 globules are seen in a field.

Note

Used as a screening test, both false positive and false negative results can occur.

- ***Determination of Total Faecal Fat—Fat Balance Test***

The patient is given a diet containing 50 to 100 gm (preferably 70 gm) of fat a day for 3 days prior to and during the period of collection. As faecal fat excretion fluctuates from day to day and if steatorrhoea is not severe, faecal fat collection can be done for 6 days.

The fatty acids in the faeces, in an aliquot after homogenization are estimated by wet method and fat excretion per day and % absorption is calculated.

Note

- Marking dyes have been used to define the beginning and end of the collection.
- Fat balance test is the most useful test and gives an indication of the degree of malabsorption.
- But the test is not done routinely in the laboratory due to foul smell and collection of faeces for 3 to 6 days is quite unpleasant job.

Interpretations

- On an ordinary diet of about 70 gm fat daily, the fat excretion per day in a normal person is 1.7 to 28 gm. Normal absorption is approximately a little more than 90%, range 95 ± 4%.
- *In steatorrhoea,* the daily excretion may be 70 to 180 gm/l and fat absorption about 50% (ranging from 15 to 85% depending on severity).

Bentley's Butter Fat Test Meal

This can be used as a "Screening Test".

Procedure

- The patient should fast for 12 to 14 hours.
- ***A fasting blood sample*** is taken and the serum separated.
- ***"Toast" meal:*** Two slices of buttered toast (0.5 gm pure butter/kg body wt) given. Unsweetened tea or coffee with milk can be given. Unsweetened orange juice (50 ml) is given along with the toast meal.
- ***A second blood sample*** is taken 2 hours later and the serum separated. The serum is diluted 1 in 10 with normal saline and light scattering intensity (LSI) in a micronephelometer is measured.

LSI value of fasted sample is deducted from the 2-hour sample to get an 'index' of the rise in blood lipids following the meal.

Interpretation

Patients with abnormal faecal fat loss, more than 18 gm/l showed a rise in LSI of less than 20 units, suggesting poor fat absorption.

- ***Urinary Oxalate Estimation***

Recently, it has been shown that ***increased excretion of oxalates can occur in malabsorption of fats.***

Possible mechanism for this increased absorption of oxalates and its urinary excretion suggested that there is preferential binding of calcium by unabsorbed fatty acids in the colonic lumen. This enhances the oxalate solubility/increased permeability of colonic mucosa.

Methods

Many methods have been evolved and used for measuring urinary oxalates—titrimetric, fluorimetric, GLC and HPLC and enzymatic methods. Of these methods, the enzymatic method has been claimed to be most suitable (oxalate oxidase method).

Interpretation

Oxalate excretion in patients with intestinal lesions and with extensive ileal resection has been found to be increased markedly 2.2 mmol/24 hours urine (normal: 0.056–0.349 mmol/24 hours urine).

b. "Tracer" Studies

The "tracer" studies are easy to carry out but require special isotope laboratory.

- ***^{131}I-Triolein Test***

Method

Lugol's iodine (20 drops) is given for 3 days prior to the test to block the thyroid iodine uptake and the patient is allowed to fast overnight. A dose of 25 to 50 μCi of ^{131}I labelled Triolein is given orally with a cup of milk.

Venous blood samples are collected at 2, 4 and 6 hours after the dose and radioactivity is measured. Total radioactivity is expressed as percentage (%) of the administered dose.

Note

Radioactivity can also be measured in 6 day stool collection (faecal excretion).

Interpretations

- ***Normal persons:*** show a peak blood rise of radioactivity of at least 9% or faecal excretion of less than 7% of the administered dose.
- ***In malabsorption of fats:*** the peak rise in blood radioactivity is much lower and the faecal excretion higher than the normal subjects.

Abnormal ^{131}I-triolein test indicates maldigestion and/or malabsorption of fats.

- ***^{131}I-Oleic Acid Test***

Indication: This test may be performed, if ^{131}I Triolein test is abnormal. The ***test will be helpful in differentiating maldigestion from malabsorption.***

Procedure

Similar to the above test.

Interpretation

- It is suggested that if ^{131}I—triolein test is abnormal and ^{131}I-Oleic acid test is normal, then there is impaired digestion and normal absorption.
- If both tests are abnormal, it indicates definitely there is malabsorption and no conclusion can be made regarding digestion.

- ***Breath Test***

Absorption of ^{14}C-labelled fat can be studied by measuring $^{14}CO_2$ in breath.

^{14}C-labelled triglyceride of octanoic acid is fed and $^{14}CO_2$ produced during metabolism of ^{14}C-labelled absorbed fat is measured in expired breath.

Interpretations

- *Normal persons:* exhales about 17.5% of the administer dose
- In malabsorption of fats only less than 4.8% is exhaled in breath.

2. Tests to Detect Malabsorption of Carbohydrates

a. Tests for Monosaccharides

Glucose tolerance test (GTT): Glucose absorption can be studied by performing a standard oral glucose tolerance test. (For details refer to Laboratory investigation of hyperglycaemia.)

Interpretations

- A rise in blood sugar of 40 mg/dl or more over the fasting level indicates normal absorption of glucose.
- A rise of blood sugar of less than 20 mg/dl, producing a "flat curve", is suggestive of malabsorption.

Note

- It is not a reliable and good test as blood sugar is influenced by many other factors besides absorption, e.g.:
  - Gastric emptying and intestinal motility
  - Presence of 'Carrier Protein' in intestinal mucosa
  - Uptake by the liver
  - Metabolism in the tissues and presence of insulin
  - Renal clearance.
- 'Flat curve' can be observed in normal subjects sometimes.

- ***D-Xylose Excretion Test***

Principle: D-Xylose is a pentose sugar, not normally present in the blood in significant amounts, hence it is preferable than glucose.

When given by mouth, it is absorbed by the jejunum and is partly (in very insignificant amounts) is metabolized to fructose-6-p in the liver. Xylose entering the systemic circulation is excreted in the urine, there being no renal threshold for it. Provided renal function is normal, D-xylose appears rapidly.

The investigation requires either urinary or plasma determination of D-xylose.

Procedure

The test is carried out on a patient after overnight fasting and has emptied the bladder completely before the test.

A dose of 25 gm or 5 gm of D-xylose is given orally. Originally, 25 gm of D-xylose dissolved in 250 ml of water being given; followed immediately by 250 ml of water.

For young children 1.1. gm/kg of body weight (up to a maximum of 25 gm) has been used. This quantity is rather unpleasant to take and rather expensive. Now some workers believe in giving 5 gm dose.

After administering xylose, all the urines passed during next 5 hours, emptying the bladder at the end of the period are collected and xylose content of the urine estimated.

A blood sample may also be collected at 1 hour after the administration of xylose to the patient. Xylose content of the blood sample is determined.

Determination of Xylose

For estimation of xylose in serum and urine, the following methods are used

- ***Gas chromatography*** (Not available in all laboratories).
- ***Colorimetric assays*** are most commonly used and can be done in hospital laboratory. Either phloroglucinol or p-bromoaniline can be used for development of the colour.

Interpretations

- If 25 gm xylose used, normal persons excrete more than 4 gm in the 5-hour period, except in persons of older age group above 65 years.
- ***Lower excretion than 4 gm in 5-hour sample indicates malabsorption;*** for older patient an excretion below 3 gm can be taken as abnormal.
- If renal function is normal, a blood xylose above 20 mg/dl should be taken as normal.
- With 5 gm dose, at least 1.2 gm of xylose should be excreted in 5 hours.

Note

The more rapid absorption from the normal jejunum is apparent if a 2-hour urine sample is used.

Ratio of excretion at 2 hours to the total excretion at 5 hours is normally greater than 0.5 and may be the most sensitive indicator of minor degrees of malabsorption.

b. Tests for Disaccharides and Disaccharidase Deficiency

- ***Disaccharides Absorption***

Principle:

Defective digestion of disaccharides in the brush-border of the jejunum can be investigated by administering a standard dose of the disaccharide and studying the plasma glucose response. Thus, lactase deficiency can be demonstrated by the poor plasma glucose rise following oral ingestion of 50 gm of lactose. Deficiency of *"maltase"* and *"sucrase"* are similarly studied using 50 gm of maltose or sucrose.

Interpretation

Normally the blood glucose levels rises by about 49 mg/dl (2.7 mmol/l) but in deficiency of the disaccharidase, increases by less than 20 mg/dl (1.1 mmol/l).

- ***Disaccharide Tolerance Test***

Principle

Disaccharidase deficiency is diagnosed by showing a "flat" disaccharide tolerance curve and normal absorption of monosaccharides.

Procedure

After an overnight fast, a fasting sample of blood is collected for fasting blood sugar. Lactose or sucrose (50 gm) is given orally dissolved in 200 ml of water. Blood samples are collected half hourly for 2 hours and blood sugar is estimated in all samples.

Interpretation

- If the disaccharide tolerance curve is "flat", a rise of blood sugar less than 20 mg/dl is obtained; the test is performed again next day, administering 25 gm each of glucose and galactose or glucose and fructose, respectively.
- The maximum blood sugar rise of more than 20 mg/dl indicates adequate disaccharidase activity, whereas a (flat) disaccharide tolerance curve with normal absorption of monosaccharides indicates specific disaccharidase deficiency.
- If the blood sugar rise is less than < 20 mg/dl with both the above tests, it suggests impaired absorption and no conclusion can be made regarding disaccharidase activity.

- ***Disaccharide Loading Test***

Administration of gradually increasing doses of a disaccharide on different days would result in diarrhoea in an individual. Subjects tolerating less than < 50 gm of lactose were considered to have lactase deficiency.

- ***"Tracer" Studies***

Breath analysis After feeding ^{14}C-lactose, $^{14}CO_2$ exhaled in breath is measured. In presence of lactase deficiency, little $^{14}CO_2$ is exhaled in the breath.

- ***Hydrogen Breath Test***

Recently, a hydrogen breath test has been used. Carbohydrates not absorbed from the small intestine is fermented by anaerobic bacteria in the colon and forms hydrogen which diffuses throughout the body. It can be measured in the breath by an electrochemical detector specific for hydrogen.

A 50 gm of disaccharide such as lactose is administered to the patient and the hydrogen in breath is monitored. A marked increase in hydrogen excretion, greater than 0.5 ml/minute, occurs if the lactose reaches the colon, indicating small intestine lesions.

Note

- Both false positive and false negative results can occur.
- *False positive result* is obtained in case of bacterial overgrowth of small intestine or due to rapid transit through small intestine.
- *False negative results* have ben reported in cases where colonic bacteria are not capable of fermenting lactose and producing hydrogen. Such an event can occur after a course of broad spectrum antibiotics.

c. Tests for Polysaccharides

- ***Starch Tolerance Test***

The test indicates the presence or absence of pancreatic amylase enzyme and thus shows whether digestion of carbohydrates is normal or impaired. In presence of pancreatic amylase, starch is broken down to maltose, isomaltose and glucose and a significant rise in blood sugar level is seen.

Procedure

To an overnight fasting subject, 50 or 100 gm of soluble starch is introduced into the stomach through a tube (to avoid action of salivary amylase).

Blood samples are collected half hourly for 2 hours like GTT. Next day, 50 or 100 gm of glucose is administered and tolerance test is done again. The maximum rise of blood sugar in both these tests is compared.

Calculation

$$\frac{\text{Maximum blood sugar rise (after glucose)} \quad \text{Maximum blood sugar rise (after starch)}}{\text{Maximum blood sugar rise (after starch)}} \quad 100$$

Interpretation

Values above 100% are suggestive of pancreatic dysfunction.

3. TESTS TO DETECT MALABSORPTION OF PROTEINS

Tests involving proteins and amino acids have been less used.

- ***Faecal Nitrogen Measurement***

Normally one quarter of the daily turnover of plasma proteins is due to their loss into the jejunum. This mainly involves albumin up to 4 gm daily, which is digested and reabsorbed during its passage along the intestine.

In pancreatic diseases, with diminished proteolytic enzymes, the digestion of secreted albumin and of dietary proteins is reduced and the patient goes into negative nitrogen balance and there is increased faecal nitrogen loss.

Interpretations

- *Normal subjects* excrete 1 to 2 gm faecal N_2 (equivalent to about 10 gm of protein) per day obtained from about 75 to 100 gm of ingested proteins and about 150 gm of proteins normally exuded in GI tract.
- Increased quantities are excreted both in small bowel and pancreatic diseases.

Protein-Losing Enteropathy

- In this condition, entry of protein into the intestine is increased and may involve other proteins besides albumin. Depending on the site and degree of protein loss, the further digestion and reabsorption may be incomplete leading to increased faecal N_2 loss.

- Moderate losses of protein may complicate:
  - Sprue syndrome
  - Colitis
  - Giant rugal hypertrophy of stomach.
- Greater losses occur in:
  - Multiple polyposis of the colon.
  - Lymphatic obstruction of the small intestine—congenital lymphangiectasia, Whipple's disease.
  - Severe venous obstruction as in constrictive pericarditis.
  - Crohn's disease.
- Altered immunological function can also produce protein loss in:
  - Infantile intestinal allergies.
  - Hypogammaglobulinaemia.

Investigations include:

- Total and differential proteins: Hypoproteinaemia, mainly hypoalbuminaemia.
- Increased faecal N_2 loss.
- "Tract" studies are more informative.

Procedure

Large number radioactive methods are available.

1. Albumin labelled with ^{131}I has been used
   Disadvantage: ^{131}I may be detached during digestion in the lumen of the gut, hence, this method is unsatisfactory.
2. Albumin labelled with ^{51}Cr or ^{3}H is found to be more suitable.
3. Polyvinyl pyrrolidone (PVP) labelled with ^{131}I.
4. Ceruloplasmin labelled with ^{67}Cu.

Out of these ^{51}Cr—labelled albumin is the best method.

Interpretations

- ***Normally*** less than 1% of the injected dose is lost in the faeces.
- ***In protein-losing enteropathy:*** faecal loss may be greater than 30% and marked fall in plasma radioactivity is seen.

4. TESTS TO DETECT MALABSORPTION OF VITAMINS

a. Test for Water Soluble Vitamins—Vitamin B_{12} and Folic Acid

(Refer to Chapter 24 laboratory investigations of macrocytic megaloblastic anaemia).

b. Test for Absorption of Fat Soluble Vitamins

"Tracer" studies involving vitamin D has been used.

- ***Vitamin A Absorption***

Procedure:

1. After overnight fasting, a fasting blood sample is drawn.
2. A dose 300,000 units of vitamin A (5 ml percomorph-liver oil) is given orally.
3. Blood samples are collected 5 and 7 hours after oral feeding.
4. Vitamin A concentration in all the samples is estimated by colorimetric assay.

Interpretations

- ***Normal:*** fasting values are between 30 and 90 μg/dl.
- ***In malabsorption***: a rise of less than 125 μg/dl indicates poor absorption.

- ***Absorption of Vitamin D***

Procedure

1. Tritium labelled vitamin D_3 is used (H^3—vit D_3)
2. A dose of 0.5 to 1 mg of H^3-vitamin D_3 of specific activity of 5 to 15 μCi per mg is administered orally with Arachis oil and 250 ml of water is given.
3. Blood samples are collected at 3, 6, 12, 24 and 36 hours (for plasma "peak" activity).
4. Faeces also collected for 6 days to determine faecal excretion of radioactivity.
5. Radioactivity is measured in plasma and faeces, the net absorption is calculated from the faecal excretion of radioactivity.

Interpretations

- *Normal:* absorption is more than 60% of the dose.
- *In malabsorption:* absorption is less than 60% of the dose.

5. TESTS TO DETECT MALABSORPTION OF MINERALS (IRON ABSORPTION)

- ***Iron Absorption***

Isotopes used: Two isotopes of Fe are used—^{55}Fe and ^{59}Fe. The later is the isotope of choice, because of shorter half life.

Procedure

A dose of 5 μCi of ^{59}Fe citrate with 5 mg of "carrier" iron is fed to a subject after overnight fasting.

The absorption of Fe can be measured by:
- *Whole body counting.*
- *Faecal excretion of radioactivity.*

Whole body counting

The total body radioactivity is measured immediately after the administration of the dose and 7 days later using a whole body counter.

Faecal excretion

The unabsorbed ^{59}Fe is measured by collecting faeces for 6 days and counting its radioactivity.

6. TESTS FOR BACTERIAL OVERGROWTH

Normal gastric secretion and the mechanical cleansing effect of peristalsis prevent bacterial proliferation in the small intestine. ***In case of stasis*** for any reason, overgrowth of organisms may occur which results in malabsorption.

Tests to Assess Overgrowth of Bacteria

- ***Bacterial Culture and Sensitivity***

In a suspected case of blind loop syndrome, small intestinal fluid may be collected with a Shiner's tube (to avoid throat contamination).

Interpretations

- A mild bacterial growth may be observed both in ileum and jejunum even in normal subjects; hence, a bacterial count by serial dilution technique must be performed.
- Bacterial counts of more than 10^3 or 10^5 per ml are considered significant. Sensitivity of the organisms to different drugs may be helpful.

- ***Thin Layer Chromatography***

In order to observe whether isolated organisms are able to deconjugate bile salts: one can look for *free bile acids* in small intestinal aspirated fluid by TLC (thin-layer chromatography).

- ***Estimation of Total Cholic Acid Levels***

Estimation of total cholic acid levels in small intestinal aspirate may help as it indicates whether bile salts concentration is reduced below the critical level for "micelle" formation.

Bile salt deficiency may result from deconjugation of bile salts by bacteria or due to an interruption of enterohepatic circulation of bile salts secondary to an ileal resection or disease.

- ***Bile Acid Breath Test***

The bile acid breath test has been used in terminal ileal disease. Conjugated bile salts pass unabsorbed into the colon where bacteria degrade them releasing glycine and the unconjugated bile salts. If the glycine moiety of glycocholic acid is labelled with ^{14}C, then the radioactivity can be subsequently measured in the breath as $^{14}CO_2$.

Metz et al combined results from the hydrogen breath test and ^{14}C glycocholate breath test to detect bacterial overgrowth in 92% cases. In hydrogen breath test using glucose as the carbohydrate source, early release of hydrogen suggests either rapid transport to the colon or bacterial overgrowth in the ileum.

Other Tests Employed for Bacterial Overgrowth

- ***Schilling test*** (Refer to laboratory investigation of macrocytic megaloblastic anaemia).
- ***Urinary indican excretion*** Some intestinal bacteria are capable of metabolizing tryp-

tophan to indoles which are absorbed by the gut and converted to indoxylsulphate (Indican) in the liver. This substance is excreted in urine and can be easily detected/measured in the laboratory.

Interpretation

Increased urinary levels of Indican are seen in patients with gut bacterial overgrowth, e.g. in blind loop syndrome.

C. HAEMATOLOGICAL AND OTHER BIOCHEMICAL LABORATORY INVESTIGATIONS

- ***Stool Examination***

A cover-slip preparation of stool in saline and iodine is examined microscopically for cysts and ova.

- ***Routine Blood Studies***
  - In all subjects—Hb, RBC count, leucocyte count—total and differential, and absolute values like PCV, MCV, MCH and MCHC should be determined.
  - ESR may be useful in conditions such as intestinal tuberculosis, regional ileitis (Crohn's disease), etc.
  - *Peripheral smear* examination is important to demonstrate hypochromia, macrocytosis, and hypersegmented multilobed polymorphs which will provide useful important diagnostic clues.

- ***Biochemical Investigations***
  - Serum iron and iron binding capacity (TIBC).
  - Serum vitamin B_{12} assay.
  - Serum folic acid, and RBC folates.

(Refer to chapter laboratory investigation of macrocytic megaloblastic anaemia, and iron deficiency anaemia).

Note

- Low values of Fe, vitamin B_{12} and folic acid in the serum indicate deficiencies of these substances which may be due to poor dietary intake or malabsorption.
- Absorption studies of these substances along with a detailed and accurate dietetic history would help in establishing the cause of the deficiency.
- ***Prothrombin time:*** may be useful, specially in bile salt deficiency in which vitmain K absorption may be impaired.
- ***Serum calcium:*** may be low, in case of impairment of vitamin D absorption and deficiency.

D. SPECIAL INVESTIGATIONS

- ***Small Intestinal Mucosal Biopsy***

In malabsorption syndrome, small intestinal biopsy could be useful for:

- Studying the shape and pattern of villi.
- Histological structure by light and electron microscopy.
- Histochemical staining.
- Enzyme estimations.
- Culture of organism.
- Autoradiography.

Interpretations

- ***Gluten-sensitive enteropathy:*** Caeliac disease and tropical sprue, which are common causes of malabsorption, result in characteristic changes in the villi of the small intestine. It is the most important investigation for diagnosing gluten-induced enteropathy which shows characteristic ***"flat stunted villi"***.
- ***Whipple's disease:*** diagnosis depends on showing abundant PAS (periodic acid-Schiff) positive material in lamina propria in a small intestinal biopsy.
- ***Protein-losing enteropathy:*** The characteristic dilated lymphatics may be observed in small intestinal biopsy.

- ***Enzyme Estimations in Mucosal Biopsy***

The diagnosis of disaccharidase deficiency can be established by estimating specific enzymes in mucosal biopsy. The presence or absence of different enzymes such as alkaline phosphatase

(ALP) can be established by specific histochemical staining.

- ***Radiological Studies***
  - ***Plain X-ray of abdomen:*** may show evidence of subacute intestinal obstruction in ileocaecal tuberculosis, intestinal stricture, biliary calculi in extrehepatic biliary obstruction or pancreatic calculi in a case of pancreatic steatorrhoea.
  - ***Barium meal and follow through***
    - ***In pancreatic carcinoma,*** widening of the duodenal loop and irregularity in medial wall of second part of duodenum seen.
    - ***Diagnosis of Crohn's disease,*** diverticulosis, etc. can be made by radiological examination.
    - Diagnosis of ***Zollinger-Ellison syndrome*** is suggested on radiological examination, on observing marked prominent gastric folds with gross distortion of mucosal pattern of upper small intestine.
    - ***Barium enema***
      - To demonstrate lesions of caecum and terminal ileum, barium enema provides much more information than that obtained with barium meal; and
      - In a case of gastrojejunocolic fistula, the abnormal tract can easily be visualized on barium enema and not by barium meal.

Tests to Detect Pancreatic Diseases

The following will be useful to detect impairment in pancreatic digestion:

a. ***Glucose tolerance test***—refer above.

b. ***Starch tolerance test***—refer above.

c. ***D-xylose excretion test***—refer above.

d. ***Faecal fat excretion***—see above.

e. ***Secretin–pancreozymin test:***
after injection of secretin and pancreozymin, levels of enzymes are estimated in blood and/or duodenal fluid collected through a double-lumen tube.

Interpretations

- Low bicarbonate level in duodenal aspirate is seen in chronic pancreatitis.
- Low volume of secretion is suggestive of obstruction to ducts, may be due to carcinoma of head of pancreas.
- In suspected case of carcinoma of head of pancreas, a positive exfoliative cytology of duodenal aspirate would be of immense value.

f. Trypsin Content of Faeces

Normal infants excrete enough trypsin in faeces to digest the emulsion containing gelatin on X-ray film. In case of cystic fibrosis, there is failure to digest the gelatin layer.

g. Radiological Studies of Pancreas

- ***Plain X-ray of abdomen:*** may show pancreatic calculi or a soft tissue shadow if there is a pancreatic cyst which can form following pancreatitis.
- ***Barium meal studies:*** may show anterior displacement of stomach or widening of the second part of duodenum.
- ***Cholecystography:*** oral/IV may detect chronic pancreatitis which may be associated with biliary calculi.
- ***Selective splanchnic (caeliac) arteriography:*** may show presence of pancreatic carcinoma by showing displacement of adjacent arteries, tumour staining by localized hypervascularity and arterial narrowing or obstruction.

- ***Retrograde Arteriography***

It may be required to diagnose cases of superior mesenteric artery insufficiency.

- ***Pancreatic Scan***

Various amino acids are utilized by pancreas for synthesis of enzymes. Methionine which contains sulphur, may be replaced by radioactive selenium. Selenium replaces sulphur of methionine with altering its properties.

A dose of about 3 to 3.5 μCi/kg of body weight of selenomethionine (^{75}Se) is injected.

Interpretations

- Radioactive selenomethionine is taken up by pancreas and makes possible of visualization of the organ.
- Very small lesions are sometimes difficult to detect and it may be difficult sometimes to say whether any lesion detected is inflammatory or malignant.

Sweat Test

The diagnosis of cystic fibrosis of pancreas can be made only by sweat analysis for sodium and chloride. Sweat can be collected by iontophoresis. Sweat Na^+ of more than 70 mEq/l and Cl^- of more than 60 mEq/l are diagnostic of cystic fibrosis of pancreas. (For details of Pancreatic function tests—refer to Chapter 6, under Organ function tests)

Flow Chart for Laboratory Investigation of a Case of Steatorrhoea is given below

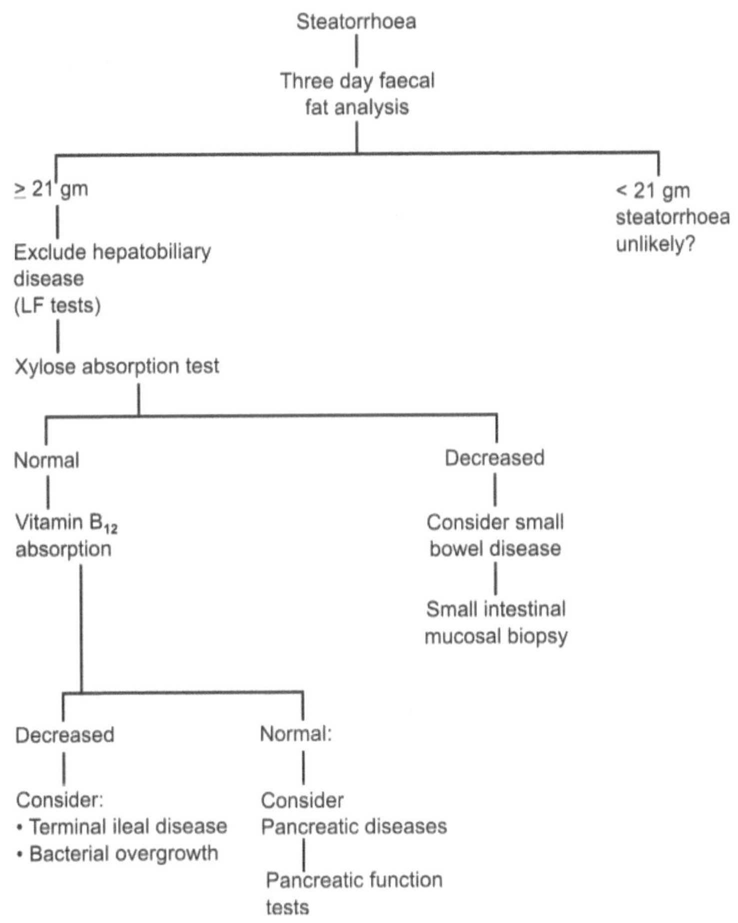

Chapter 19

Obesity

INTRODUCTION

It is difficult to define obesity—various definitions have been given.

"Anyone who is more than 20% above the 'Standard' weight for people of the same age, sex and race must generally be considered to be at least overweight."

Alternatively,

"Obesity is that physical state in which the amount of fat stored in the body is excessive."

"Obesity is due to excess of adipose tissue and is defined as that body weight over 20% above mean ideal body weight."

It is still not clear whether obesity represents a disease process or a symptom, a common clinical manifestation of a group of disorders, like diabetes, hypertension and certain endocrine disorders. But though it may be a symptom, it commands the medical attention and accorded as the status of a serious condition due to its implications and associations with certain diseases.

IMPORTANCE OF OBESITY

Obese persons are more prone than the average populations to certain disease processes. They are:

- *Diabetes mellitus:* Type II (maturity-onset)
- *Cardiovascular disorders:* hypertension, angina of efforts, widespread atherosclerosis, varicose veins and thromboembolism.
- *Liver diseases:* prone to develop fatty liver, cholelithiasis and cholecystitis.
- *Physical consequences of too much fat*
  - bronchitis;
  - alveolar hypoventilation associated with massive obesity eventually leading to CO_2 retention (obesity hypoventilation syndrome or **"Pickwickian syndrome"**);
  - backache, arthritis of hips and knee joints, flat feet; and
  - hernias, ventral and diaphragmatic.
- *Metabolic diseases:* like gout (hyperuricaemia).
- *Skin disorders:* intertriginous dermatitis. Intertrigo is quite common in the folds below the breasts and in the inguinal regions.
- ***Gynaecological disorders***
  - amenorrhoea, oligomenorrhoea;
  - toxaemia of pregnancy; and
  - endometrial carcinoma.
- *Surgical postoperative complications* Surgical "risks" in general is greater in obesity.
- *Industrial, household and street accidents:* Obese persons are susceptible to these accidents.

TYPES OF OBESITY

Immediate cause of obesity is always a positive energy balance, but there are many ways in which the balance may be tilted towards the positive side. Thus obesity is often divided into **2 types:**

- ***Exogenous obesity.***
- ***Endogenous obesity.***

1. Exogenous obesity

Overfeeding and gluttony with less physical activity. Many people overeat than the calorie requirements either because they are too fond of their foods which is a pleasure, or quite often because they are unhappy, foods give them solace.

2. Endogenous obesity

There may be one or more endogenous factors: endocrinal, metabolic, hypothalamic lesion.

Pathologically, the types of obesity are:

- ***Hyperplastic type.***
- ***Hypertrophic type.***

a. Hyperplastic type

This type is a life long obesity characterized by an increase in adipose cell number as well as increase in adipose cell size. ***Fat distribution is usually peripheral as well as central.*** Long term response to treatment is not good. After weight reduction, adipose cell size may shrink ***but the increased number of cells persist.***

b. Hypertrophic type

It is seen in adults after twenty years of age ***(adult onset type).*** It is characterized by hypertrophy of adipose tissue cells without increase in adipose cells number. There is increase in cell size only. ***Fat distribution is usually central.*** The energy requirements of the body diminish with the advancing age and if there is no corresponding reduction in eating habits, a ***"middle-aged spread" is the natural result. Long term response to treatment is fairly good.***

CAUSES

Obesity is most commonly due to overeating than the caloric requirement. Obesity can be encountered with other diseases, viz. certain metabolic disorders, and endocrine disorders. Thus, the causes of obesity as listed below, though may not be all complete but encompasses the more common and certain uncommon syndromes which have been reported.

1. ***Genetic influences***
2. ***Physiological***
    - Overeating than caloric requirement
    - Pregnancy
    - Postmenopausal women
    - Use of oral contraceptives for prolonged periods.
3. **Metabolic**
    - Diabetes mellitus.
    - Hyperlipidaemic states specially, Type-IV and Type V.
4. ***Hypothalamic injuries or abnormalities* (e.g. Prader-Willi syndrome)**
5. ***Miscellaneous and endocrine disorders***
    - Hypothyroidism
    - Cushing's disease and Cushing's syndrome
    - Pseudohypoparathyroidism
    - Islet cell tumour (insulinoma)
    - Polycystic ovary syndrome
    - Laurence-Moon-Biedl syndrome
    - Fröhlich syndrome
    - Acromegaly.

PATHOGENESIS

Genetic and Other Factors in Obesity

Age: Immoderate accumulation of adipose tissue may occur at any age, but is more common in middle life. Minor degrees of corpulence, 10 to 15% above optimal weight are the rule rather than the exception after the age of 30 years.

Sex: Adult women are more prone to obesity as compared to men. The normal fat content of an average young woman, approximately 15% of body weight, is twice that of young men of comparable age. Women in menopausal period become usually obese. Obesity is also more frequent in pregnancy and women on oral contraceptives.

- ***Genetic factor:*** obesity occurs much more frequently among the members of certain families than among others. A genetic factor may be identified in many cases but its mode of transmission and operation is still not known.

- ***Psychological factors:*** Psychological factor also plays an important role. Obese persons are often psychologically imbalanced. Peoples who are suffering from anxieties, worries, and under constant tension or are frustated, they eat more to compensate.
- ***Hypothalamic factor:*** **Two mechanisms** within the hypothalamus appear to regulate food intake:
  - If certain **lateral centres** are bilaterally destroyed, aphagia results.
  - When the ***medially controlled centres*** are bilaterally destroyed, the lateral "feeding" areas are freed of their usual regulatory checking action and hyperphagia occurs. The individual eats more than requirements and obesity results.

The exact site of the hunger sensation accompanying hypoglycaemia is not well understood. Persons with so-called ***"pituitary obesity"*** presumably suffer from a hypothalamic disturbance. It has been established that experimental pituitary destruction does not cause obesity unless the hypothalamus is also injured.

- ***Epidemic encephalitis:*** may be followed by the development of obesity, and in such cases hypothalamic lesions have been found which resemble those known to cause experimental obesity.
- ***Endocrine factors:*** Certain endocrinal disorders may predispose to obesity:
  - ***Frohlich's syndrome:*** is characterized by hypogonadism and obesity has been considered the result of hypopituitarism. In adiposogenital dystrophy, the excessive fat accumulation may result from hypothalamic disturbance, but its typical distribution is characteristic of hypogonadism, which may result from pituitary insuffiency.
  - ***Cushing's syndrome:*** (Adrenocortical hyperfunction): is often associated with an increase in body fat mainly confined to the head, neck and trunk (***truncal obesity and "buffalo hump"***), but spares the limb. It is often associated with a gain in weight.
    Although a low BMR cannot explain the usual type of obesity, hypothyroidism may be associated with gain in weight, partly due to water retention in tissues and partly to fat storage; which is evident in particular sites stated above.
  - ***Functional or organic hypoglycaemia (Hyperinsulinism):*** is frequently associated with abnormal hunger leading to excessive food intake and obesity. Hyperinsulinism may aggravate the disability by promoting lipogenesis and inhibiting lipolysis.
  - ***In pregnancy:*** endocrine factors play part in increasing weight and producing obesity.
  - ***Hypothyroidism:*** diminished BMR and en-ergy expenditure may be associated with gain in weight and obesity.
  - ***Hypogonadism:*** In man as well as in animals, removal or destruction of the gonads by diseases predisposes to obesity. Many women show such changes and gain in weight after the menopause. The adiposity characteristic of hypogonadism involves chiefly the breast, abdomen, hips and thighs.

The endocrine disorders do not cause the obesity as such, but may favour its development by increasing food intake or decreasing energy expenditure or both. Localization of fat deposits is, however, specifically influenced by certain abnormalities of the internal secretions.

Metabolic Changes in Obesity

Various metabolic abnormalities observed in obesity are not permanent in nature. They are induced with weight gain and are reversible with weight reduction.

1. Changes in Fat Metabolism

- ***Serum triglyceride level:*** Increased TG level (hypertriacylglycerolaemia) is seen characteristically in obesity. This may be explained partly due to associated hyperinsulinism seen in obese patients. Studies have shown a good correlation between hypertriacylglycerolaemia and hyperinsulinisim.

- ***Serum cholesterol level:*** In obesity associated with Type IV and Type V hyperlipoproteinaemias, alongwith hypertriglyceridaemia, there may be slight to moderate hypercholesterolaemia. As such, serum cholesterol levels are less closely related with obesity, but statistically significant relationship do exist. It may be ***explained partly by the increased cholesterol production rate in relationship of degree of obesity.*** It is supported by the fact that cholesterol gallstones are more common in obese individuals.
- ***Mobilization of FFA:*** As obesity is usually associated with hyperinsulinaemia, it is expected to play a part in lipogenesis.

Fatty acid mobilization from adipose tissue appears to be less affected and is considered to be normal in obesity.

- ***Lipoprotein lipase activity:*** Lipoprotein lipase brings about the delipidation of TG of circulating chylomicrons and VLDL. It appears to be sensitive to the availability of insulin and its activity has been found to be increased in adult-onset type of obesity (hypertrophic type). Increased activity of the enzyme would lead to increased FFA assimilation in adipose tissue and thus it can lead to increased fat deposition, in adipose tissue.

2. *Changes in Carbohydrate Metabolism*

Obesity is associated with hyperinsulinaemia. The β-cells of Islet of Langerhans of pancreas are stimulated to produce more insulin. The nature of the stimulus is not known which may be hormonal or neuronal or by some specific amino acids or fatty acids. Hyperinsulinism may aggravate obesity by promoting lipogenesis and inhibiting lipolysis. Prolonged hyperinsulinism in obesity might lead to the exhaustion of β-cells in those individuals who are genetically susceptible to diabetes mellitus.

Insulin resistance is associated with obesity. The obesity has been found to be associated with fewer numbers of insulin "receptors", on adipose tissue, liver and muscle. A high blood insulin level (hyperinsulinaemia) decreases the number of insulin receptors on target cell membrane, probably ***through internalization of the "insulin-receptor complex"*** into the cell and thus decreases the insulin sensitivity of the target tissues, thus contributing, to insulin resistance and impaired glucose utilization by the cells.

3. *Changes in Acid-base Status*

Massive obesity may be ***associated with alveolar hypoventilation leading to CO_2 retention.*** PCO_2 may be high ↑ and this can bring about certain personality changes, fatiguability, dyspnoea and somnolence, called as ***"obesity-hypoventilation syndrome" (Pickwickian syndrome).***

4. *Energy Metabolism in Obesity*

BMR as ordinarily determined, is usually normal in obese subjects. Their energy expenditure per unit mass is the same as in mormal people. It appears that since BMR of an obese person is normal and his surface area large, his total O_2 consumption must be greater than normal. It may be as much as 25% more than that of normal persons of the same age. The individual uses more oxygen, burns fuel and yet continues to store fat.

CLINICAL FEATURES

Most of the obese patients are asymptomatic. When obesity is marked, exertional dyspnoea, depression, somnolence and easy fatiguability are likely to occur. Marked obesity may be associated with alveolar hypoventilation leading to CO_2 retention (PCO_2↑) which may account for above features. Many of the symptoms attributed to obesity actually result from an associated disorder like DM or endocrinopathy, rather than from obesity *"per se."*

Symptoms

The more common symptoms seen in obese individuals are as follows:

- Fatigue/tiredness on exertion.
- Exertional dyspnoea.
- Weakness, malaise.
- ***Symptoms of reactive hypoglycaemia*** like weakness, palpitation, sweating, often seen in obese and adult-onset diabetics about 3 to 5 hours after meals.
- Excessive weight gain in spite of normal or reduced calorie intake, frequent steroid therapy, and in Cushing's disease or syndrome.
- Excessive hunger found in obesity associated with pregnancy, women taking oral contraceptives, steroid therapy, adult onset DM, etc.

Signs

Obesity "Per se" may produce some physical findings, but most of the signs seen in obese individuals are primarily related to associated underlying disorders like endocrinopathy.

- ***Pink striae*** are commonly seen over abdomen, thighs, buttocks, breasts, particularly in young women, pink colour usually disappears leaving shiny and white striae.
- When obesity is massive, ***exertional dyspnoea*** and tachypnoea may be seen.
- ***Intertrigo*** is quite common in the folds below the breast and in the inguinal regions.
- ***Plethora*** involving the cheeks and neck is not unusual.
- ***Blood pressure*** is usually normal. Sometimes systemic hypertension may be present due to associated disorders like DM.
- Occasionally ***ankle oedma*** may be noted.
- With certain endocrinopathies associated findings may be of help in diagnosis (see below).

LABORATORY INVESTIGATION

Can be discussed as follows:

- ***To establish the presence of obesity.***
- ***To find out the cause of obesity.***

A. TO ESTABLISH THE PRESENCE OF OBESITY

No laboratory method is available to establish obesity. This can be ascertained from the physical examination of the patient. Obesity can be diagnosed from the age, sex, height and weight. ***A person can be considered as obese if his weight is more than 20% above the "standard" weight for people of the same age, sex and race.***

Overweight is defined by international standards as having a body mass index (BMI) of 25 and above. ***People with a BMI of 30 are considered obese.***

BMI is calculated by dividing height in metres squared by weight in kilograms (kg)

$$\text{BMI} = \frac{(\text{Height in metres})^2}{\text{Weight in kg}}$$

For example:

A person who is 5 feet 9 inches in height (1.75 metres) and weighs 155 pounds (70 kg) has a BMI of 23, which is considered as normal and healthy. At 169 pounds (76 kg) such a person would have a BMI of 25 and is overweight.

A variety of methods for assessment of total body fat have been used for research purposes. These are not available routinely.

- body density determination.
- determination of total body water.
- total body potassium (^{40}K).
- distribution of fat soluble gases.

In addition to above, anthropometric measurements like limb and trunk diameters and circumferences and skin-fold thickness have been used.

B. TO ESTABLISH CAUSE OF OBESITY

After ascertaining that a person is obese, the cause of obesity may be investigated.

- **Clinical Features**

A detailed physical examination is important and certain findings, if present, may indicate the associated disorders. Obesity if associated with:

- ***"Overt" symptoms like polyuria, polydipsia, polyphagia*** indicate presence of maturity-onset diabetes mellitus.

- ***Presence of xanthomata, xanthelasma and arcus senilis*** suggest hyperlipoproteinaemias type IV/V.
- ***Short stature/stocky build, a round facies, brachydactylia and history of tetany*** suggest pseudohypoparathyroidism.
- ***Hypogonadism*** typically seen in hypothalamic obesity syndromes.
- ***Truncal obesity, buffalo hump, moon facies, plethora, purpura, weakness*** suggest Cushings' syndrome/disease.
- ***Puffiness of face and extremities, thickenning and drying of skin ("coarse" skin), falling of hairs specially from eyebrows, yellowish tinge of skin due to carotenaemia, a delayed return of deep tendon reflexes*** seen in myxoedema.
- ***Hirsutism*** may occur in polycystic ovary syndrome.
- ***Excessive growth of the hands, feet and jaw*** are typical of acromegaly.

b. Routine Laboratory Investigations

- ***Urine Analysis***

Routine examination and deposits. Presence of sugar in urine point to DM.

- ***Blood Sugar Estimation***

  - ***Fasting blood sugar estimation*** should be carried out. A high fasting blood sugar would indicate DM.
  - ***Post prandial glucose tolerance test*** may be adequate in most cases to exclude DM.
  - ***A 5-hour glucose tolerance test*** may be indicated in patients with symptoms of reactive hypoglycaemia to document the hypoglycaemia.

(For details refer to laboratory investigation of hypoglycaemia.)

- ***Serum Calcium Level***

Low serum calcium (hypocalcaemia) is frequently encountered in pseudohypoparathyroidism.

(Refer to laboratory investigation of hypocalcaemia.)

- ***Serum Uric Acid Estimation***

Serum uric acid must be estimated primarily to obtain a baseline value and also because hyperuricaemia frequently occurs with restricted calorie intake and after weight loss. Increased serum uric acid level is also found with obesity of hyperlipoproteinaemias type IV and V.

- ***Estimation of Total Cholesterol and Triacylglycerol (TG)***

Fasting total cholesterol and fasting triglyceride (triacylglycerol) would be helpful in case of hyperlipoproteinaemias.

(For details refer to laboratory investigation of hyperlipoproteinaemias.)

High cholesterol level would also suggest myxoedema in which hypercholesterolaemia is characteristically seen.

- ***Thyroid Function Tests***

The following tests may be required as routine tests to establish hypothyroidism:

- ***Serum T_3, T_4 estimation***
- ***T_3 resin uptake***
- ***Serum TSH.***

(Refer to laboratory investigation of hypothyroidism and thyroid function tests.)

- ***Other Ancillary Routine Investigations***

Following ancillary investigations may be helpful.

- *X-ray chest*
- *ECG*

Note

- As a rule, above mentioned laboratory tests are usually normal in patients of exogenous obesity who have not been on a dietary regimen. Only abnormality which may be found in exogenous obesity is increase in serum TG which is frequently elevated when obesity is marked.
- Psychiatric consultation may be specially valuable in planning treatment and determining prognosis in patients with serious weight problems.

c. Special Laboratory Investigations

In patients in whom clinical features and routine laboratory studies suggest the possibility of an underlying or associated disorder/ systemic disease, like DM or endocrinopathies, additional special laboratory investigations will be required to establish the diagnosis.

- ***Demonstration of Thyroid Autoantibodies***

When routine analysis of T_3, T_4 and TSH shows abnormality and if hypofunction of gland is suspected, tests for thyroid autoantibodies should be carried out.

(For details refer to Chapter Thyroid Function Tests.)

- ***Complete Lipid Profile***

If TG and cholesterol are high, a complete lipid profile must be carried out, as obesity is associated with Type IV and Type V hyperlipoproteinaemias.

For complete lipid profile and for clinical features and biochemical profile in Type IV and Type V hyperlipoproteinaemias—refer to the Chapter on Laboratory Investigation of hyperlipoproteinaemias.

- ***Fasting Insulin and Blood Sugar Determinations***

Both these parameters should be measured serially during a 72-hour fast if hyperinsulinism is suspected. Insulin assays may also be helpful in the evaluation of patients who exihibit symptoms of reactive hypoglycaemia during glucose tolerance tests.

(Refer to Chaper on Laboratory Investigation of Hypoglycaemis).

- ***Estimation of Serum PTH***

Serum PTH assay will be of immense value in diagnosis of pseudohypoparathyroidism. The level is immeasurable or low in idiopathic and surgically induced hypoparathyroidism.

The typical clinical features as mentioned above, alongwith hypocalcaemia and high serum PTH would be diagnostic of pseudohypoparathyroidism associated with obesity.

(Refer to Chapter Laboratory Investigation of Hypocalcaemia.)

- ***Estimation of Growth Hormone***

Growth hormone should be measured in association with a glucose tolerance test, if acromegaly is being considered as a cause in obesity. Growth hormone levels are measured while fasting, and at one and two hour intervals after glucose administration.

- ***Overnight Dexamethasone Suppression Test (Screening Test)***

If truncal adiposity, moon facies, buffalo hump, plethora, weakness are present and clinically suggestive of Cushing's syndrome or disease, then an overnight dexamethasone suppression test should be performed, as a screening test.

- A plasma cortisol level is estimated in a blood sample at 8 a.m. on the day of the test.
- Dexamethasome 1.0 mg is given at midnight.
- The plasma cortisol level is again determined on a sample of blood drawn at 8 a.m. the next morning.

Interpretations

- ***Normally,*** the administration of dexamethasone causes a reduction in the plasma cortisol level to 5 to 7 µg/dl or less.
- If the plasma cortisol level is ***not suppressed*** by this test, and Cushing's syndrome or disease is suspected, further evaluation of adrenocortical function would be necessary.

(Refer for details—Chapter on Adrenocortical Function Tests and Laboratory Investigation of Hypercortisolism).

- ***Other Hormone Assays***

Measurement of plasma free testosterone, urinary testosterone, plasma FSH and LH and determination of urinary 17-oxosteroids and testosterone excretion following dexamethasone and chorionic gonadotropin administration may be of help in those cases of obesity in which polycystic ovary syndrome, hyperthecosis ovarii or ovarian neoplasm is suspected.

d. Other Ancillary Specific Investigations

- ***Pulmonary function tests and blood gas analysis*** may be required, if alveolar hypoventilation leading to CO_2 retention along with clinical features like daytime somnolence, personality changes, exertional dyspnoea, fatigue, ***(Pickwickian syndrome)*** are present. Characteristically, in such case, PCO_2 values may be consistently above 48 mm of Hg.
- ***Skull X-rays and if required, CT scanning*** *and* ***arteriography*** may be indicated when infiltrative pituitary-hypothalamic disease or Cushing's disease is suspected.
- ***Pelvic ultrasound and CT scanning*** may be indicated in ovarian disorders, viz. polycystic ovary syndrome, or ovarian neoplasms or hyperthecosis ovarii.

Chapter 20

Polyuria

INTRODUCTION

Polyuria is difficult to define, but a useful working definition is, *"a daily urine output in excess of three litres* (average output in healthy adult is 1.5 to 2 litres), ***particularly if combined with polydipsia or nocturia or both."***

Implications: Polyuria *per se* is not hazardous, provided the lost fluid and solutes are replaced. It may occur in association with normal and pathologic states. Polyuria may become deleterious if losses of fluid and electrolytes are excessive and not replaced correctly. In that event hypotension and cardiovascular collapse may then occur.

CAUSES

Causes of polyuria are conveniently divided into **four main groups**.

- ***Psychogenic—compulsive water drinking (water diuresis)***
- ***Central diabetes insipidus—produces water diuresis***
- ***Nephrogenic diabetes insipidus***
- ***Solute diuresis.***

1. Psychogenic-Compulsive Water Drinking (Water Diuresis)

Polyuria may sometimes be the result of compulsive water drinking, called psychogenic polydipsia. It is characterised by:

- a personality disorder, usually associated with psychic disturbances;
- the presence in middle aged females;
- involves the primary intake of excessive quantities of fluid resulting in suppression of ADH secretion; and
- water intake and polyuria fluctuates from day to day.

Biochemically:

- typically both plasma and urine osmolalities are ***low;***
- there is a lack of responsiveness to arginine vasopressin (AVP);
- occasionally, dilutional hyponatraemia $[Na^+]\downarrow$; and
- rarely water intoxication.

2. Central Diabetes Insipidus

There is ***deficient ADH secretion.*** The condition is also called neurogenic, central or cranial and hypothalamic diabetes insipidus (HDI). This disorder represents:

- a complete or partial defect in the pituitary secretion of ADH (vasopressin) in response to osmoregulatory factors;
- impaired renal concentrating ability resulting in polyuria;
- increased fluid intake by thirst mechanisms prevent severe dehydration, in case the thirst centre is abnormal severe dehydration can occur;
- incidence of HDI-1 in 25000 cases; and
- destruction of > 80% ADH secreting neurons produces HDI. Injury to neurohypophysis may produce transient HDI.

Causes of HDI

a. ***Hereditary form*** can occur, transmitted as autosomal dominant.
b. ***Idiopathic (30% cases),*** in which no cause is known.
c. ***Acquired (70% cases)***
   - Neoplasms.
   - Head injury.
   - Post surgical—after brain surgery.
   - Autoimmune disorders.
   - Infections and granulomas.
   - Ischaemic/hypoxic disorders.

Biochemically:

- plasma hyperosmolality ↑—mild in nature;
- urine—dilute with low sp gr and low osmolality; and
- unresponsive to arginine vasopressin (AVP).

3. Nephrogenic Diabetes Insipidus (NDI)

The condition is ***due to a failure of the kidney to respond to normal or increased concentration of ADH.*** In majority, ADH is incapable of increasing cyclic AMP level in renal tubular epithelial cells.

Causes

The condition can be due to following causes.

a. ***Hereditary form***—inherited as X-chromosome-linked trait, mostly affects males.
b. ***Idiopathic***—no cause is known.
c. ***Acquired:***

- ***Renal diseases:*** The inability to concentrate urine adequately may result in obligatory polyuria. The most common causes:
  - chronic renal failure, particularly if associated with interstitial disease;
  - recovery from acute renal failure;
  - polycystic disease of kidney; and
  - acute pyelonephritis.
- ***Metabolic disorders:*** These include:
  - hypokalaemia;
  - hypercalcaemia;
  - amyloidosis; and
  - multiple myelomatosis.
- ***Drug induced diseases:*** Drugs include:
  - lithium;
  - demeclocycline;
  - barbiturates;
  - potent diuretics; and
  - methoxy-flurane anaesthesia.

Biochemically:

- Plasma osmolality—normal or increased;
- Urine is dilute with low sp gr and low osmolality; an inability to concentrate urine ade-quately with fluid restriction; and
- Lack of responsiveness to vasopressin (ADH).

4. Solute Diuresis

Polyuria may respresent an appropriate physiologic response to osmolar/sodium loads.

• *Osmolar Loads*

Osmolar loads may result in excretion of isotonic urine. The following are some of the examples of solute loads that may produce osmotic diuresis and polyuria.

a. ***Glycosuria:*** in uncontrolled diabetes mellitus.
b. ***Mannitol:*** administration.
c. ***Urea:***
   - increased production—hyper catabolic states;
   - administration of urea; and
   - renal diseases—chronic renal failure, postobstruction, post acute tubular necrosis.
d. ***Hyperalimentation therapy*** with amino acids or glucose.

• *Sodium Loads*

Sodium loads that are accompanied by increased water intake may result in sodium diuresis and the excretion of isotonic urine. This may occur as follows:

a. High dietary intake of sodium-rare (increased intake)

b. Administration of excessive quantities of salt and water IV or tube feedings ***(iatrognic).***
c. Rapid resorption of oedema fluid.
d. Increased renal loss, e.g.:
    - diuretic therapy, renal salt losing nephritis;
    - renal tubular acidosis; and
    - mineralocorticoid deficiency.

LABORATORY INVESTIGATION

A. History and Clinical Examination

Before entering into laboratory investigations in a case of polyuria, ***a proper history taking and clinical examination is essential.***

A general clinical examination and history to exclude drug therapy like:

- Lithium administration in psychiatric cases.
- Any history of potent diuretic therapy.
- Rule out any administration of solute or fluid loads or both.
- A psychogenic polydipsia as possible cause of polyuria by proper history and a review of fluid and electroyte balance.
- Any possibility of diabetes mellitus from family history and clinical examination. For this a qualitative Benedict's test on urine and a fasting blood glucose may be helpful.

B. Urinary Osmolality

First and ***most important crucial test*** is to determine urinary osmolality by osmometer. This one single test can differentiate two major causes of polyuria.

a. **Water diuresis.**
b. **Salt diuresis.**

Normal urine osmolality
Osmotic limits—50 to 1200 mosm/kg.

Normal random specimen of urine in healthy adult with average fluid intake 300 to 900 mosm/kg.

Remarks

- If urinary osmolality is <200 mosm/kg, it is water diuresis.
- If urinary osmolality is ~300 mosm/kg or greater, it is solute diuresis.

1. Water Diuresis

Urine osmolality <200 mosm/kg.
Possibilities are following.

- Psychogenic polydipsia (compulsive water drinking).
- Central diabetes insipidus (HDI).

The above two conditions are differentiated by either:

a. ***Water deprivation test*** by attempting to elicit ADH secretion by water deprivation.
b. ***DDAVP test*** administration of DDAVP, renal conservation of water occurs.

Methodology

a. Water Deprivation test

- patient can drink overnight;
- a light breakfast is allowed without tea/ or coffee;
- no smoking prior to or during the test;
- the test lasts for 8 hours (usually 0800 to 1600 hours), during which no fluids are allowed, only some dry food may be permitted; and
- urine is collected **hourly** (with no preservative), volume is measured and osmolality determined.

b. DDAVP test

- DDAVP, 2 μg, IM may be given immediately on completion of water deprivation test when it is indicated, and
- urine is collected each hour for 4 hours for osmolality determination.

Note

The patient may drink water but no more than twice the volume excreted during the water deprivation test, is allowed for next 24 hours due to danger of water overload.

Inferences

1. ***With water deprivation test***
   - If the urinary osmolality exceeds 800 mosm/kg, the test is stopped and the patient is considered normal. Patients with a normal pituitary-ADH-renal axis will be able to concentrate their urine indicating psychogenic polydipsia (compulsive water drinking).
   - Patients with HDI will only be able to achieve urine osmolalities below 600 mosm/kg, usually more than 200 mosm/kg. The test is continued until the urinary osmolality "reaches a plateau (two consecutive urinary osmolality" values with a difference of less than 30 mosm/kg).
2. At this point, water deprivation test comes to an end. A blood sample in heparinised bottle should be collected for a plasma osmolality determination and then SC injection of 5 units of soluble AVP (arginine vasopressin) or 20 μg DDAVP IM given and urine samples collected hourly for urinary osmolality determination.

Ratio of Urine/Plasma Osmolality

Ratio of urine/plasma osmolality will be of great help to differentiate HDI-severe and partial type from NDI (nephrogenic diabetes insipidus).

Normally, ratio of urine to plasma osmolality in a random urine sample ***(with average fluid intake)*** varies from 1.0 to 3.0.

Remarks

- A urine: Plasma osmolality ratio of more than 1.0 and an increase in the urine osmolality, after AVP or DDAVP injection, of at least 50% or in excess 800 mosm/kg indicate severe HDI.
- A urine: Plasma osmolality ratio of more than 1.0 and an increase in urine osmolality after AVP or DDAVP by 60 to 70% or osmolality in excess of 800 mosm/kg indicate partial HDI.

Differentiation of HDI and NDI

- These two can be differentiated by water deprivation test followed by AVP or DDAVP test as stated above.

  A urinary osmolality that does not reach 600 mosm/kg at any point during the test period and shows no increase, i.e. unresponsive to AVP test is diagnostic of **"nephrogenic diabetes insipidus (NDI)"**.
- ***Estimation of plasma ADH:*** Both HDI and NDI can also be differentiated by estimation of plasma ADH.

  Normal value: Plasma ADH in normal healthy adult with normal intake of water varies from 0.35 to 1.94 ngm/l (0.32 to 1.80 p.mol/L).

  Specimen collection: Blood should be collected in chilled tubes containing EDTA. Specimen is sent to laboratory in ice, centrifuged at 4°C within 30 minutes of collection. Separated plasma is stored at 20°C until analysed.

  Inference
  - ***In HDI,*** plasma ADH is decreased or may be absent.
  - ***In NDI,*** plasma ADH may be normal or slightly to higher side of normal.

2. Solute Diuresis

Urine osmolality is ~300 mosm/kg. If the urine osmolality during polyuria is ~300 mosm/kg or between 300 and 600 mosm/kg, then a solute diuresis is probable. In such an event, other laboratory investigations are required:

- ***For Diabetes Mellitus***

a. Urine should be analysed for glucose. Qualitative Benedict's test for presence of glucose.
b. Blood-for fasting blood sugar.
c. If required full GTT should be done.

- ***Serum and Urinary Sodium [Na^+]***

Serum and urinary Na^+ should be estimated in suspected cases of:

- Diuretic therapy.
- Salt losing nephritis.

- ***Blood Urea and Serum Creatinine***

Estimation of blood urea and serum creatinine should be done:

Flow Chart for Laboratory investigation of a case of polyuria

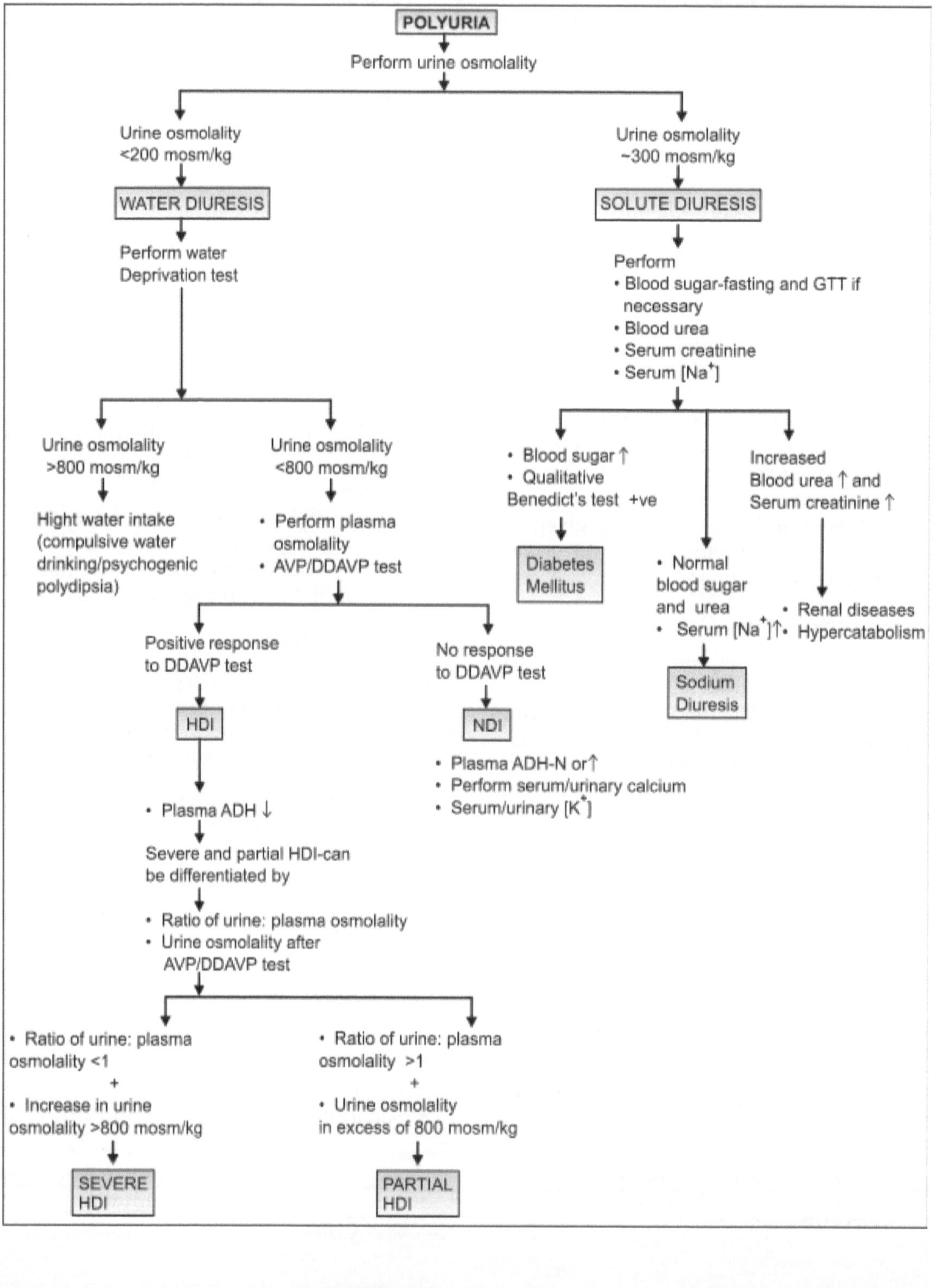

- In renal diseases.
- Post acute tubular necrosis.
- Obstructive nephropathy

In these cases, the diagnosis would have been suspected during the clinical work-up.

c. Miscellaneous Other Laboratory Tests

Certain other laboratory and clinical investigations will be required for aetiological diagnosis of HDI and NDI.

- ***For HDI***
  - Look for evidence of neoplasms.
  - Evidence of any infection/granuloma.
  - Autoimmune conditions.
- ***For NDI***
  - Serum and urinary potassium for evidence of hypokalaemia.
  - Serum and urinary calcium for hypercalaemia.
  - For multiple myelomatosis
    - total and differential proteins;
    - serum electrophoresis for monoclonal gammopathy; and
    - Bence Jones, protein in urine.

Chapter 21

Haemolytic Transfusion Reaction

INTRODUCTION

A haemolytic transfusion reaction may be defined as the occurrence of signs of red cells destruction either of donor cells or of recipient following a blood transfusion, the most obvious signs being haemoglobinuria and jaundice.

TYPES OF HAEMOLYTIC TRANSFUSION REACTION

Two types of red cells destruction have been recognized:

- *Intravascular*
- *Extravascular*

A. Intravascular Destruction

In this type, rupture of the red cells occur within the blood stream, inside the lumen of blood vessel, with consequent liberation of free Hb in plasma. There is a ***rapid haemolysis, characterized by:***

- ***Haemoglobinaemia***
- ***Methaemalbuminaemia***
- ***Haemoglobinuria***
- ***Little or no jaundice.***

This condition is characteristically seen in ABO incompatibility.

B. Extravascular Destruction

In this type, the intact red blood cells are removed from the blood stream by the cells of the RE system. There may be little or no destruction of red cells within the blood stream. There is a ***slow haemolysis, characterized by:***

- ***Hyperbilirubinaemia***
- ***Jaundice***
- ***Little or no Hb in plasma.***

This condition is characteristically seen in Rh incompatibility and in transfusion of aged stored blood.

Fate of Liberated Hb Within Blood Stream

Plasma normally contains a protein called **haptoglobin (Hp).** It is a glycoprotein in nature and is synthesized in liver. It binds free Hb—average approximately 100 mg free Hb/100 ml of blood. The binding capacity varies with different phenotypes. Three genotypes are Hp^1/Hp^1, Hp^2/Hp^1, and Hp^2/Hp^2, corresponding phenotypes being 1-1, 2-1, 2-2.

Combining power is greatest with type 1-1 (approximately, 136 mg/dl), intermediate with type 2-1 and least with type 2-2. Bound Hb circulates as ***"Hp-Hb stable complex"***. As the molecule is large it cannot be excreted through kidney but it is subsequently destroyed by RE system.

When binding capacity of haptoglobin is saturated, free Hb circulates in the plasma. Some of this free Hb can bind with albumin to form "methaemalbumin". After IV destruction of RB Cells, methaemalbumin can be detected in plasma after 5 hours and remains detectable for 24 hours or more depending on the severity.

When the amount of free Hb reaches about 25 mg/dl or more it is excreted in urine producing ***"haemoglobinuria"***.

Methaemalbumin can be detected by a simple and sensitive test called ***Schumm's test***.

Note

Methaemalbumin is not detectable in plasma of normal healthy individual, hence ***detection of methaemalbumin is diagnostic of intravascular red cells destruction.***

CAUSES OF HAEMOLYTIC TRANSFUSION REACTION

1. Incompatible Blood Transfusion

- ***ABO Incompatibility***

This is the most common cause and should be considered first. Mainly it is ***intravascular haemolysis*** characterized by haemoglobinaemia, haemoglobinuria and little or no jaundice. Destrunction of recipient's red blood cells occurs by antibodies present in donor's plasma which are lytic.

Rapid process and ***usually results in a more severe and serious reaction*** and needs immediate attention.

- ***Rh Incompatibility***

It is ***mainly extravascular destruction*** of RBCs by RE cells and is characterized by hyperbilirubinaemia and jaundice. It may be associated with little or no haemoglobinaemia and haemoglobinuria and is a comparatively slow process.

D +ve donor's cells when transfused to a D -ve recipient having anti-D antibodies, the donor cells are destroyed.

- Other abnormal antibodies present in recipient's plasma viz. anti-E, anti-C, anit-Kell, anti-fya, anti-S, etc. (rare cause).

2. Other Causes

a. Simulated IV Haemolysis

If enough of free Hb is transfused into the circulation, the recipient may develop haemoglobinaemia and haemoglobinuria and thus IV haemolysis may be simulated and suspected. Appreciable amount of free Hb may be transfused in following conditions:

- Transfusion of over-heated blood;
- Transfusion of frozen blood which has been thawed;
- Transfusion of grossly infected blood; and
- Blood transfused "under pressure" through narrow gauze needle.
  - ***Transfusion of over-heated blood:*** Blood gets haemolyzed at a temperature of 50°C or more. Hence, accidents can occur when a bottle of blood is placed in a vessel of hot water with the intention of warming the blood to body temperature.

    Note

    As a rule blood should not be warmed before transfusion.
  - ***Transfusion of frozen blood:*** Blood is stored in refrigerators. If it is not correctly regulated and monitored and if the temperature goes below – 3°C, the blood may freeze. Such frozen blood when thawed may be severely haemolyzed.
  - ***Transfusion of infected blood:*** Blood which is grossly contaminated may be haemolyzed and some bacteria produce haemolysins and destroy red cells.
  - ***Blood transfused "under pressure":*** If blood is transfused through a narrow-gauze needle under pressure, red blood cells may get ruptured and significant amount of haemolyzed blood may be transfused.

b. Osmotic Lysis of Red Cells

True IV destruction may be produced by osmotic lysis of red blood cells. Haemolytic transfusion reactions have sometimes been observed in recipients receiving transfusion of whole blood passed through a bottle containing 5% glucose and/or 0.225% saline.

c. Injection of Water into Circulation

It is a rare cause. Water may gain entrance into the circulation during irrigation of bladder in transurethral prostatectomy. If the patient is receiving blood transfusion same time, haemoglobinura may be detected and transfusion is blamed.

- ***Transfusion of Aged Stored Blood***

It produces extravascular haemolysis with hyperbilirubinaemia and jaundice.

CLINICAL FEATURES

A haemolytic transfusion reaction may be associated with alarming symptoms with development of shock or with none at all depending on the severity of haemolysis.

Three stages of haemolytic transfusion reaction can be recognized:

1. Stage of Haemolytic Shock

Onset: Appears often during the course of blood transfusion, sometimes even after 50 to 100 ml of blood have been given. In others, onset is delayed until more than 500 ml blood is transfused.

Symptoms and Signs

Complaints of:
- Throbbing in head and headache.
- Aching in the lumbar region, a constant feature.
- Breathlessness.
- Shaking chills may be present accompanied by fever.
- Abdominal pain, pain in chest, precordial oppression, nausea and vomiting are common.
- Circulatory collapse with hypotension followed by recovery from shock, the features of circulatory collapse recede and the patient feels better.
- Haemoglobinaemia and haemoglobinuria follows.

This phase of apparenet recovery is temporary.

Special Feature in This Stage

- ***Haemorrhagic tendency*** In occasional cases, a haemorrhagic tendency develops. This may sometimes be the first manifestation of haemolytic reaction. It is characterized by ***"persistent oozing"*** from the surgical site.

  Cause: Due to IV coagulation in the recipient caused by thrompoplastin like activity from haemolyzed red cells. Widespread IV coagulation results in excess utilization of coagulation factors required for clotting leading to:
  - hypoprothrombinaemia;
  - hypofibrinogenaemia; and
  - thrombocytopenia.

Note

A haemolytic reaction may be masked, if the patient is under anaesthesia. Possibility of haemolytic reaction to be considered when there is:
- a sharp rise in pulse rate;
- a sharp fall in BP;
- flushing; and
- sweating or bleeding which is difficult to control.

2. Stage of Renal Insufficiency

The stage of haemolytic reaction is followed by renal insufficiency. This stage is characterized by rapidly increasing retention of N_2, convulsions /and drowsiness, a rising BP, followed by stupor and coma. The renal insufficiency starts suddenly after a week or less of onset of oliguria.

3. Stage of Salt-Losing Diuresis

If the patient survives, from 8th to 16th day, tubular recovery/regeneration starts which is characterized by:
- Copious diuresis.
- Severe dehydration unless salt and water are supplied.
- Recovery.

I "Reaction shock" (Haemolytic shock) (1st day)	*II Renal insufficiency (1st to 12th day)*	*III Salt-losing diuresis (8th to 16th day)*
• IV haemolysis • Sudden onset • Chills or rigor • Fever • Pain in lumbar region • Hypotension • Dyspnoea and cyanosis • Mental confusion • Haemoglobinaemia	• Tubular damage (lower nephron nephrosis/or haemoglobinuric nephrosis) • Oliguria • Hypertension • Azotaemia • Haem casts • Hyperpotassaemia (Hyperkalaemia) • Decreased serum Na, Cl, Ca and CO_2 combining power • Rising titres of agglutinins • Cryptagglutinoids	• Tubular recovery/ regeneration • Copious diuresis • Severe dehydration unless salt and water supplied • Recovery

Summary of Clinical Features

As per **Muirhead and Co-workers** summary of clinical features is tabulated as given above in the box.

ACTIONS TO BE TAKEN ON SUSPICION OF A HAEMOLYTIC REACTION

1. ***Stop the blood transfusion.***
2. A sample of *venous blood* should be collected from a vein well away from the transfusion site. Avoid haemolysis during blood sample collection.
   - Part of the blood to be collected in heparinized bottle or in 3.8% sodium citrate.
   - Part of the blood to be put in a sterile plain bottle without any anticoagulant.

   This constitutes the ***"Post transfusion sample"*** required for investigation.
3. Instruction should be given to collect the next specimen of urine passed by the recipient. This constitutes the ***"Post transfusion urine sample"***.
4. Donor's blood bottle to be preserved and kept in the refrigerator, for certain tests.

SPECIMENS TO BE SENT TO THE LABORATORY FOR INVESTIGATION

1. ***Pretransfusion sample of blood*** of the recipient.
2. ***Post transfusion sample of blood*** of the recipient.
3. Post transfusion sample of urine of the recipient.
4. Left out portion of the donor's blood.

Pretransfusion sample of the blood of recipient helps in investigation in three ways:
- Recipient's full blood group can be rechecked.
- Presence of blood group antibodies can be determined with certainty. After transfusion of incompatible blood, all or almost all antibodies may be adsorbed on the transfused cells.
- Can compare the colour of serum/plasma of pretransfusion sample with post transfusion sample.

LABORATORY INVESTIGATION

Laboratory investigation can be discussed under ***two stages:***

- ***Demonstration of occurrence of increased blood destruction*** Evidences for haemolysis.
- ***The demonstration of the cause of the increased haemolysis (Evidences for cause of haemolysis).***

A. EVIDENCES OF HAEMOLYSIS

Evidences of haemolysis can be of the following types:

a. Clinical evidences
b. Laboratory evidences
   - Recipient's blood (Post transfusion sample)
   - Recipient's urine (Post-transfusion urine)
   - Donor's left out blood.

a. Clinical Evidences

These are very variable, there may be haemolytic shock or other extreme may be symptomless (if very slow drip).

Other features are:

- Chills associated with fever.
- ***Lumbar pain is characteristic.***
- Occurrence of ***'haemoglobinuria'*** as an immediate sequel of the transfusion or occurrence of jaundice after about 10 to 12 hours of blood transfusion are strong indications of haemolysis.
- In very severe cases, oliguria may be present and may even be followed by suppression of urine and signs and symptoms of renal failure.

b. Laboratory Evidences

1. **Recipient's blood—post transfusion sample**

- ***Microscopic Examination***

A small drop of recipient's blood should be placed on a slide and allowed to spread out under a cover-slip and examined under microscope.

Remarks

If incompatible blood has been transfused and not yet entirely destroyed, ***small clumps of agglutinated donor cells may be seen.***

- ***Examination of Haemoglobinaemia***

Centrifuge a portion of heparinized or citrated blood and in supernate, look for:

- Evidence of free Hb (Pink colour).
- Any increase in bilirubin (Yellow coloration).

Note

- Compare with pretransfusion sample
- The amount of free Hb in plasma should not exceed 5 mg/dl normally. Such an amount cannot be detected by ordinary hand spectroscope.

Naked eye examination

About 20 to 30 mg/dl of free Hb gives "faint pink" colour to plasma and an amount 100 mg/dl or more give difinite "red" colour.

Such quantities can be detected by hand spectroscopy.

- ***Detection of Methaemalbumin***

When the plasma contains free Hb, detectable by NE, it is usually pointless to look for methaemalbumin.

For detection of methaemalbumin:

- In practice, ordinary hand spectroscopy is quite satisfactory. α-band of methaemalbumin lies at 623-624 mμ, in red part of the spectrum. (cf-methaemoglobin—the band is seen at 630 mμ).
- ***Schumm's test*** More sensitive test for methaemalbumin.

  Method: one volume of plasma, taken in a test tube is covered with layer of ether, and 1/10th volume or slightly more concentrated ammonium sulphide is run and then shaken.

  The aqueous layer is examined spectroscopically. If methaemalbumin is present, a sharp band is seen at 558 mμ due to formation of a haemochromogen.

Note

Schumm's test can be positive at about 6 hours after transfusion and remains positive for about 24 hours.

- ***Plasma Haptoglobin Level***

Normal values: Mean normal plasma haptoglobin is about 90 mg/dl but there is wide variation.

In haemolytic state: values are grossly decreased and may be absent in severe cases. ***Low or absent values in the absence of any hepatic disease indicate strong haemolysis.***

- ***Serum Bilirubin and van den Bergh Reaction***

Estimation of serum bilirubin is helpful in extravascular type of haemolysis. An indirect van den Bergh reaction and increased serum bilirubin (hyperbilirubinaemia) is found.

2. Examination of Recipient's Urine

There are **three characteristic findings:**

- Haemoglobinuria in intravascular haemolysis.
- Urobilirubinuria in extravascular haemolysis.
- Hemosiderin in urine.

(a) Haemoglobinuria

- ***Naked Eye Examination***

When urine is ***alkaline,*** most of the Hb will be present as oxy-Hb and the urine specimen will be dark red in colour. If the urine is ***neutral*** or ***acid,*** methaemoglobin will be formed and the urine specimen will appear brown or black.

- ***Spectroscopic Examination***

Presence of oxy-Hb and methaemoglobin can be confirmed by spectroscopic examination of the sample.

- Bands of oxy-Hb lies at 578 $m\mu$ (α-band) and 540 $m\mu$ (β-band) in the yellow and green part of the spectrum, respectively.
- α-band of methaemoglobin lies at 630 $m\mu$ in the red part of the spectrum.

(b) Urobilirubinuria

Increased urobilin excretion if present can be demonstrated by Schleisinger's test.

(c) Haemosiderin in Urine

In patients with chronic haemoglobinaemia, haemosiderinuria is a constant feature. It is invariably found when plasma free Hb concentraction exceeds 25 mg/dl.

Method

- Contrifuge 15 ml of recipient's urine.
- Resuspend the sediment in 1 ml of supernate.
- Add an equal volume of 5% HCl
- It is followed by addition of 0.5 ml of 10% of potassium ferrocyanide in water.

Remarks

- When there is gross haemosiderinuria, deep blue granules/particles are seen.
- If these are not obvious, centrifuge the sample, the blue granules can be seen in the tip of the centrifuge tube.
- Sediment on examination microscopically will demonstrate—***blue granules in renal epithelium.***

Note

The centrifuged deposit of the recipient's urine in haemoglobinuria will contain practically no RBC or a few only.

B. TO FIND OUT THE CAUSE OF HAEMOLYSIS

Cause of Haemolysis

- Tests on Donor's blood
- Tests on Recipient's blood (Both pre and post transfusion samples)

1. Common Tests for Both

Regroup donor and recipient, repeat cross matching and perform a direct Coombs' test.

- ***ABO Incompatibility***

The samples of blood from donor and recipient should be re-grouped as regards ABO system, both agglutinogens in the Red blood cells and agglutinins in serum to be checked. The possibility of an ABO incompatibility is more common and should first come to mind and be excluded.

- ***Rh Incompatibility***

Next Rh-incompatibility should be considered. The clinical history, previous transfusions, family history, number of pregnancies may be suggestive.

Note

If the donor is found to be Rh +ve (D +ve) and the recipient Rh -ve (D -ve), the patient's serum must be examined for Rh D antibody.

- ***Coombs' Test***
    - Indirect Coombs' test will be found most reliable single test for this.
    - At the same time, a direct Coombs' test should be performed on the post transfusion sample of blood. If the patient's serum contains Rh antibody, and there are some surviving Rh +ve cells, the direct Coombs' test will be positive.

- ***Cross-Matching***
    - *Repeat direct matching test:* A suspension of the donor's red cells should be tested against the *"Pre-transfusion sample"* of the recipient's serum in saline, in 25% albumin, and antiglobulin test.

      The above may show straight way that some gross error has been committed. Occasionally the antiglobulin test reveals incompatibility that has been missed by a test in albumin.
    - If the results of the above tests are negative or doubtful, a cross-matching using trypsinizsed or papainized donor cells should be set up and incubated at 37°C.

- ***Detection of Abnormal Antibodies***

Finally identification of abnormal antibodies other than anti-Rh like anti-Kell, anti-S, anti-fya, anti-E to be looked for though it is rare.

Note

- The three antibodies anti-Kell, anti-S and anti-fya have all been shown to be capable of causing haemolytic reaction.
- The identification of an abnormal antibody other than anti-Rh demands a panel of donors whose full blood groups are known. If such a panel is not available, it is wise to submit the blood sample to a reference laboratory which can do it.

2. TESTS ON DONOR'S BLOOD

- ***Age and Volume of Blood***

Age of the blood and volume given should be noted. The significance of this is that stored blood show definite ***increase in red cells fragility towards the end of third week of storage*** and in some patients having liver diseases, large volume of transfusion of such aged blood, though compatible, can ***produce extravascular haemolysis*** with ***hyperbilirubinaemia, jaundice*** and ***urobilirubinuria.***

- ***Transfusion of Infected Blood***

Infection is a cause of haemolysis in stored blood and in order to be able to exclude, proceed as follows:

- **Smell**—a foul odour in grossly contaminated blood.
- A ***"hanging drop"*** preparation may help to demonstrate the presence of organisms.
- Examination of a stained smear may be helpful.
- Requisite amount of blood to be taken out from the bottle with a sterile pipette and inocculated to sterile broth and sent for culture.

- ***NE Evidence of Haemolysis***

Look for haemolysis in a centrifuged sample of donor's blood. If haemolysis is present, enquire, whether blood bottle was overheated or whether blood was frozen and subsequently haemolyzed on thawing.

- ***Tests to Prove Damage by Donor's Plasma***

Haemolysis of patient's red blood cells may take place due to immune anti-A or anti-B being

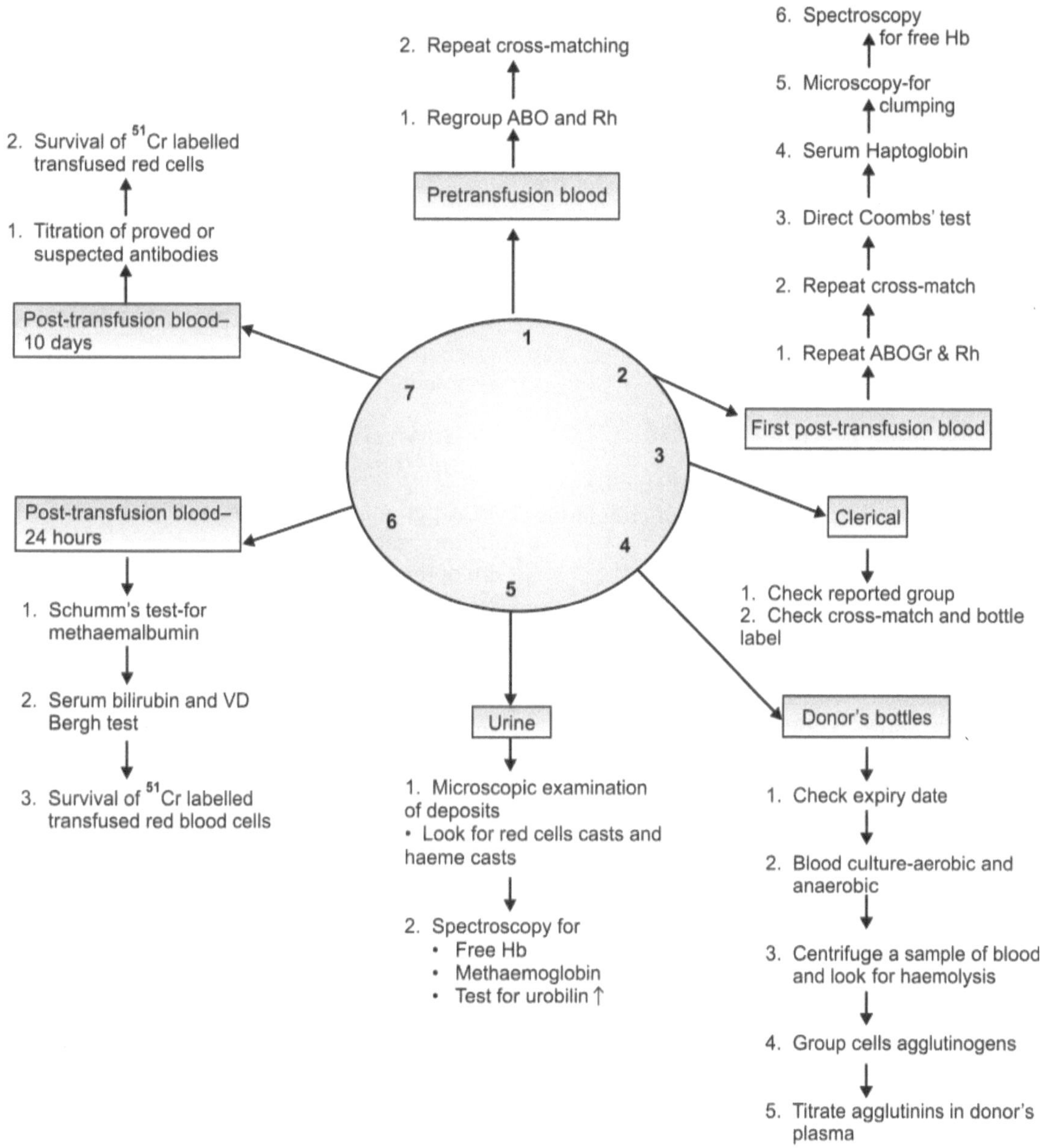

Fig. 21.1: Schematic representation of laboratory investigation

transfused viz. if group 'O' blood being given to group A or B recipient. Titres of anti-A and anti-B of the transfused plasma should be ascertained and also tests carried out for anti-A or anti-B haemolysins.

Note

If group O blood has, in fact, been given to group A or B recipient and if the donor's blood is suspected then osmotic fragility of the recipient's blood should be measured and, a stained blood film should be examined.

Inference

An increase in osmotic fragility and the presence of spherocytes are pointers to the haemolytic reaction being due to the transfusion of immune anti-A or anti-B or presence of haemolytic antibodies.

3. Tests on Recipient's Blood (Post Transfusion Sample)

- ***Antiglobulin Test (Coombs' test)***

A direct antiglobulin test will probably be +ve, if incompatible donor cells are still circulating in relatively large number.

- ***Infected Blood—Blood Culture***

If there is any suspicion that infected donor's blood associated with haemolysis is the cause of the reaction, a blood culture from the recipient is also indicated.

- ***Titration of Anti-A and Anti-B in Recipient's Serum***

If the patient is not seen until after the incident and if no donor's blood is available, the cause of ***an incompatible transfusion may be revealed by an increase in the titre of an iso-antibody present in the patient's serum.***

Example

A manifold rise in anti-A titre in a group B subject, which reaches a peak one to two weeks after transfusion, is a clear indication that the recipient had received group 'A' blood.

- ***Survival Study of Donor's Cells by ^{51}Cr***

In a patient who has recovered from a transfusion reaction, it is now possible to tag a few ml of the blood believed to be incompatible, and to follow accurately its survival after IV injection and thus to confirm or refute its incompatibility.

A schematic representation of investigation to be done in a suspected haemolytic transfusion reaction is depicted in Figure 21.1.

Chapter 22

Haemolytic Anaemia

INTRODUCTION

A haemolytic anaemia is characterised by shortened lifespan and an increase in the rate of red cells destruction.

Note

- Normally "effete" red cells undergo lysis at the end of their lifespan of 100 to 120 days within the cells of RE system in the spleen and elsewhere like bone marrow and liver ***(extravascular haemolysis)*** and Hb is not liberated into the plasma in appreciable amounts.
- In haemolytic anaemia, the red cells lifespan is shortened (accelerated haemolysis). In majority, the haemolysis takes place within the bloodstream **(*IV haemolysis*)**—plasma Hb rises and may be associated with ***haemoglobinaemia*** and ***haemoglobinuria***. On the other hand, in some types of haemolytic anaemia, the increased haemolysis is predominantly extravascular **(*EV haemolysis*)** and the plasma Hb is barely raised.

The clinical and laboratory phenomena of increased haemolysis reflect the nature of the haemolytic mechanism, where the haemolysis is taking place and the response of the bone-marrow to the anaemia resulting from the increased haemolysis, viz.:

- ***Erythroid hyperplasia; and***
- ***Reticulocytosis.***

CAUSES

Premature destruction of red cells may occur from ***two fundamental defects***:

- ***Intracorpuscular (intrinsic) abnormality of red cells.***
- ***Extracorpuscular (extrinsic) abnormality of red cells.***

A. Intracorpuscular (Intrinsic) Defects

- The fault lies in the red cells themselves.
- Normal compatible red cells when transfused to such a patient survive for a normal span of life, but the patient's red cells when transfused into a normal healthy recipient are destroyed prematurely.

Intracorpuscular defects may be of two types:

- *Congenital*
- *Acquired*

1. Congenital

- ***Membrane Defects***
  - Hereditary spherocytosis.
  - Hereditary elliptocytosis.
- ***Haemoglobin Defects***
  - Haemoglobinopathies:
    - Hb-S (Sickle cell disease)
    - Other abnormal haemoglobins like Hb-C, Hb-M, etc.

- Thalassaemias
  - β-thalassaemia (Thalassaemia major).
  - α-thalassaemia like Hb-H disease, Bart's Hb.
- ***Double heterozygous disorders*** Hb S—β-thalassaemia.

• ***Enzymic Defects***

- Non-spherocytic congenital haemolytic anaemia.
  - Due to deficiency of G-6-PD.
  - Due to deficiency of pyruvate kinase (PK-deficiency).
  - Other enzymes like hexokinase deficiency.
  - Drug-induced haemolytic anaemia and Fabism.

2. *Acquired*

Paroxysmal nocturnal haemoglobinuria (PNH).

B. Extracorpuscular (Extrinsic) Defects

In these the fault is not with RB cells, the fault lies in plasma ***due to the development of an abnormal haemolytic mechanism.*** Normal compatible red cells when transfused to such a patient are ***destroyed prematurely,*** but the patient's cells when transfused to a normal recipient survives normal lifespan. ***Extrinsic defects are acquired.***

2. Acquired Causes

• ***Immune Mechanisms***

Autoimmune acquired haemolytic anaemias are:

- Either due to ***"warm antibody";*** or ***"cold"*** antibody.
- Paroxysmal cold haemoglobinuria (PCH).
- Haemolytic disease of the newborn (HDN).
- Incompatible blood transfusion.
- Drug-induced haemolytic anaemia.

• ***Non-immune Mechanisms***

- Mechanical haemolytic anaemia:
- Cardiac haemolytic anaemia.
- Microangiopathic haemolytic anaemia.
- March haemoglobinuria.

• ***Miscellaneous Causes***

- Haemolytic anaemia due to direct action of chemicals/drugs.
- Haemolytic anaemia due to infection.
- Associated with burns.
- Poisoning: Lead poisoning.

LABORATORY INVESTIGATIONS

Laboratory investigation of a case of suspected haemolytic anaemia may be discussed **in three steps as follows.**

- ***To establish that anaemia is present.***
- ***To find out the evidences for haemolysis.***
- ***To detect the mechanism or the underlying cause (defect).***

A. TO ESTABLISH THE PRESENCE OF ANAEMIA

Presence of anaemia may be suggested by the following:

1. History

- Weakness and easy fatiguability.
- Passing of pink coloured urine.
- Complaining of jaundice.

2. Physical Examination

- Look for pallor/and yellow colouration of conjunctivae.
- Splenomegaly/and hepatomagaly.
- Leg ulceration/pigmentation.
- Lymph node enlargement (Lymphadenopathy).
- Evidence of purpura.

3. Certain "Basic" Laboratory Tests

- Hb-estimation.
- Total RB cells count.
- Haematocrit.
- Red cells indices specially MCHC
- Peripheral smear examination

Note

For laboratory confirmation of anaemia, the haematocrit and measurement of Hb concentration are the most practical and reliable tests available.

- Red cells indices are helpful for morphologic grouping of anaemia.
- Calculations of MCV and MCH require a red cell count and this may carry considerable error unless electronic counter is used.
- MCHC is the most reliable of the red cell indices, since it is based on the haematocrit and Hb value, which carry comparatively less error.

B. EVIDENCES FOR HAEMOLYSIS

Examination of peripheral blood smear and certain laboratory tests will point to the presence of haemolysis.

1. Haematological Evidences

- ***Peripheral Blood Smear***

A peripheral blood smear may reveal changes which may strongly suggest the haemolytic nature of the anaemia.

a. Examination of an Unstained Smear

- ***Heinz bodies:*** may be seen as refractile objects in dry unstained films, if the illumination is cut down by lowering the microscope condenser. They can also be seen by dark-ground illumination or phase contrast microscopy.

Interpretation

Finding of Heinz bodies in man suggests chemical poisoning, drug intoxication, presence of unstable Hb like Hb Köln or in G-6-PD deficiency.

b. Examination of a Stained Smear

- ***Basophilic or polychromatophilic macrocytes*** with or without normoblasts suggest augmented erythropoiesis associated with haemolysis or haemorrhage.

Other findings indicative of haemolysis are:

- abnormally shaped red blood cells ***(poikilocytes)***;
- presence of ***ovalocytes*** or ***elliptocytes;***
- presence of sickle cells—sickle cell disease;
- presence of ***spherocytes*** which can be *hereditary* spherocytosis or acquired type; and
- presence of red cell fragments ***(schistocytes)***
- ***Target cells:*** A prominent feature of haemoglobinopathies, particularly Hb-C. Also seen in β-thalassaemia, with liver diseases and sometimes Fe-deficiency anaemia.
- ***Microcytosis*** and ***stippling*** suggests thalassaemia or lead poisoning rather than Fe-deficiency.
- ***Inclusions for Hb-H*** and presence of malarial parasites in red blood cells.

(For details of peripheral smear—see below)

- ***Reticulocyte Count***

- A relatively accurate index of effective red cells production when it is expressed in absolute numbers.
- Range of reticulocyte count in health—
  Adults **and** ***children:*** 0.5 to 2.5%.
  Infants (full term, cord blood): 2 to 6%.
- ***In absolute numbers,*** the normal reticulocyte count in health is about 50 to 100 × $10^9/l$
  - A 3 to 6 fold increase in the corrected or absolute reticulocyte count indicates an optimal increase in erythropoiesis, in response to blood loss due to increased red cells-destruction.

Note

- ***Reticulocytosis is a characteristic feature of haemolytic anaemia.***

- It is to be noted that decreased numbers may be found with severe haemolytic anaemia of autoimmune type.

- ***Bone Marrow Smear***

Bone marrow smear examination will ***show increased erythropoiesis***

In normal subjects: erythroid: myeloid ratio is 1:3.

In haemolytic anaemia: erythroid to myeloid ratio is increased.

2. Biochemical Evidences

- ***Serum Bilirubin and VD Bergh Reaction***

In haemolytic anaemia, the total serum bilirubin is frequently elevated, but usually not more than 4 mg/dl, predominantly in the indirect reacting fraction (unconjugated bilirubin).

  - ***VD Bergh reaction*** is usually indirect positive due to predominance of unconjugated bilirubin.

- ***Faecal and Urinary Urobilinogen***

In the absence of liver disease, an increase in the urinary urobilinogen is strongly suggestive of a haemolytic process, but a normal value cannot be used as evidence against haemolysis. Presence of increased amounts of faecal urobilinogen is a good pointer to increased destruction of circulating red blood cells.

- ***Plasma Free Hb***

Normal range is 1 to 4 mg/dl. The ***concentration of plasma free Hb is raised in haemolytic anaemia,*** where there is rapid destruction of the red blood cells inside the lumen of the blood vessel ***(IV haemolysis).*** Marked increase of free Hb is seen in mismatched blood transfusion, black water fever, haemolytic disease of the newborn (HDN), paroxysmal cold haemoglobinuria (PCH), and paroxysmal nocturnal haemoglobinuria (PNH).

Mild to moderate increase is seen in sickle cell anaemia, homozygous β-thalassaemia and acquired haemolytic anaemia.

(For fate of free Hb after intravascular haemolysis—see Investigation of haemolytic transfusion reaction).

- ***Demonstration of Presence of Hb in Urine (Haemoglobinuria) and Haemosiderin in Urine (Haemosiderinuria)***

See under—investigation of haemolytic transfusion reaction.

- ***Presence of Methaemalbumin in Plasma and Schumm's Test***

See under—Investigation of haemolytic transfusion reaction.

- ***Plasma Haptoglobin (Hp) Level***

Plasma haptoglobin binding capacity with free Hb differs with the phenotype of Hp (see under—Investigation of haemolytic transfusion reaction). It is demonstrated by paper electrophoresis and consists of haptoglobin (α_2-globulin) and heme-binding globulin-haemopexin.

It usually measures 50 to 150 mg/dl, with heme-binding globulin contributing less than 10 mg/dl. Depletion of haptoglobin occurs with haemolytic diseases when red cells survival is half of the normal. ***A binding capacity less than 20 mg/dl is strongly suggestive of a haemolytic process.*** (Exception—genetic absence of Hp and in liver diseases).

- ***Enzyme Studies***

Intravascular haemolysis is usually accompanied by an elevation of serum lactate dehydrogenase (LDH) and aspartate transaminase level (S-GOT). Estimations of these two enzymes may be useful.

- ***Red Cells Survival Studies With ^{51}Cr***

Where facilities are available red cells survival studies with ^{51}Cr will be helpful.

The above laboratory investigations alongwith history and clinical findings will establish the haemolytic nature of the anaemia.

C. LABORATORY INVESTIGATION TO DETECT THE MECHANISM/OR UNDERLYING CAUSE

As discussed above, the mechanism of excessive destruction of red cells are either:

(a) Intrinsic intracorpuscular defects or
(b) Extracorpuscular defects.

To differentiate the above two, the ideal test is Coombs' test.

• *Coombs' Antiglobulin Test*

A positive Coombs' test indicates extracorpuscular defect, as extracorpuscular haemolytic disease is frequently associated with an anti-erythrocyte antibody which is demonstrable by the direct Coombs' test.

Note

A positive Coombs' test means that only the red cells are coated with gamma globulin, it does not necessarily imply that haemolysis is present. ***A negative Coombs' test is consistently found in the haemolytic anaemias associated with intrinsic red cells defects.***

• Measurement of Survival of ^{51}Cr Labelled Compatible Normal Red Cells

If facilities available, it is a very sensitive method for distinguishing intracorpuscular defects. ***The lifespan of the ^{51}Cr labelled normal donor cells is normal in patients with intracorpuscular defects but is shortened in those with extracorpuscular defects.***

Once the differentiation is done to ***two main groups,*** then laboratory tests should be performed to establish the underlying cause of each group.

I. Laboratory Tests in Respect of Coombs' Negative Haemolytic Anaemias— Intrinsic Red Cells Defects

Suggested laboratory investigations to be considered are:

- *Peripheral blood smear re-examination*
- Tests for osmotic fragility (including incubation) and autohaemolysis.
- Demonstration of sickling and Hb-S.
- Haemoglobin electrophoresis for other abnormal Hbs.
- Measurement of Hb A_2 and Hb F.
- Screening for heat-unstable Hb.
- Incubated sample for Heinz body formation or precipitation of unstable Hb.
- ***Tests to demonstrate PNH:*** Urinary haemosiderin and sucrose lysis test, if +ve, acid haemolysis test (Ham's test).
- ***Enzyme screening*** for G-6-PD and pyruvate kinase (PK) deficiencies.

Note

All the above tests should not be performed at once. Peripheral smear should be re-examined carefully as this may provide excellent clues to the cause of haemolysis (RB Cells defect)

1. Peripheral Blood Smear

- ***Spherocytes:*** Increased numbers of spherocytes with only mild to moderate anisocytosis, suggest strongly ***hereditary spherocytosis.***

  In most cases, blood smears of parents and siblings will detect at least one other similar case.
- ***Sickling:*** It may be seen in smear occasionally indicating the need for sickle cell preparation and Hb electrophoresis for demonstration of Hb-S.
- ***Target cells:*** Presence of many target cells with little or no anaemia is strongly indicative of ***haemoglobinopathies*** specially Hb-C disease.
- ***Neutropenia:*** It is seen characteristically in later stages of ***paroxysmal nocturnal haemoglobinuria (PNH)*** which may be associated with ***hypochromasia*** and ***microcytosis*** due to continued loss of Fe because of haemoglobinuria.
- ***Basophilic stippling:*** It is commonly seen in ***thalassaemias*** and greatly helps in distinguishing this disease from Fe-deficiency which produces an otherwise similar smear.

Note

Basophilic stippling best detected at high magnification in the large polychromatophilic red cells suggestive of abnormal RNA.

- ***Howell-Jolly bodies:*** These are seen characteristically in the red cells after splenectomy. But in late stages of sickle-cell disease, due to repeated splenic infarctions when autosplenectomy has taken place, these may be seen.

- ***Red cell inclusions:*** Presence of red cells inclusions, which can be seen with methylene blue stain ***indicate presence of abnormal unstable haemoglobins*** like Hb-Köln and Hb-Zürich.

Once the peripheral smear is examined thoroughly, ***it is likely to suggest, along with the history/and clinical findings, a specific disease, then additional laboratory tests should be made to support the diagnosis.***

2. Tests for Osmotic Fragility Including Incubation and Autohaemolysis

Increased osmotic fragility is characteristic of ***hereditary spherocytosis.***

Note

- Increased osmotic fragility is also observed with spherocytosis associated with Coombs' positive haemolytic anaemia.
- Spherocytosis and increased osmotic fragility indicate presence of immune antibodies in Coombs' positive haemolytic anaemia.
- ***Osmotic fragility after incubation of 37°C:*** It is done mainly for differentiation between congenital non-spherocytic haemolytic anaemia-Dacie Type I and Type II (PK deficiency).

Interpretations

- Osmotic fragility is normal in Type II (PK deficiency) and greatly increased after incubation at 37°C for 24 hours.
- ***Autohaemolysis:*** When normal defibrinated blood is incubated under sterile conditions at 37°C, little haemolysis occurs within 48 hours.

  The rate of haemolysis is ↑ increased in:
  - Hereditary spherocytosis;
  - Type II congenital non-spherocytic anaemia (PK deficiency); and
  - PNH (paroxysmal nocturnal haemoglobinuria).
- ***Autohaemolysis after addition of glucose:*** Hereditary spherocytosis is the likely diagnosis if addition of glucose significantly decreases auto-haemolysis. On the other hand, in P-K deficiency, haemolysis is not decreased by addition of glucose.

3. Demonstration of Sickling and Hb-S

Sickle cells preparation, to demonstrate sickling of red blood cells, and Hb-electrophoresis are done for the confirmation of diagnosis of sickle cell disease.

Sickling in Whole Blood

The Sickling phenomenon may be simply demonstrated in a thin wet film of blood sealed between slide and cover slip by means of petroleum jelly/or paraffin wax mixture to ***produce O_2 deficiency*** and seen under microscope. ***Sickling develops in the various types of sickle cell disease and also in Hb-S trait.***

Interpretations

- ***In homozygous Hb-S disease or Hb-S-C disease or Hb-S/β-thalassaemia,*** marked sickling is usually visible after incubation for one hour or less at 37°C and filamentous forms like "sickles" are seen.
- ***In Hb-S trait,*** the process is slower and the changes are less severe and incubation for 12 hours may be required to show the changes.

Note

Sickling can be hastened by the addition of reducing agents like sodium dithionate in the blood.

- ***Hb electrophoresis:*** Can be done in cellulose acetate, pH 6.5 and citrate agar electrophoresis, pH 6.0 to demonstrate Hb-S.

4. Haemoglobin Electrophoresis for Abnormal Haemoglobins

Haemoglobin electrophoresis can be done as stated above, to find out and differentiate other haemoglobins.

It is performed specially for the measurement of Hb A_2 and Hb-F in suspected β-thalassaemia. Elevations of one or both is seen in this disease and alongwith history and other clinical findings confirm the diagnosis.

Note

Failure to detect any rise in Hb A_2 and Hb F does not exclude the possibility of thalassaemia.

Other Tests-for Hb A_2 and Hb-F

a. A raised Hb A_2 is characteristic in heterozygous β-thalassaemia for the diagnosis of β-thalassaemia traits.
   Two methods are available for Hb-A_2:
   - ***Cellulose acetate electrophoresis (pH 8.9)*** as stated above, and eluted into buffer and the % Hb A_2 calculated by measuring and comparing the absorbance of Hb A_2 eluate and an eluate prepared from the remaining haemoglobins.
   - ***Micro chromatography*** can also be used for estimation of Hb A_2

     Normal range: of Hb A_2 has been given as 1.5 to 3.5% (Mean 2.5 ± 0.15%).

     Hb A_2 is usually raised in β-thalassaemia and range varies from 4.0 to 7.0%.
b. ***Hb-F may be estimated by several methods other than electrophoresis,*** all of which are *based on its resistance* ***to denaturation at alkaline pH.***
   - ***Alkali denaturation test:*** For small amounts of Hb-F, below 10 to 15%, method using NaOH is reliable, whilst for levels over 50% and in cord blood, the method of Jonxis and Visser is preferable.
   - ***Immunological methods:*** More recently, immunological methods have been devised to measure Hb-F by immunodiffusion and by enzyme-linked immunoassay (ELISA method). RIA methods have been evolved and proved to be most accurate.

     Normal Hb-F

     In infants aged 1 year, the level of Hb-F should not be more than 1%. The normal range for healthy adults is 0.2 to 1.0%.
c. ***Demonstration of Intracellular Hb-F in RB Cells:***
   Two techniques have been widely used for measuring intracellular Hb-F distribution.
   - ***Acid elution test:*** It is most frequently used. The identification of RB cells containing Hb-F depends upon the fact that they resist acid-elution to a greater extent than do normal cells. RB cells containing Hb-F appear as isolated, darkly stained cells amongst a background of pale staining ghost cells (normal RB Cells) under the microscope.
   - ***Immunofluorescent technique:*** It is more sensitive method and uses specific anti-Hb-F antibodies. Immunofluorescent labelling is capable of detecting cells with as little as 0.5% Hb-F.

5. Screening for Heat Unstable Hb

If there is suspicion of an ***unstable Hb haemolytic anaemia (UHbHA),*** a firm diagnosis depends on demonstration in the laboratory that Hb is abnormally unstable.

Points for demonstration of unstable Hb:
- The clinical picture itself may provide clues, e.g.
  - Presence of cyanosis due to methaemoglobinaemia.
  - Presence of anaemia and jaundice.
  - Passing of dark brown to almost black urine due to excretion of dipyrroles *(dipyrroluria).*
- ***Careful inspection of peripheral smear*** can suggest diagnosis of UHbHA, specially if splenectomy has been done.

Note

The ***presence of many Heinz bodies in the blood of a haemolytic anaemia patient after splenectomy strongly suggests unstable Hb.***
- ***Auto haemolysis:*** In a patient of haemolytic anaemia in whom the spleen has not been removed, ***autohaemolysis test may provide an important pointer to the presence of UHbHA.***

Note

If ***an unstable Hb*** is ***present,*** the ***serum may appear brown or opaque after incubation for 48 hours.***

Explanation: The above is due to presence of methaemoglobin and Heinz bodies.

If a smear is made and stained with methyl violet, numerous Heinz bodies may be seen.

- ***Starch gel electrophoresis at pH 8.6:*** Some unstable haemoglobins migrate in the position of Hb-S, or just in front of Hb A_2. In some cases, free α-chains can be seen to migrate towards cathode.

Methods to demonstrate Hb unstability

The following *two methods* are used:

- ***Heat instability test***
- Isopropanol precipitation test

a. ***Heat instability test:*** When Hb solution is heated, the secondary and tertiary structures are broken including van der Waals bonds and the Hb molecule becomes less stable. Under suitable controlled conditions, ***such unstable Hb get precipitated, while the normal Hb remains in solution.***

Remarks

- Normal control haemolysate may give faint cloudiness after one hour.
- ***Unstable Hb shows marked precipitation after one hour*** and ***gross flocculant precipitation seen after two hours.***

b. ***Isopropanol precipitation test:*** When Hb is dissolved in isopropanol, which is more nonpolar than water, Hb molecule becomes less stable due to weakening of the bonds. This results in precipitation of unstable Hb as compared to normal Hb which remains in solution.

Remarks

- ***Normal control:*** Shows faint cloudiness only after 30 minutes.
- ***Unstable Hb:*** Undergoes precipitation at 5 minutes and gross flocculant precipitate develops by the end of 30 minutes.

6. Incubated Sample for Heinz Body Formation or Precipitation of Unstable Hb/Other Red Cell Inclusions

The most important red cells inclusions to be looked for in the haemoglobinopathies are:

- ***α-chain inclusions*** in β-thalassaemia major.
- ***Hb H inclusions*** in α-thalassaemias.
- ***Heinz bodies*** in unstable Hb diseases—in chemical poisoning, drug intoxication and in G-6-PD deficiency.

Note

- Precipitated α-chains are found in the cytoplasm of nucleated red cell precursors of patients with β-thalassaemia major. Similar to Heinz bodies, they stain readily supravitally with methyl violet and appear usually as irregularly shaped bodies close to the nucleus of normoblasts.
- ***Hb H Inclusions develop in Hb Bart's hydrops faetalis syndrome and in Hb H disease.***

Method

Mix 2 volumes of fresh blood added to any anticoagulant with 1 volume of 1% New Methylene blue in saline. Incubate the mixture at 37°C for one hour. Make a film of the suspension and when dry examine microscopically unfixed. The inclusions appear as multiple greenish blue bodies.

- ***Heinz bodies*** are insoluble denatured globin chains. They may be demonstrated in the peripheral blood of patients if the blood is kept at 37°C for 24-48 hours. Methyl violet or brilliant cresyl blue can be used for demonstration of both α-chain inclusions and Heinz bodies.

7. Tests to Demonstrate PNH

Number of tests are available to demonstrate PNH.

a. Screening Tests for PNH:

- Heat resistance test.
- Sucrose lysis test.
- Cold antibody lysis test.
- Inulin test.

b. Confirmatory Test—Acidified Serum Test (Ham's Test)

If PNH is suspected, the first test should be an examination of urine for Hb and urinary sediment to be examined for haemosiderin followed by sucrose lysis test.

If the haemosiderin and sucrose lysis test are +ve, the diagnosis of PNH should be confirmed by acidified serum test (Ham's test).

Mechanism of Haemolysis of PNH Cells:

- Haemoglobinaemia and haemoglobinuria is ***intermittent*** in PNH.
- PNH red cells are unusually susceptible to lysis by complement.
- In Ham's test, complement is activated via the alternative pathway.
- In sucrose lysis test, a low ionic strength is thought to lead to the binding of IgG molecules non-specifically to the cell membrane and to the subsequent activation of complement via the classical sequence.
- In all the tests, ***PNH cells undergo lysis because of their greatly increased senstivity to lysis by activated complement.***

Note

- The sucrose lysis test is based on the fact that red cells absorb complement components from serum at low ionic concentrations. PNH cells due to their great sensitivity undergo lysis but normal red cells do not.
- The RB Cells in some cases of leukaemias and myelosclerosis may show some lysis (less than 10%) but in such cases, Ham's test is usually negative.
- The final confirmatory test for PNH is Ham's test. The test is specific for PNH red blood cells.
- Only condition which may show +ve Ham's Test is rare congenital disorder "congenital dyserythropoietic anaemia, CDA Type II or HEMPAS".
- ***Other important additional biochemical features shown by PNH red cells*** are:
  - Diminished activity of red cells enzyme ***"acetylcholinesterase"*** ↓
  - Deficiency of a special protein called ***"decay accelerating factor" (DAF),*** considered normally to protect red cells, leucocytes and platelets from damage by complement.
  - **Glycophorin α** present in RBC membranes of PNH patients have been found to be abnormal.
  - PNH neutrophils have been found to be deficient in the enzyme alkaline phosphatase (ALP).

"HEMPAS" differs from PNH in following respects:

- HEMPAS red cells show lysis in only a proportion of normal sera (<30%).
- They do not show lysis in patients own acidified sera.
- Sucrose lysis test is always -ve.

8. Enzyme Screening for G-6-PD and PK Deficiency

a. Red cells enzyme deficiencies do not produce any characteristic morphologic abnormalities in the peripheral blood smear examination.

b. An enzyme deficiency should be suspected if the problem appears to be intracorpuscular (Coombs' negative) and no other causes of intracorpuscular haemolytic disorders are found.

c. G-6-PD deficiency is comparatively more common than PK deficiency. G-6-PD deficiency most frequently associated with haemolysis which is episodic and related to exposure to oxidant drugs or infection.

d. A number of ***"screening tests"*** for G-6-PD deficiency are available. They are:
   - Methaemoglobin reduction test,
   - Ascorbate-cyanide screening test,
   - Fluorescent screening test,
   - Methaemoglobin elution test.

e. G-6-PD assay can be performed if any of the screening test (mentioned under d) is positive.

   The activity of the enzyme is assayed by following the rate of production of NADPH, which unlike $NADP^+$, has a peak of UV light absorption at 340 mμ.

Note

- It is to be noted that the screening tests may not show any abnormality during the haemolytic episodes as many young red cells may be present.

- Under above circumstances, the test should be repeated several months after recovery to confirm diagnosis.

f. Pyruvate kinase (PK) deficiency is much rarer and less common than G-6-PD deficiency. ***Unlike G-6-PD deficiency, it is usually associated with chronic haemolysis.***

Enzyme assay for red cells PK for the confirmation of the diagnosis is becoming more readily available and can be set up in a laboratory. Suspected PK deficiency patient invariably shows reticulocytosis due to chronic haemolysis and in such a case if PK level is below normal range, such patient can be considered PK deficient.

g. ***Additional laboratory test for G-6-PD deficiency is glutathione stability test.***

Interpretations

- ***In normal subjects,*** incubation of red blood cells with oxidizing drugs like acetyl phenyl hydrazine has little effect on G-SH content of red cells, since its oxidation by the oxidant drug is reversed by ***"glutathione reductase",*** which, in turn, relies on G-6-PD for a supply of NADPH.

  Hence, in G-6-PD deficient patients the stability of G-S-H is significantly decreased.

- ***In normal adults,*** red cells G-SH is lowered by not more than 20% by incubation with the oxidant drug acetyl phenyl hydrazine. On the other hand, **in G-6-PD deficient patients, it is lowered by more than 20%,** viz. in heterozygotes the fall may be 50% or more, whilst in homozygotes, the fall is more and may be totally lost.

II. Laboratory Tests in Respect of Coombs' Positive Haemolytic Anaemias—Extracorpuscular Defects

In a suspected case of haemolytic anaemia of extracorpuscular defects, the suggested laboratory investigations are follows:

- Study of peripheral smear.
- Plasma Hb, plasma Hp, urinary Hb and haemosiderin to be checked for evidence of IV haemolysis.
- Specific immunohaematology tests in addition to Coombs' test:
  - Warm and cold antibodies,
  - Donath-Landsteiner antibodies.
- RA factor and antinuclear antibody test (ANA) in suspected cases of collagen diseases.
- Fibrinogen and fibrin-spilt products in suspected case of IV coagulation.
- Other investigations, if any, to detect underlying infections, neoplasms and other disorders.

Note

- Choice of laboratory investigations to be done in evaluation of extracorpuscular defect will depend to some extent on clinical features.
- History and physical examination will be more helpful in evaluating these disorders than compared to intracorpuscular defects (hereditary disease).

1. Peripheral Smear Examination

- Presence of ***red-cells fragmentation (Schistocytes)*** suggests disseminated IV coagulation.

Note

Fragmentation of red cells are also seen in other conditions characterised by mechanical damage to the red cells.

- Presence of abnormalities of leucocytes and platelets may indicate presence of leukaemias and also in disseminated IV coagulation.
- Spherocytosis, neutropenia and varying degrees of thromocytopenia may be found in collagen diseases like systemic lupus erythematosis (SLE).
- Malaria parasites may be seen in red blood cells in case of malaria which may be associated with haemolysis.

2. Plasma Hb, Hp, Urinary Hb and Haemosiderin

When IV haemolysis is suspected because of presence of red cells fragmentation in peripheral blood smear or because of occurrence of haemoglobinuria without haematuria, absence or diminished plasma haptoglobin (Hp); elevation of free Hb in plasma; positive Schumm's test for methaemalbumin and presence of urinary free Hb/and/or haemosiderin, confirms the diagnosis.

Note

Mechanical injury to red blood cells in the feet of distant runners produces ***"march haemoglobinuria"*** which can produce the above changes.

3. Other Immunohaematological Tests

In addition to the positive Coombs' test, certain other immunohaematological tests can be done to characterise the protein coating of the damaged red blood cells.

All Coombs' positive haemolytic disorders may be classified into ***"warm"*** and ***"cold"*** agglutinins type and fall under autoimmune haemolytic anaemia (AIHA).

a. Autoimmune Haemolytic Anaemia (AIHA)

Causes

1. ***Idiopathic:*** Where no cause is known.
2. ***Secondary or symptomatic types:*** Associated with:
   - Other autoimmune diseases, like SLE, rheumatoid arthritis.
   - Malignant diseases of lymphoreticular system, like lymphomas.
   - Atypical pneumonia **(*Mycoplasma*).**
   - Viral pneumonias.
   - ***Infectious mononucleosis***
   - Paroxysmal cold haemoglobinuria (PCH).
   - Drug-induced haemolytic anaemia.

Diagnosis of AIHA: Depends primarily in demonstration of the autoantibodies. Thermal characteristic of the antibody is extremely important. Auto antibodies associated with AIHA are separated into ***two categories*** de-pending on their ***thermal characteristics:***

1. ***"Warm" antibodies:*** Which are able to combine with their corresponding red cell antigens at 37°C.
   - Commonest type of warm antibody is an IgG immunoglobulin.
   - Many IgG autoantibodies have Rh-specificity.
   - IgA and IgM warm autoantibodies are much less common and when present, they are usually formed in addition to IgG autoantibody.
2. ***"Cold" antibodies:*** Cannot combine with antigen at 37°C, but form an increasingly stable combination with antigen as the temperature falls from 30°C to 2 to 4°C.
   - ***Cold autoantibodies are always IgM type.***
   - These antibodies can produce chronic IV haemolysis *in vivo*, the intensity of which is influenced by the ambient temperature, the condition is referred as ***"cold haemagglutinin syndrome/disease" (CHAD).***
   - Haemolysis is due to the destruction of the red blood cells by complement which is bound to the red cell surface by the antigen-antibody reaction which occur in the blood vessels of exposed skin if the temperature is less than 30°C.

b. ***If PCH is suspected-look for a specific cold antibody called "Donath-Landsteiner antibody."***

Perform Donath-Landsteiner test—direct and indirect.

- ***DL antibody of paroxysmal cold haemoglobinuria differs from other cold antibodies in that—***
  - it is IgG type;
  - has different specificity;
  - it is, far more lytic to normal red cells in relation to its titre than are anti-i or anti-I antibodies; and
  - it has well-defined specificity within the P blood group system namely anti-P.

The disease is characterised by episodes of brisk IV haemolysis and haemoglobinuria following exposure to cold.

4. Collagen Diseases

Connective tissue diseases specially SLE and less frequently rheumatoid arthritis (RA) are commonly associated with the presence of antibodies against the patient's own red cells, and thus with a positive Coombs' test. Hence, ***tests for rheumatoid factor (RA factor) and ANA (antinuclear antibody) test should be performed on every patient with Coombs' positive haemolytic anaemia.***

Note

- A negative ANA test result does not rule out the possibility of SLE, as the haemolysis may precede long before other manifestations of the disease appear.
- ***ANA test should be repeated at frequent intervals.***

5. *IV Coagulation*

When IV coagulation is suspected, the following tests help:

- Fibrinogen assay.
- Assay of fibrinogen degradation products.

Note

1. The findings of
   - decreased fibrinogen level ↓;
   - + thrombocytopenia;
   - +presence of red cells fragments (Schistocytes) in peripheral smear; and
   - +an increase in fibrin-spilt products,

   strongly suggests this disroder.
2. Other clotting factors, viz. prothrombin, factor X, etc. also may be low.
3. Prompt diagnosis and anticoagulant therapy are required to save the patient from fatal disseminated IV coagulation.

All Coombs' positive haemolytic anaemia, are considered as "idiopathic", if no underlying cause is found. Thus, the diagnosis of idiopathic AIHA is made by exclusion only.

But all these cases must be followed-up for a number of years as such cases may later on turn up as collagen diseases/or a lymphoreticular disease like lymphomas.

Flow Chart for laboratory investigation of a case of haemolytic anaemia

Once it is established that anaemia is present and it is haemolytic in nature, the laboratory investigations should be directed to find out the cause.

The most crucial and important test to differentiate intrinsic red cells defect from extrinsic defect is by Coombs' test

Suspected haemolytic anaemia

↓

Perform Coombs' test (If facilities available ^{51}Cr labelled red cells survival may be done)

A. Coombs' test negative (-ve)

↓

Indicate red cells intrinsic defect

↓

Consider
- Membrane defects
- Hb defects
- Enzyme defects
- Acquired PNH

B. Coombs' test positive (+ve)

↓

Indicate extrinsic defect

↓

Consider
- AIHA
- Collagen diseases
- IV Coagulation

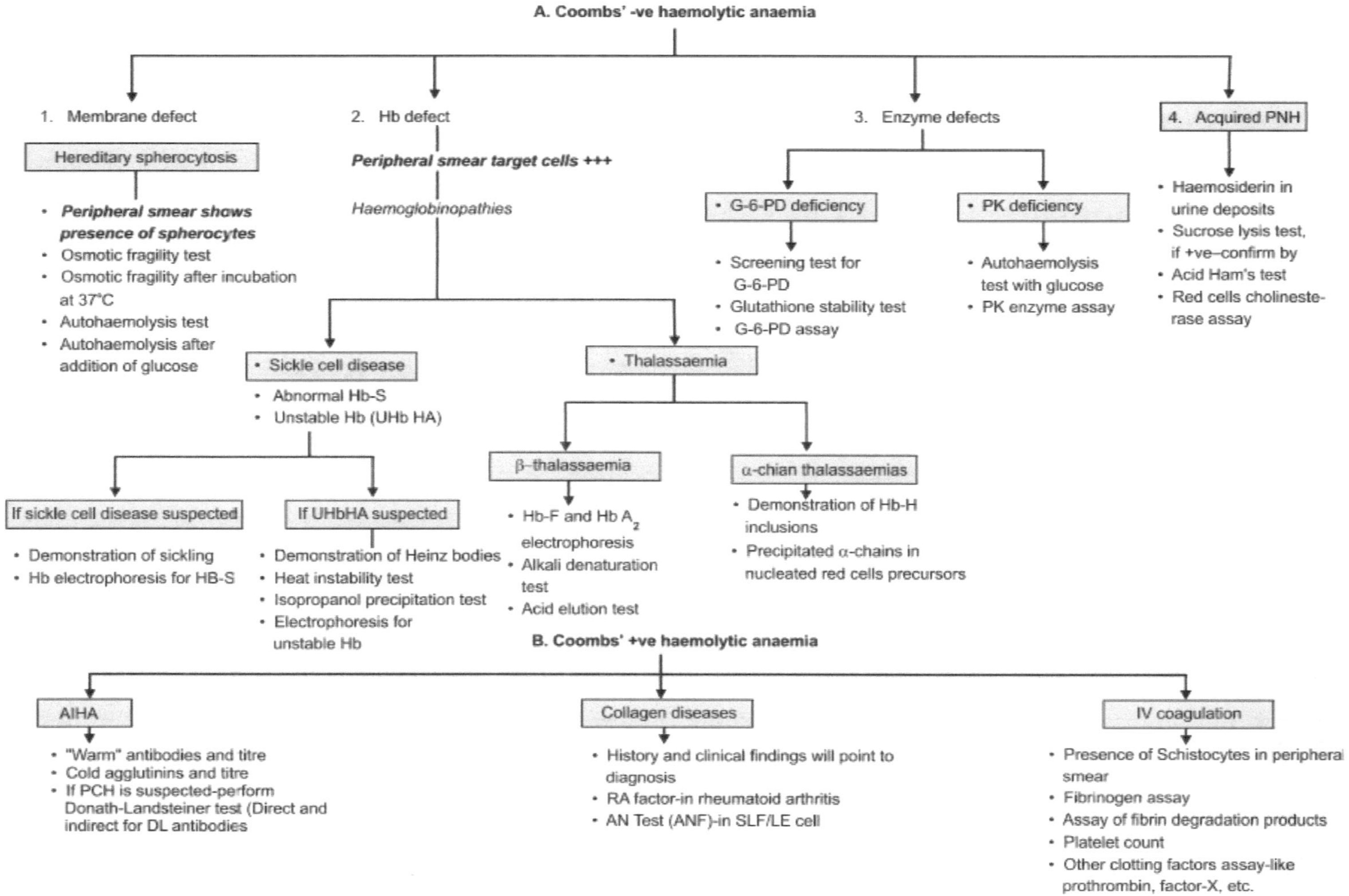
A. Coombs' -ve haemolytic anaemia
1. Membrane defect
Hereditary spherocytosis
• Peripheral smear shows presence of spherocytes
• Osmotic fragility test
• Osmotic fragility after incubation at 37°C
• Autohaemolysis test
• Autohaemolysis after addition of glucose
2. Hb defect
Peripheral smear target cells +++
Haemoglobinopathies
• Sickle cell disease
• Abnormal Hb-S
• Unstable Hb (UHb HA)
If sickle cell disease suspected
• Demonstration of sickling
• Hb electrophoresis for HB-S
If UHbHA suspected
• Demonstration of Heinz bodies
• Heat instability test
• Isopropanol precipitation test
• Electrophoresis for unstable Hb
• Thalassaemia
β-thalassaemia
• Hb-F and Hb A_2 electrophoresis
• Alkali denaturation test
• Acid elution test
α-chian thalassaemias
• Demonstration of Hb-H inclusions
• Precipitated α-chains in nucleated red cells precursors
3. Enzyme defects
• G-6-PD deficiency
• Screening test for G-6-PD
• Glutathione stability test
• G-6-PD assay
• PK deficiency
• Autohaemolysis test with glucose
• PK enzyme assay
4. Acquired PNH
• Haemosiderin in urine deposits
• Sucrose lysis test, if +ve–confirm by
• Acid Ham's test
• Red cells cholinesterase assay
B. Coombs' +ve haemolytic anaemia
AIHA
• "Warm" antibodies and titre
• Cold agglutinins and titre
• If PCH is suspected-perform Donath-Landsteiner test (Direct and indirect for DL antibodies
Collagen diseases
• History and clinical findings will point to diagnosis
• RA factor-in rheumatoid arthritis
• AN Test (ANF)-in SLF/LE cell
IV coagulation
• Presence of Schistocytes in peripheral smear
• Fibrinogen assay
• Assay of fibrin degradation products
• Platelet count
• Other clotting factors assay-like prothrombin, factor-X, etc.

Chapter 23

Iron Deficiency Anaemia

INTRODUCTION

Iron deficiency produces anaemia which is ***hypochromic microcytic*** in nature. It is the most common type of anaemia in India. It occurs in all ages, but is specially, common in females in child bearing age. Hence, it is necessary to diagnose and evaluate such cases early and institute the treatment. It has been estimated that 20% of the world's population is iron deficient. Iron deficiency is always secondary to an underlying disorder usually chronic occult blood loss.

Iron deficiency anaemia develops when the supply of iron is insufficient for the requirements of Hb synthesis. It is only when the tissue stores are exhausted that the supply of iron to marrow becomes inadequate for Hb synthesis and hypochromic microcytic anaemia develops.

PATHOGENESIS: MAJOR FACTORS

Major factors involved in pathogenesis of iron deficiency anaemia are as follows:

- ***Inadequate dietary intake/absorption***
- ***An increased physiological demand for iron***
- ***Pathological blood loss (chronic/occult blood loss)***

1. *Inadequate Intake*

Inadequate intake may result from either

- nutritional deficiency (dietary intake), or
- impaired absorption

Nutritional deficiency as a result of an inadequate intake is of particular importance in infants and young children. It may also occur in adults due to:

- Poor economic status
- Anorexia in alcoholics
- Pregnancy
- Impaired absorption
- Gastrectomy or gastroenterostomy
- Tropical sprue or caeliac disease in children/or adults

2. *Increased Physiological Demand*

Increased demand of iron occurs in:

- Children during period of growth
- In women during reproductive period of life. Physiological need incresases during this period due to—
  - repeated pregnancies, and
  - menstrual loss.

3. *Pathological Blood Loss*

Chronic blood loss from pathological lesions may cause iron deficiency at all ages and in both sexes. It is of great importance in adult males and females in menopause. In this group, it is not due to any physiological cause.

CAUSES OF IRON DEFICIENCY ANAEMIA

1. Females in Reproductive Period of Life

Major aetiological factors in this group areas follows:

- ***Menstrual Blood Loss***

Average monthly loss from menstruation is 15 to 28 mg of Fe. Associated menorrhagia and metrorrhagia aggravates anaemia.

Pregnancy: Each pregnancy requires about 500 to 600 mg of Fe for the foetus and to cover blood loss during parturition

Situation is aggravated by:

- Repeated pregnancies with poor dietary intake and miscarriages.
- Associated pathological blood loss.
- Deficient dietary intake.
- Chronic aspirin ingestion.

Iron deficiency anaemia is more common in women of lower economic status, probably due to inadequate intake of foods rich in Fe such as meat, liver, kidney, eggs, and green vegetables

2. Infants and Children

Major aetiological factors of anaemia in infants and children are as follows:

- Deficient diet and inadequate intake.
- Impaired absorption due to caeliac disease/ sprue.
- Increased demand for growth.
- Prematurity-diminished iron stores at birth.
- Infections.

3. Adult Males and Post Menopausal Women

Mainly due to chronic blood loss due to pathological lesions. Main aetiological factors in this group of subjects are given below.

- Bleeding from peptic ulcers.
- Haemorrhoids (bleeding piles).
- Uterine bleeding (pathological lesion).
- Oesophageal varices.
- Hookworm infection is the most common cause in India.
- Ulcerative colitis.
- Malignancies:
  - carcinoma of stomach
  - carcinoma of colon

Haematuria, haemoptysis, haematemesis, repeated epistaxis are other uncommon causes of iron deficiency anaemia.

LABORATORY INVESTIGATIONS IN IRON DEFICIENCY ANAEMIA

Laboratory investigations in iron deficiency anaemia involve **three steps:**

- ***To establish anaemia is present and it is hypochromic microcytic type.***
- ***To establish that the anaemia is of iron-deficiency.***
- ***To determine the cause of anaemia.***

A. TO ESTABLISH THE PRESENCE OF ANAEMIA AND ITS NATURE

1. History and Clinical Features

- Onset of iron deficiency anaemia is usually insidious.
- Symptoms common to all anaemias like weakness, fatigue, lassitude, dyspnoea on exertion, and palpitations.
- Pallor of skin and mucous membranes is common; with more severe anaemia the sclera is pearly white.
- In females, it is due to excessive menstrual loss.

2. Routine Blood Examination

- ***Red Cells Indices***

Hb: Diminished concentration of Hb in microcytic red cells-low Hb-mild to moderate, depending on severity.

RB cells: Red cells count is reduced to a lesser degree than Hb and the count may be near normal when Hb reduction is 8 to 9 gm%.

Colour index: It is reduced, usually less than 0.9.

MCV: Usually reduced, less than 80 cμ and ranges from 55 to 74 cμ depending on the severity of anaemia.

MCH: It is reduced, usually less than 27 μ μgm and ranges, from 15 to 21 μμg depending on the severity.

Note

The co-existence of B_{12} and folic acid deficiency may result in finding of normal MCV and MCH in spite of depleted Fe stores.

MCHC: It is reduced in parallel with MCV. It is usually less than 30 to 32%. Variation varies from 25 to 30%.

3. Peripheral Smear

- ***RBCs***

RBCs are ***hypochromic*** and there is gross ***anisocytosis*** and ***poikilocytosis.*** Majority of red cells are smaller than normal and a few, are tiny ***microcytes.*** A small number of slightly macrocytic cells, often ***polychromatic,*** are commonly present.

Elliptical forms: are common and elongated *pencil-shaped cells* may be seen.

Target cells: are present commonly in small numbers.

Normoblasts: are uncommon, but occasionally appear in small numbers in severe anaemia.

"Ring" or "Pessary" cells: are seen in severe cases. Extremely large area of central pallor surrounded by a small rim of Hb concentrated at periphery.

- ***WBCs***

The total and differential count of WB cells are usually normal.

- ***Platelet Count***

Usually normal may be slightly increased in bleeding conditions, if associated.

- ***Reticulocyte Count***

Usually normal or reduced. It may be slightly raised, from 2 to 5%, specially after any associated haemorrhage.

B. TO ESTABLISH IRON DEFICIENCY

1. History

Proper history may reveal a common cause of Fe deficiency.

2. Clinical Examination

The following findings may be suggestive of Fe deficiency.

- ***Koilonychia:*** In long standing Fe deficiency anaemia and in severe cases, the nails become concave or spoon shaped. The condition is known as koilonychia and when present strongly suggests Fe deficiency anaemia. The finger nails become thin, lustreless, become brittle and show longitudinal ridges.
- ***Atrophic glossitis:*** Tongue shows atrophy of papillae, resulting in a pale, smooth, shiny/glazed atrophic tongue. When present it is suggestive of Fe deficiency anaemia; but it may be present in other conditions also, like macrocytic megalobastic anaemia.
- ***Sclera:*** It may show pearly white colour. It is typical of Fe deficiency anaemia but not pathognomonic.
- ***Angular stomatitis:*** It is the redness, soreness and cracking which sometimes develop at the angles of the mouth. But it is not characteristic feature and may be due to associated vitamins deficiency, specially riboflavin (vitamin B_2).

3. Iron Studies

- ***Serum Iron Level***

In normal healthy subjects, serum iron level ranges:

- ***in males:*** 120 to 140 μg/dl; and
- ***in females:*** 90 to 120 μg/dl

In Fe deficiency anaemia, serum iron level will be reduced.

Note

Tests for serum Fe are performed on serum or heparinized plasma

Caution: No EDTA, oxalate or citrated plasma be used as they can bind Fe and give lower value.

Principle of serum assay: Iron is released from its protein binder, transferrin, by addition of a protein-denaturing solution (usually a mixture of trichloracetic acid and HCl). After centrifugation, a reducing agent such as ascorbic acid, thioglycolic acid or hydroxylamine is added to convert Fe (ic) to Fe (ous). The Fe(ous) complexes with a chromogenic agent, such as bathophenanthroline or ferrozine, to form a highly coloured complex. The coloured complex is quantitated spectrophotometrically.

The absorbance is directly roportional to concentration.

Note

The assay is not influenced by slight haemolysis, but markedly haemolyzed samples should be rejected.

- ***Measurement of (TIBC) Total Iron Binding Capacity***

Total amount of the Fe which can bind to the transferrin in 100 ml of serum is called total iron binding capacity (TIBC).

In normal subjects, it ranges from 300 to 360 μg/dl, irrespective of sex (both males and females).

In Fe deficiency anaemia: total iron binding capacity (TIBC) is grossly increased ↑.

Note

It is the ***crucial*** and ***most important*** test to differentiate ***Fe deficiency hypochromic microcytic anaemia from other causes of hypochromic*** microcytic anaemia (see below) in which TIBC is either normal or reduced.

Principle of assay: In TIBC assay, a known excess of Fe (ic) is added to serum, to completely saturate the endogenous transferrin. After reaction, the ***unbound Fe (ic)*** is removed with $MgCO_3$ or an anion-exchange resin. After centrifugation, the supernatent is assayed as for serum Fe. Requirements are same as serum Fe assay.

- ***Saturation of Fe Binding Protein***

It is calculated by dividing the serum Fe value by the TIBC and expressed as %

$$\frac{\text{Serum Fe}}{\text{TIBC}} = \%$$

Normal range is 30 to 40 %

Average normal=33% saturated, i.e., iron binding protein is about 1/3 saturated.

- ***Unsaturated or Latent Iron Binding Capacity***

The fraction of the iron binding protein to which Fe is not attached is known as the "unsaturated or latent iron binding capacity".

SUMMARY

In Fe deficiency anaemia, the following are the findings:

- Serum Fe is reduced ↓, values usually ranging from 15 to 60 μg/dl.
- TIBC is increased ↑, sometimes up to 500 μg/dl or even more.
- Unsaturated iron binding capacity is thus increased ↑.
- Per cent saturation of the iron binding protein, is decreased ↓, values commonly being about 10%.

- ***Serum Ferritin Assay***

This is an important and crucial assay, since ferritin levels very closely mimic iron-stores, ***this assay is an indicator of early deficiency.***

Principle of assay: Ferritin tests are performed on serum. Several methods are available based on an antigen antibody reaction. Essentially, the sample is incubated with anti-ferritin (attached to a bead or magnetic particle). The ferritin in serum is complexed with the anti-ferritin antibody. A second antibody is then added, which is labelled with ^{125}I or horse radish peroxidase. After separation of the bead or magnetic particle from the excess unreacted second antibody, the bead or particle is counted in a gamma counter, or if the assay is ELISA type, reacted with substrate and the product is quantitated via absorbance readings. Appropriate "standards" and "controls" are included each time the assay is run.

Note

- There are variations in each kit and each laboratory should establish its own reference range.
- The assay is **not** influenced by iron contamination, lipaemic samples, or interferance from Hb or bilirubin.
- One problem faced is that chronic diseases, e.g. rheumatoid arthritis; viral hepatitis; hepatic injury; and malignancies will result in normal ferritin levels in serum.
- Another aspect of ferritin assay to be noted is that the half life of ferritin is 6 days.
- Some clinicians have used this assay as an indicator of early protein-energy malnutrition (PEM).

- ***Free Erythrocyte Protoporphyrins (FEP)***

In Fe deficiency, the protoporphyrins accumulate in red cells as there is insufficient Fe to combine with it to form heme. (Last step of heme synthesis is blocked by Fe deficiency.)

- *Normal range:* is 20 to 40 μg/dl
- *In Fe deficiency:* FEP values are increased, usually ranging from 100 to 600 μg/dl

Principle of assay: The assay specimen should be either heparinized or EDTA whole blood. Free erythrocyte protoporphyrin is extracted from erythrocytes and its concentration is measured in a fluorimeter.

Note

- FEP determinations should be done routinely in paediatric practices as a "screening test" for both Fe deficiency and Pb poisoning.
- Lead poisoning, common in children, also results in failure to complete heme synthesis.
- An alternative to FEP is zinc protoporphyrin assay (ZPP), which requires no extraction steps. Basically the concentration of ZPP in capillary or venous blood is measured in a haematofluorimeter

- ***Serum Transferrin Receptor Assay***

Serum transferrin receptor is assayed with the ELISA technique using monoclonal antibodies. This test has been found to detect Fe deficiency reliably after body stores of Fe are depleted.

Note

- Serum receptor levels are an indicator of mild Fe deficiency of recent onset.
- Studies have shown that ***the serum ferritin is the most sensitive index of Fe status when there are residual iron stores, whereas the serum receptor is more sensitive when there is functional iron deficiency.***
- Because of the reciprocal relationship between serum receptor and ferritin measurements, the ratio of receptor ferritin indicates the Fe-status.

CONCLUSION: ROLE OF Fe STUDIES IN Fe DEFICIENCY STATUS

Three phases of Fe deficiency can be recognized. Position of Fe studies during these three phases are as follows:

1. Stage of Fe Storage Depletion

This phase is not usually recognizable by the patient and normally does not elicit a medical examination.

Serum ferritin falls during this phase and is the only good indication of possible Fe deficiency. Many women of child bearing age remain in this phase for years.

2. Stage of Iron Deficiency

The iron stores are very close to exhaustion. The serum ferritin is low ↓. TIBC is increased ↑ and transferrin saturation is low ↓. Erythropoiesis is slowed due to unavailability of Fe to make Hb. FEP increases ↑ and Hb concentration falls ↓ to the lowest limit of normal Hb values.

3. Stage of Fe Deficiency Anaemia

At this phase, there is ***clinically definite anaemia***. Serum ferritin levels may continue a slow decline. Transferrin saturation continues to fall. TIBC increases further and FEP increases ↑ to upper limit of reference range. Hb concentration continues to drop ↓, Hb is less than normal reference range.

Note

- To be classified as Fe-deficiency anaemia, a low Hb and a documented abnormal serum ferritin or Fe studies result must be present.
- ***It is extremely important to determine iron levels in all patients, with hypochromic microcytic anaemia, since there are diseases—thalassaemias and sideroblastic anaemias which show hypochromic microcytic anaemia. Iron administration may be hazardous and can lead to iron overload in these conditions.***

CHARACTERISTIC BONE MARROW CHANGES

Bone marrow smear can be examined which will show characteristic changes, pointing to Fe deficiency anaemia.

- ***Erythroid hyperplasia*** increase being mainly in the more mature forms. ***Predominant cells*** are polychromatic normoblasts seen characteristically, which are usually smaller than normal ***"micronormoblasts"***. ***Cytoplasmic ripening*** seems to lag behind nuclear condensation, so that nucleus often appears **"pyknotic"** or almost pyknotic, despite the fact that cytoplasm is still polychromatic
- ***Granulopoiesis:*** is normal.
- ***Megakaryocytes:*** are present in normal numbers.

- ***Bone Marrow Haemosiderin***

Estimation of bone marrow haemosiderin is a more reliable indicator. Examination of both unstained fresh marrow preparations and films stained with K-ferrocyanide shows that Fe is either absent or present only in minute amounts.

Normally, Fe is stored in RE cells as haemosiderin which may be seen as golden-yellow granules in normal unstained marrow smear or as blue granules following staining with K-ferrocyanide. ***Presence of haemosiderin in marrow rules out Fe deficiency anaemia.***

Note

In Sideroblastic anaemia pathological "ring" sideroblasts are seen.

C. TO DETERMINE THE CAUSE OF ANAEMIA

The cause of Fe deficiency anaemia varies with the ***age*** and ***sex*** of the patient.

1. History and Physical Examination

Proper history taking and careful consideration of clinical features establishes the cause in many cases, but further investigations are often necessary.

Main causes to be looked into discussed below.

(a) In Infants and Children

Dietary: Major caustive factor is inadequate dietary intake of Fe (nutritional) which fails to meet increased demands of growth.

Prematurity: Inadequate antenatal store.

Other causes

- Blood loss.
- Infections.
- Impaired absorption as in caeliac disease.
- Congenital abnormalities of GI tract.

(b) Females in Reproductive Period of Life

Menstrual history: Chiefly menorrhagia and metrorrhagia.

Pregnancies: Numbers of pregnancies and interval/and miscarriages.

Nutritional status

- Blood loss from GI tract.
- Chronic aspirin ingestion.

(c) Adult Males and Post Menopausal Women

Principal aetiological factor is chronic blood loss, in addition to inadequate nutrition.

Hookworm infection: most common in India, specially in patients from rural areas.

Presence of haemorrhoids (piles).

Haematemesis/malaena.

Blood loss from GI tract due to peptic ulcer, malignancies.

Chronic aspirin ingestion.

2. Iron Studies

In patients with low serum Fe, **most crucial test will be TIBC**, which will indicate the cause.

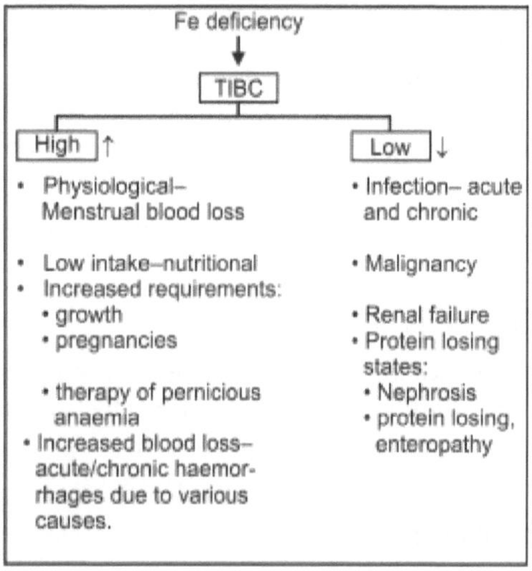

3. Special Investigations

The disorders in which particular investigations are specially helpful are given in brackets.

A. *Investigations Commonly Required*

- ***Stool examination:*** Routine examination
  - for ova e.g. hookworm ova (HW anaemia) and
  - for blood using benzidine or O-Tolidine. Precautions are to be taken before carrying out the test. ***Repeat three times*** if necessary, before declaring as negative.
- ***Urine examinations:*** Microscopic examination for haematuria
- ***Barium meal:*** For peptic ulcar, carcinoma of stomach.
- ***Barium enema:*** For carcinoma colon and caecum, ulcerative colitis.
- ***Barium swallow:*** For oesophageal varies.
- ***Colonoscopy/or Sigmoidoscopy:*** For carcinoma rectum, ulcerative colitis.
- ***Proctoscopy:*** For haemorrhoids.

B. *Investigations Occasionally Required*

- ***Chest X-ray:*** Disorders causing haemoptysis.
- ***Cystoscopy and pyelography:*** For disorders causing haematuria.
- ***Liver function tests:*** (For cirrhosis liver)—total and differential protein and A:G ratio.
- ***Iron-absorption studies:*** With the help of ^{59}Fe, one can determine—
  - rate of absorption of Fe from GI tract;
  - rate of disappearance of ^{59}Fe from the plasma; and
  - rate of "turnover" of plasma Fe indicates the extent of activity of erythropoietic marrow.
- ***Oncogenic markers:*** CEA for colorectal cancer; CA 50-in gastrointestinal cancer; and CA 72-A in gastric and colorectal cancer.
- ***Other tests:*** For collagen diseases
  - Rheumatoid factor for rheumatoid arthritis. LE cell demonstration for SLE.
  - Antinuclear antibodies in SLE.

DIFFERENTIAL DIAGNOSIS OF HYPOCHROMIC MICROCYTIC ANAEMIA

The majority of cases of hypochromic microcytic anaemia are due to Fe deficiency. Hypochromic anaemia is also commonly encountered in disorders in which the morphological abnormality is not due to unavailability of Fe but due to a block in Fe utilization or globin synthesis in the red cell precursors.

Other Causes of Hypochromic Anaemia

- Anaemia of chronic infections.
- ***Thalassemia,*** both major and minor—hypochromia is one of the characteristic feature.
- ***Sideroblastic anaemia.***
- ***Anaemia of renal insufficiency.***
- ***Anaemia associated with collagen diseases,*** viz. rheumatoid arthritis, SLE.
- Anaemia of disseminated malignancy and malignant lymphomas.

Note

- With the exception of thalassemia major (β-thalassemia) and some sideroblastic anaemias, the hypochromia associated with

Table 23.1: Differentiation of hypochromic anaemia by biochemical parameters

	Serum Fe	*TIBC*	*Saturation of TIBC*	*Serum ferritin*	*Marrow haemosiderin*	*Hb* *Hb A_2*	*HbF*
• ***Iron deficiency anaemia***	Decreased↓	Increased↑	Decreased↓	Decreased↓	Absent	Normal	Normal
• ***Simple microcytic anaemia (chronic infection)***	Decreased↓	Decreased↓ or Normal	Decreased↓ or Normal	Increased↑ or Normal	Normal or Increased↑	Normal	Normal
• ***β-thalassemia (thalassemia major)***	Increased↑	Decreased↓	Increased↑	Normal	Increased↑	Normal or Increased↑	Increased↑
• ***Thalassaemia minor***	Normal or increased ↑	Normal	Normal or increased ↑	Normal	Normal or increased ↑	Increased ↑	Normal or increased ↑
• ***Sideroblastic anaemia***	Increased↑	Decreased↓ or Normal	Increased↑	Increased↑ or Normal	Increased↑ *pathological "ring" sideroblasts characteristic*	Normal	Normal

others is seldom as marked as in severe Fe deficiency. Usual problem is to distinguish between hypochromia due to these disorders and hypochromic anaemia of mild to moderate degree due to Fe deficiency.

- The establishment of an accurate diagnosis in the hypochromic anaemia is of great importance in ensuring correct treatment. The administration of Fe to a patient with a hypochromic anaemia due to a cause other than Fe deficiency is not only unhelpful but may be dangerous as it increases body Fe stores leading to "iron overload".

Differentiation of these conditions by Fe studies and other biochemical studies is shown in Table 23.1.

Flow Chart for Investigation of hypochromic microcytic anaemia

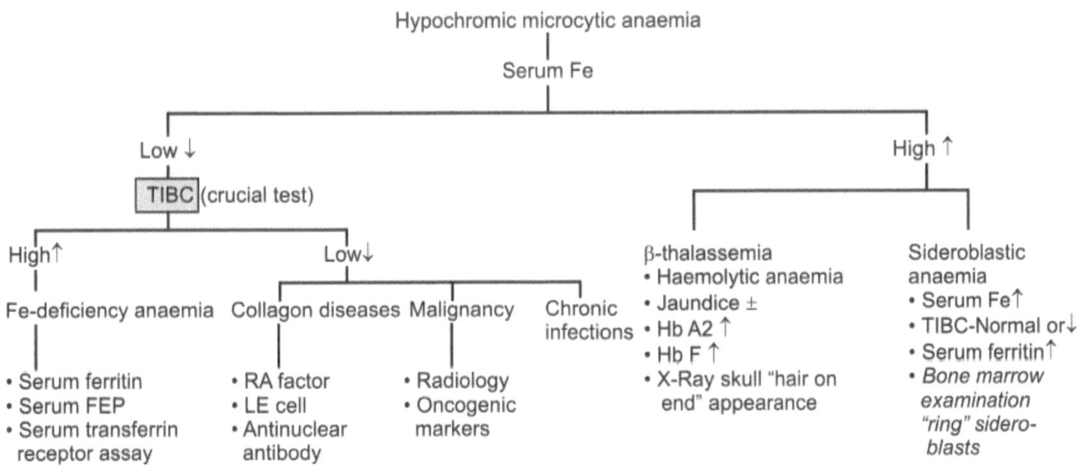

Chapter 24

Macrocytic Megaloblastic Anaemia

INTRODUCTION

Macrocytic anaemia is defined as an anaemia in which the mean corpuscular volume (MCV) is increased. Most authorities agree that the MCV in excess of 100 fl. is abnormal and such red cells are macrocytic.

Note

When routine haemogram shows an increased MCV, the presence of macrocytosis must always be suspected.

Such cases must be confirmed by examination of peripheral smear carefully which can throw light on the type of macrocytic anaemia and its cause.

TYPES

Macrocytic anaemias are divided into ***two main types*** depending on the type of erythroid precursors present in bone marrow smear, which can be normoblastic reaction or megaloblastic.

- ***Normoblastic macrocytic anaemia characterised by normoblastic erythropoiesis.***
- ***Megaloblastic macrocytic anaemia characterised by megaloblastic erythropoiesis.***

A. Normoblastic Macrocytic Anaemia

These are associated with various well defined disorders. ***They do not respond to either vitamin B_{12} or folic acid therapy*** and only respond, when the underlying disease process is alleviated or cured.

B. Megaloblastic Macrocytic Anaemias

These are usually deficiency diseases, resulting from deficiency of either vitamin B_{12} or folic acid or both. Mechanism producing the deficiency of B_{12} or folic acid varies with the underlying associated disorders. The ***anaemia responds well to administration of the deficient substance, i.e. vitamin B_{12} or folic acid.***

Megaloblastic anaemia are characterised by distinctive cytological and functional abnormalities in peripheral blood and bone marrow cells due to impaired DNA synthesis. Megaloblasts are abnormal in function as well as in appearance, with the result that the mature red cells formed from them are abnormal in size and shape, ***the most important prominent abnormality is "macrocytosis".***

CAUSE OF MACROCYTOSIS

Macrocytosis is caused by the presence of reticulocytes or mature red cells of increased size or both, in the peripheral blood. Reticulocytes are slightly larger than normal mature red cells, and when present in increased numbers in peripheral blood produces a mild to moderate degree of macrocytosis. In a well-stained peripheral smear they have a ***slight, diffuse basophilic tint.***

I. Megaloblastic Anaemias Due to Folic Acid Deficiency

Causes of Folic Acid Deficiency

- ***Inadequate or decreased intake of folic acid or*** (nutritional deficiency).
- ***Impaired absorption of folic acid from intestine*** (malabsorption syndrome):
  - tropical sprue and
  - caeliac disease.
- ***Increased demand***

Pregnancy—Marginal deficiency is likely to become overt in presence of increased demand in the body.

- Other associated disorders, viz.—
  - leukaemia and lymphomas;
  - haemolytic anaemia;
  - carcinoma;
  - inflammatory disorders; and
  - sideroblastic anaemia, etc.
- ***Drugs: Folate antagonists***—inability to utilise folic acid due to the presence of antagonists.

Important drugs

- Those which inhibit the enzyme ***"dihydrofolate reductase".***
  - Methotrexate.
  - Pyrimethamine.
  - Trimethoprim.
- Other drugs—mechanism not known clearly.
  - oral contraceptives,
  - anticonvulsant drugs, like phenytoin-used for treatment of epilepsy. 50% of patients, receiving phenytoin may develop folate deficiency on prolonged treatment. Subnormal folate level in serum, red cells and CS Fluid have been found.

Clinical Manifestations of Macrocytic Megaloblastic Anaemia Due to Folate Deficiency

Two cardinal features are:

- Macrocytic megaloblastic anaemia.
- Glossitis.

Note

Folate deficiency does not produce subacute combined degeneration of spinal cord as seen with vitamin B_{12} deficiency. Occasional case may show peripheral neuropathy.

II. Macrocytic Megaloblastic Anaemia Due to Vitamin B_{12} Deficiency

Causes of Vitamin B_{12} Deficiency

- ***Inadequate dietary intake:*** Nutritional deficiency is not common but a rare cause. Vitamin B_{12} reserve is good. Human body contains 2000 to 5000 µg vitamin B_{12} and has a daily requirement of about 2 µg. ***Vegeterians are likely to develop.***
- ***Impaired absorption***

1. ***Gastric causes***
   - Lack of intrinsic factor
     - Pernicious anaemia (autoimmune factors)
   - Gastrectomy (total or partial).
2. ***Intestinal mucosal defect***
   - Lesions of small intestine
   - Caeliac disease
   - Tropical sprue.
3. ***Parasitic infestation: Like fish tapeworm infestation (Diphyllobothrium latum)***
4. ***Drugs:***
   a. A number of drugs can impair vitamin B_{12} absorption. They include:
      - PAS (para-aminosalicylic acid)
      - Cimetidine
      - Cholestyramine
      - Neomycin
      - Colchicine
      - Phenformin and metformine, etc.

   b. ***Prolonged exposure to the anaesthetic agent nitrous oxide*** may result in megaloblastic changes in bone marrow as well as peripheral smear.
5. ***Congenital megaloblastic anaemia:*** Though rare, but of clinical interest. Defects can be in vitamin B_{12} absorption, transport or in metabolism.

They include:
- Familial selective vit B_{12} malabsorption.
- Congenital intrinsic factor deficiency.
- Inherited transcobalamine II deficiency.
- Methylmalontic acidaemia and acciduria.

Clinical Features of Megaloblastic Anaemia Due to vitamin B_{12} Deficiency

Three important features of vitamin B_{12} deficiency due to any cause are:
- Macrocytic megaloblastic anaemia.
- Glossitis.
- ***Subacute combined degeneration of the spinal cord*** and peripheral neuropathy.

Note
- Above may occur singly or in combination.
- Anaemia may be less.
- Neurological abnormalities more common with pernicious anaemia than in megaloblastic anaemias due to other causes.

Nieweg's Hypothesis

Deficiency of folic acid is not accompanied by neurological lesions but B_{12} deficiency is accompanied with neurological lesions, viz. subacute combined degeneration of the cord and peripheral neuropathy but, folic acid deficiency and B_{12} deficiency produces megaloblastic anaemia, why?

This is explained by Nieweg's hypothesis

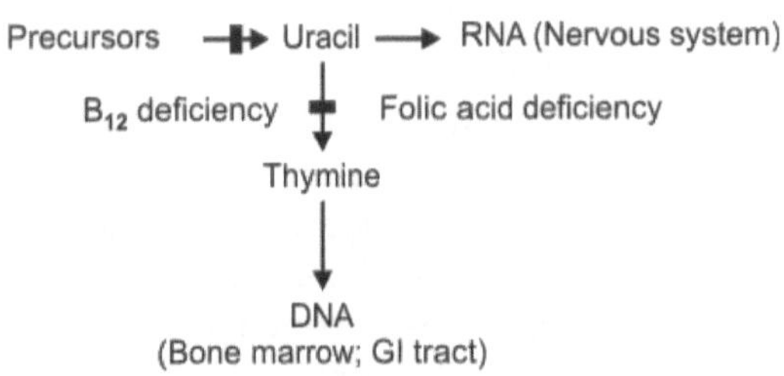

Nieweg's hypothesis postulates that folic acid is concerned with DNA metabolism. This explains how a deficiency of folic acid would produce bone marrow and GI changes unaccompanied by neurological lesions.

On the other hand, a deficiency of vitamin B_{12} would cause neurological lesions as a result of impairment of RNA synthesis as well as changes in bone marrow and GI tract due to impairment of DNA synthesis (as shown above).

Mechanism of Megaloblastic Anaemia

- ***Main Cause***

Decreased production of mature red blood cells. The anaemia results from failure of the megaloblastic bone marrow to compensate for a moderate reduction in red cell lifespan. This is due to interference with marrow function due to lack of haemopoietic factors.

- ***Haemolytic Element***

Decreased production is also partly due to:
- Death in marrow of some of abnormal megaloblasts and precursors (intramedullary destruction or haemolysis).
- Peripheral haemolytic element:

Red cells survival studies, have shown presence of mild haemolysis, due to both intracorpuscular and extracorpuscular causes.

Biochemical Basis of Megaloblastic Change

Main biochemical change common to both vitamin B_{12} and folic acid deficiency is a block or impairment of DNA synthesis. This impairment is due to the fact that deoxyuridylate cannot be methylated to form thymidylate in the DNA synthetic pathway. Methyl (CH_3) group is supplied by the folic acid coenzyme, the "biochemically active" form, methylene-F.H_4. Deficiency of folic acid due to any cause cannot form methylene-F.H_4 so that supply of CH_3 group stops.

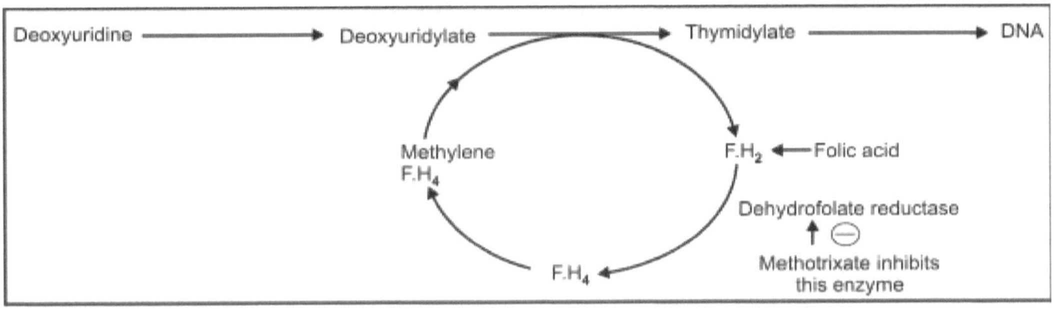

PERNICIOUS ANAEMIA

This is the principal form of macrocytic megaloblastic anaemia due to B_{12} deficiency. It is also called ***Addisonian anaemia*** (recognised by Addison's in 1855).

Fundamental defect is the ***failure of secretion of intrinsic factor (IF)*** by the stomach due to permanent atrophy of gastric mucosa. In absence of IF, vitamin B_{12} (extrinsic factor from diet) is not absorbed resulting in B_{12} deficiency and pernicious anaemia.

Types: It can occur in ***two*** forms:

- ***Adult type:*** in middle and older age group, more than 40 years.
- ***Juvenile type:*** usually occurs after 10 years of age.

Family history is usual and clinical manifestations and pathogenesis is same in both. Pathogenesis of gastric atrophy is not very clear. ***Current evidences point that it is the end-result of a complex interaction between genetic and autoimmune factors***

1. *Genetic factors*

Points in favour

- Runs in family (10% of patients show that more than one family member is affected).
- Blood group A is more susceptible in patients and in relatives.
- Definite racial tendency.
- Certain physical characteristics common, e.g. fair skin and blue eyed persons.
- Incidence of low serum B_{12} levels, other autoimmune diseases and presence of gastric autoantibodies more in relatives.

Summary of Pathogenesis

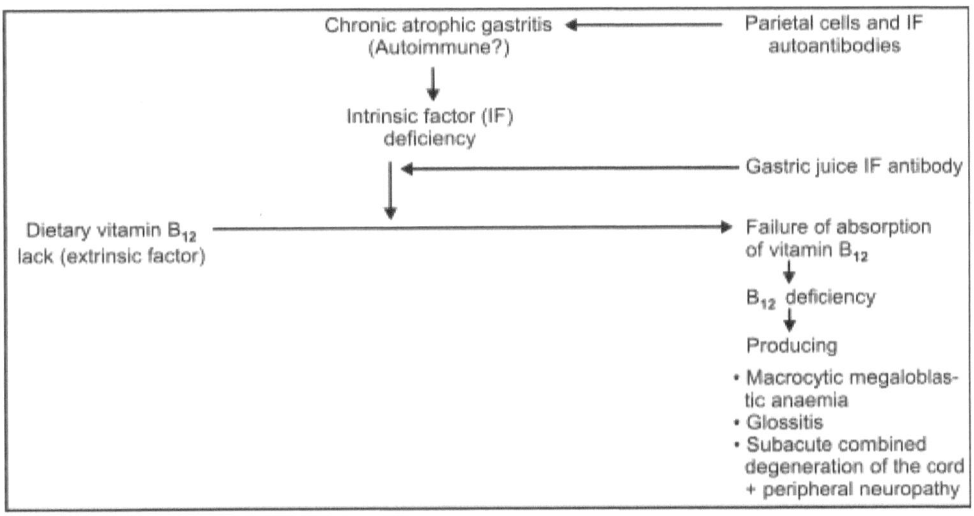

2. ***Autoimmune factors:*** Consensus of opinion favours as autoimmune disorders

Points in favour:

- More frequently found with other autoimmune disorders, viz. Spontaneous adult myxoedema, Hashimoto's thyroiditis, hyperthyroidism, rheumatoid arthritis, systemic lupus erythematosus (SLE), etc.
- Demonstration of gastric parietal cell autoantibodies in serum and gastric juice.
- Demonstration of intrinsic factor antibodies.

Note

It is claimed that these autoantibodies are responsible for atrophy of gastric mucosa.

LABORATORY INVESTIGATION

When confronted with a suspected case of macrocytic megaloblastic anaemia, laboratory investigations have to be carried out to confirm the diagnosis.

It can be considered in **three steps** as follows:

- ***To establish the presence of anaemia and its macrocytic nature.***
- ***To establish that the anaemia is megaloblastic.***
- ***To establish the cause:***
  a. Nature of deficiency—B_{12} or folic acid or both.
  b. Cause of deficiency.

A. INVESTIGATIONS TO ESTABLISH ANAEMIA AND ITS MACROCYTIC NATURE

1. Clinical History

- *Age and sex:* Pernicious anaemia occurs in middle aged and older age groups, usually in females above 40 years (except juvenile type). If the age group is less, then look for other causes of B_{12} or folic acid deficiency.
- *Family history:* Pernicious anaemia occurs in families—amongst relatives.
- *Diarrhoea/steatorrhoea:* To be looked for caeliac disease/tropical sprue.
- *Dietary habits:* Consumption of alcohol and inadequate nutrition.
- **Pregnancy**
- *Abdominal operations:* History of partial or total gastrectomy.
- *Drugs:* Administration of anticonvulsants, oral contraceptive agents and dihydrofolate reductase inhibitors, etc.

2. Physical Examination

- *Pallor/anaemia:* The symptoms common to all forms of anaemia are present in most cases, like weakness, easy fatiguability. Anaemia may be slight or absent in some cases. As onset is insidious, the anaemia is usually moderately severe when the patients presents.
- *Glossitis:* It is present in 25% of cases and occurs in both B_{12} and folic acid deficiency. Occasionally antedates symptoms of anaemia by months. Whole of mouth and throat may be involved causing burning pain in deglutition. Tongue becomes smooth and shiny, loss of papillae.
- *Nervous system involvement:*
  - ***Does not occur in folate deficiency*** may be occasional peripheral neuropathy.
  - Nervous system involvement—peripheral neuropathy (40% cases) and presence of subacute combined degeneration of the cord are characteristic of B_{12} deficiency.
- *General nutritional state:* Look for any evidences of specific nutritional deficiencies or other diseases.

3. Full Blood Examination (Complete haemogram)

- *Hb level:* Usually low but may be normal depending on the severity and ranges from normal value to as low as 3.0 g/dl.

Commonly, level ranges from 7.0 to 9.0 g/dl when the patient is first seen.

- ***RBCs count:*** Low, it is nearly 3.0 millions per cumm. In severe cases, it may come down to even 1.0 to 1.5 million/cumm.

- ***Absolute values***

MCV: ***It is always increased and is proportional to degree of anaemia.*** Usually greater than 95 cμ. Ranges from 110 to 140 cμ in moderately severe anaemia. In severe anaemias, values up to 160 cμ may be obtained.

MCH: It is normal, ranges from 33 to 38 μμ gm.

MCHC: It is normal but, because of the increased size of the red blood cells, MCHC may be increased.

Note

- MCV may be normal or reduced if there is co-existing disorder causing red cells microcytosis.
- Occasionally the Hb level is normal, only abnormality found is macrocytosis with an elevated MCV.

- ***Leucocyte count***

Total WBCs count: Reveals usually **leucopenia** with associated **neutropenia**. There is relative lymphocytosis. Total WBC count varies from 3000 to 5000/cumm, shift to left is characteristically seen.

Differential WBC count: *Shows* neutropenia with relative lymphocytosis. ***Hypersegmented neutrophils are always present (macropolycyte is characteristic).***

- ***Platelet count:*** Moderate thrombocytopenia is usual, with the platelet count ranging from 100,000 to 150,000/cumm. Occasionally, it may be lower than this, specially with severe anaemia and can cause haemorrhagic manifestations.
- ***Reticulocyte count:*** In the untreated patient, rarely more than 2%. Reticulocytes are slightly larger than abnormal mature red cells. In well-stained films they have a slight, diffuse basophilic tint.
- ***Peripheral smear examination:*** Characteristic feature is the presence of macrocytic red blood cells, many of which are ***oval in shape (oval macrocytosis).***
- In untreated patient:
  - ***anisocytosis***
  - ***pearshaped poikilocytes;*** and
  - ***a few polychromatic and stippled cells are common.***

A small number of nucleated red cells and cells containing ***Howell-Jolly bodies*** and ***Cabot's rings*** are often seen. ***Neucleated red cells may be typical megaloblasts,*** particularly when anaemia is severe.

Large hypersegmented polymorphs are characteristic and usually present. Occasionally large polymorph with nucleus containing up to 8 to 9 lobes may be seen ***(macropolycyte).***

Note

- The importance of hypersegmented polymorphs in the diagnosis of megaloblastic erythropoiesis with minimal or no anaemia has been re-emphasised by **Herbert.**
- Finding of more than 3 five-lobed neutrophils per 100 neutrophils or a substantial increase in neutrophils with 4 lobes (normally 15 to 25%) in a peripheral smear suggests the possibility of incipient megaloblastic anaemia.
- ***Lobe average*** is determined by counting total number of nuclear lobes in 100 neutrophils and dividing by 100.

Normal average: is about 3. ***An increased lobe average with oval macrocytosis and pancytopenia is pointer to macrocytic megaloblastic anaemia.***

B. TO ESTABLISH THAT THE ANAEMIA IS MEGALOBLASTIC

- ***Peripheral smear:*** As discussed above.
- ***Bone marrow examination:*** Bone marrow aspiration usually yields a large number of fragments. The fragments and cell trails are ***hypercellular.***

  Hyperplastic fragments show complete or partial replacement of fat by marrow cells.
- ***Erythropoiesis*** is intensively active and predominantly megaloblastic, shows a

"shift to left" with an increased proportion of more primitive cells.

- ***Megaloblasts*** are larger than erythroblasts, with an increase in cytoplasm and nuclear size at every stage of development. Chromatin network is more than open, being arranged in a fine reticular fashion, to give a stippled appearance. There is ***"dissociation of cytoplasmic and nuclear maturation"***, the maturation of the nucleus lags behind that of the cytoplasm. ***Megaloblastic erythropoiesis*** is characterised by an increase in the proportion of more primitive cells ***("maturation arrest")***. ***Promegaloblasts*** and ***basophil megaloblasts*** may be 50% of total erythroblasts.
- ***Granulopoiesis:*** It is ***also active*** but the ***myeloid: erythroid ratio is reduced*** or ***even may be reversed*** (normal M:E ratio = 3:1). "Giant metamyelocyte, called giant stab cell is seen approximately 30 mμ in diameter, and has large U-shaped nucleus.
- ***Megakaryocytes:*** are either normal or slightly increased; nuclear multisegmentation of megakaryocytes is seen.
- ***Iron stain of marrow*** shows large amounts of iron in the fragments and in reticulum cells throughout the cell trails. Abnormal sideroblasts are increased, but 'ring' sideroblasts are not found.
- ***Marrow culture:*** Chromosomal abnormalities, like chromosomal breakage, are found in marrow culture.

C. TO ESTABLISH THE NATURE/CAUSE OF THE DEFICIENCY

After establishing the macrocytic megaloblastic anaemia, one should now find out the cause/ and nature of deficiency.

Nature of deficiency: Is it due to vitamin B_{12} deficiency or folate deficiency or both?

1. ***For establishing vitamin B_{12} deficiency:*** following tests are required.
   - Serum vitamin B_{12} assay.
   - Urine:
     - Methyl malonic acid (MMA)
     - Valine loading test.
2. ***For establishing folic acid deficiency*** following tests are required:
   - Serum folate assay.
   - Red cells folate assay.
   - Urine—FIGLU test.
   - Folic acid clearance test.

1. For Vitamin B_{12} Deficiency

- ***Serum Vitamin B_{12} Assay***

The finding of a low serum vitamin B_{12} level is an essential prerequisite for the diagnosis of pernicious anaemia.

Methods

- Microbiological assay.
- Radioimmunoassay.

a. Microbiological Assay of B_{12}

Principle: The serum to be assayed is added as a source of B_{12} to a medium containing all other essential growth factors for a B_{12} dependant micro-organism. The medium is then inocculated with the micro-organism and the amount of B_{12} in the serum is determined by comparing the growth as estimated turbidimetrically, with the growth produced by a standard amount of B_{12}.

Two micro-organisms used are:

- *Euglena gracilis*
- *Lactobacillus leichmanii*

Euglena assay is more sensitive and specific.

Interpretations

- ***Normal values: By Euglena gracilis assay*** is 140 to 900 μμg/ml (average—approximately 350 μμg/ml).
- A value of less than 100 μμg/ml invariably indicates B_{12} deficiency.
- Patients with pernicious anaemia-usually shows level less than 50 μμg/ml.
- Erythropoiesis usually becomes megaloblastic, when serum concentration falls below 80 to 100 μμg/ml.

b. Radioisotope Assay of B_{12}

Requires an isotope laboratory which is not available in routine clinical laboratory.

Principle: Assay involves isotope dilution of non-radioactive serum vitamin B_{12} by adding ^{57}Co labelled B_{12}. A carrier with B_{12} binding capacity is then used to adsorb a portion of the mixture of radioactive and non-radioactive B_{12}. The free and bound forms of the vitamin are separated and the quantity of radioactive B_{12} adsorbed to the binding substance is measured.

By comparing the measurements of a series of standard of known B_{12} content, the B_{12} level of the unknown is calculated.

Note

Most radioisotope assay methods yield higher vitamin B_{12} levels than microbiological assay.

Interpretations

- ***Normal range:*** is 165 to 684 ng/l.
- ***In B_{12} deficiency:*** levels below 130 ng/l are seen.

- ***Competitive Protein Binding Assay***

See under folic acid assay.

Urinary Assays

- ***Methyl Malonic Acid (MMA) in Urine***

Methylmalonyl CoA is formed during the metabolism of propionic acid as follows:

- Coenzyme form of B_{12} participates in the isomerization of methylmalonyl CoA to succinyl CoA.
- In vitamin B_{12} deficiency, the conversion does not take place and methylmalonyl CoA accumulates and leads to increased excretion of methylmalonic acid (MMA) in urine.

2. For Folic Acid Deficiency

- ***Serum Folic Acid Assay***

a. Microbiological Assay

Principle: Folic acid activity of serum is due mainly to the presence of a folic acid coenzyme, 5-methyl-tetrahydrofolate (5-methyl FH_4). This compound is microbiologically active for *Lactobacillus casei,* which is used in the assay of folic acid activity in serum.

(Principle is similar to microbiological assay of B_{12}).

Interpretations

- ***Normal value:*** by *L. casei* assay is 5 to 20 mμg/ml.
- ***Megaloblastic anaemia*** due to folic acid deficiency: shows a value less than 4.0 mμg/ml.
- ***In pernicious anaemia*** due to B_{12} deficiency: the value is not lowered, ranges from 4.0 to 27 mμg/ml.
- Level in the range of 4 to 6 mμg/ml are less decisive and may not be associated wth clinical or cytological features of folate deficiency.

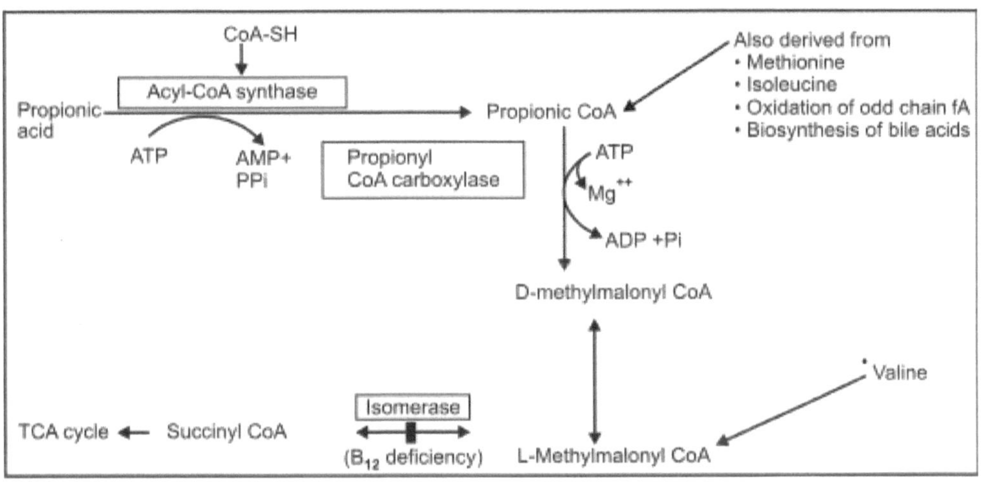

b. Radioisotope Assay

The assay is based on similar principles to that of radioisotope B_{12} assay, and uses labelled PGA or methyl-FH_4 and a folate binding protein purified from cow's milk.

Note

Concurrent Folic Acid and B_{12} Assay

Recently-kits are available which permit concurrent assay of both folic acid and B_{12} by competitive protein binding.

c. Red Cell Folate Assay

Red blood cells contain 20 to 50 times more folate as compared to serum. ***Red cell folate level is usually a more reliable indicator of tissue folic acid stores than the serum folic acid.***

Method
Both microbiological or RIA method can be used.

Interpretation

Normal levels with microbiological assay range from 160 to 640 µg/l and with radioisotope assay from 199 to 795 µg/l.

Note
- Low red cell folate levels are seen in patients of megaloblastic anaemia due to folate deficiency.
- In severe pernicious anaemia: subnormal values may be seen, thus lacks specificity.

d. Folic Acid Clearance Test

Principle: Rate of clearance from the plasma of a standard IV dose of folic acid (PGA) has also been used in the assessment of folic acid deficiency. Only a small proportion of injected dose of folic acid is excreted in the urine, so that the rate of clearance from the plasma is a measure of the uptake of folic acid by tissues.

Method
- Blood samples are taken at 3, 15 amd 30 minutes after the administered dose, and the serum folic acid (PGA) levels are measured by microbiological assay with *Str faecalis* which responds to PGA but not to the naturally occurring folic acid material in serum.

Interpretation

- Rapid clearance of folic acid is found in folic acid deficiency.

e. "FIGLU Test" (Histidine Loading Test)

Principle: In the metabolism of the amino acid histidine, formimino glutamic acid (FIGLU) is an intermediate product.
- "FIGLU" is converted to glutamic acid. This step requires active form of folic acid, tetrahydrofolate (FH_4) as a coenzyme. In folic acid deficient patients, this reaction cannot be carried out and as a result "FIGLU" accumulates in the blood and excreted in urine.
- ***Thus "FIGLU" excretion in urine is an index of folic acid deficiency.*** When a "loading" dose of histidine is given, the excretion of "FIGLU" in urine is increased further ***("Histidine loading test").***

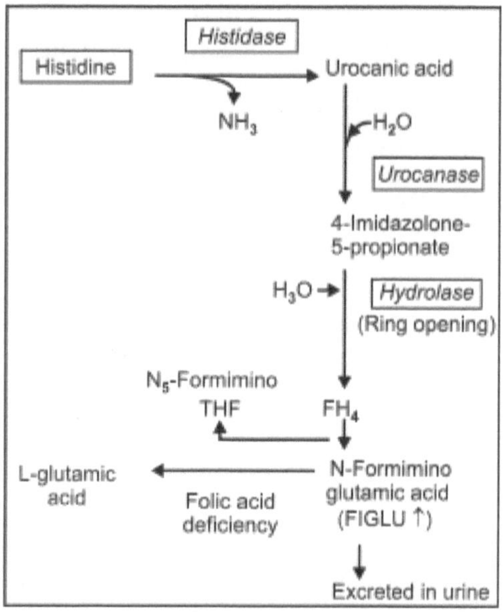

Method

- After administering 20 gm of L-histidine to the patient "FIGLU" excretion in 6 hours urine is estimated.
- "FIGLU" can be measured by semiquantitative method using high voltage electrophoresis and conventional voltage electrophoresis.
- More recently, quantitative estimation by spectrophotometric method is available.

Interpretations

- *In folic acid deficiency:* "FIGLU" excretion in urine is positive.
- Other conditions where it can be positive are
  - cirrhosis of liver; and
  - in some severe cases of vitamin B_{12} deficiency.

D. TO ESTABLISH THE CAUSE OF DEFICIENCY

1. Nutritional

- Megaloblastic anaemia resulting from nutritional causes is usually due to folate deficiency.
- Cases of combined folate and B_{12} deficiency may be seen in tropics.
- B_{12} reserve in body is more.
- Folic acid content of food is low in relation to minimum daily requirement.
- Causes to be looked for:
  - Poverty.
  - Strict vegetaranians.
  - Alcoholics.

2. Vitamin B_{12} Absorption Studies—"Radio Tracer"

a. Urinary excretion ("Schilling" test).
b. Faecal excretion.
c. Hepatic uptake.
d. Whole body counting.
e. Plasma radioactivity.

Principle: Absorption of vitamin B_{12} can be measured by the use of radioactive B_{12}. Vitamin B_{12} is a cobalt compound and can be labelled with the following isotopes of cobalt.

- **^{60}Co (half-life 5 years)**
- **^{56}Co (half-life 77 days)**
- **^{57}Co (half-life 270 days)**
- **^{58}Co (half-life 71 days)**

^{58}Co labelled B_{12} is preferred as the half-life is lowest and radiation dose to the subject is reduced. The physiological limit of vitamin B_{12} absorption is 2 μg and as the oral dose of vitamin B_{12} administered increases the amount absorbed and excreted also increase but the per cent absorption decreases.

Method

To an overnight fasting subject, 1 μg of vitamin B_{12}, containing 1 μci of radioactivity is administered in 20 to 50 ml of water by mouth. The subject is starved for another 2 hours.

The absorption of vitamin B_{12} can be measured by 5 different ways. They are:

a. Urinary Excretion (Shilling's Test)

With oral dose of ^{58}Co-labelled B_{12} as above. 1 mg ("flushing" dose) of non-radioactive ("cold") vitamin B_{12} is injected IM. Urine passed in next 24 hours is collected (any urine passed before giving the labelled B_{12} is discarded.) Radioactivity of this urine and of a "standard" is measured.

Calculation

The per cent of dose excreted in the urine is calculated as follows:

Table 24.1: Differentiation of vitamin B_{12} and folic acid deficiency

Deficiency	*Serum assay*		*Red cells folate*	*Urinary excretion*	
	B_{12}	*Folic acid*	*assay*	*FIGLU*	*MMA*
• B_{12} deficiency	↓	N or ↑	N	N or ↑	↑
• Folic acid deficiency	N	↓	↓	↑	N

$$\frac{\text{Total counts/min in 24 hours urine}}{\text{Counts/min in standard (Test dose)}} \times 100$$

Interpretations

- *Normal urinary excretion:* It is greater than 15% of the test dose.
- In patients with ***pernicious anaemia*** or with vitamin B_{12} deficiency with intestinal malabsorption or other causes is less than 5%.

Note
- Most widely used test due to simplicity.
- Low values may be found in renal diseases.
- Not highly reproducible method.
- Administration of 1 mg of B_{12} ("cold") is unphysiological and changes the clinical status of the patient.

b. Faecal Excretions

The unabsorbed B_{12} is measured by collecting faeces for 6 days and measuring its radioactivity.

Interpretations

- *Normal subjects:* Absorb more than 50% of the dose administered.
- *Decreased absorption:* It is observed in pernicious anaemia and after total/partial gastrectomy.

Note
- An accurate quantitative method.
- Prolonged collection of faeces for 6 days is tedious.
- Not suitable for outpatient.

Modification of the Test

The test is modified by administering an unabsorbable "marker", ^{51}Cr-labelled chromic oxide alongwith. A mixture of 5 μci of ^{51}Cr labelled B_{12} is administered ***orally*** to fasting subject. By counting the activities of ^{51}Cr and ^{58}Co in a sample of faeces passed after 24 hours, it is possible to calculate vitamin B_{12} absorption with reasonable accuracy.

c. Hepatic Uptake

Unabsorbed portion of test dose is completely excreted in faeces after 7 days and the absorbed materials is stored in liver which can be assessed by surface scintillation counter.

Note
- Relatively simple method.
- Collection of excreta avoided.
- Satisfactory for outpatient.
- Duration is lengthy.
- Liver diseases/anatomical variations of liver can affect.

d. Whole Body Counting

Based on the fact that absorbed B_{12} is stored in the organs (e.g. liver) for a long time and is not rapidly excreted from the body, total activity in the body of the subject is measured by means of a whole body counter, immediately after the administration of the dose and 7 days later, when all the radioactivity is presumed to be excreted out in faeces.

Note
- Collection of stool/urine avoided.
- With sensitive counters very small quantities of radioactivity may be used.

e. Plasma Radioactivity

Peak radioactivity in the blood is observed in samples collected at 8 to 12 hours after the administration of the dose. The blood levels may be used to judge absorption but the test is unreliable because of the low count rate in blood sample.

Note

- For normal absorption of B_{12}, an adequate intrinsic factor (IF) secretion by parietal cells of gastric mucosa and a normal ileum are obligatory. Vitamin B_{12} absorption will, therefore, be impaired in gastric mucosal and/or ileal lesions.
- If absorption of B_{12} is poor, the test should be repeated after a week, alongwith

intrinsic factor. A dose of 40 mg of intrinsic factor (IF) or 25 ml of normal human gastric juice to be given alongwith the labelled B_{12}.

3. Folic Acid Absorption Studies

The absorption of folic acid can be measured by:

- Radioactive method by using ^3H-folic acid
- Microbiological assay by using stable folic acid.

1. *Radioactive Method Using ^3H-Folic Acid*

About 50 to 100 µci of ^3H- folic acid is administered ***orally*** to a fasting subject and the absorption of folic acid is measured by:

- *Faecal excretion.*
- *Urinary excretion.*

a. Faecal Excretion

Unabsorbed ^3H-folic acid is measured by collecting faeces for 6 days and counting the radioactivity. Measurement of ^3H in faeces can be made only by counting ^3H_2O produced by oxidation of faeces (i) by oxidation by wet method; or (ii) with combustion bombs. The radioactivity is then measured in a liquid scintillation counter. Absorption is calculated by subtracting the excreted activity from the dose fed.

Interpretations

- ***Normal subjects:*** absorb more than 50% of the dose administered.
- ***In folic acid deficiency:*** absorption less than 50% of the dose administered.

Modification

Similar to B_{12}, a double "tracer" method by using an unabsorbed "marker" such as ^{51}Cr labelled chromium oxide can be used alongwith ^3H folic acid.

b. Urinary Excretion

After feeding ^3H folic acid, the absorbed radioactivity can be flushed out by injecting 15 mg of "cold" folic acid IM.

Interpretations

- ***Normal subjects:*** excrete more than 25% of the dose in 24 hours urine.
- ***In folic acid deficiency:*** excretion is less than 25% of the dose in 24 hours urine.

Advantage

The advantage of the ^3H folic acid method is that absorption can be measured with a physiological dose of folic acid.

2. *Microbiological Assay*

a. On Blood

Method

After an overnight, fast, inject 15 mg of folic acid IM daily for 3 days so that tissues get saturated. Thirty six hours after the last injection, 40 µg/kg folic acid is given orally. Blood samples are collected in the fasting state and at 1 and 2 hours after the administration of the dose. The folic acid activity is measured using *streptococcus faecalis—R.*

Interpretations

- ***Normal subjects:*** show a rise of at least 40 mµg/ml in any of the two samples.
- ***Folic acid deficient patients:*** do not show the rise.

b. Urinary Excretion

Five mg of folic acid is given subcutaneously on the first day. A similar dose is given *orally* next day.

Using *Streptococcus faecalis—R* by microbiological assay, folic acid activities assayed on 24 hours urine samples on both days.

Interpretation

- If less than 1.5 mg of folic acid is excreted in 24 hours urine after the oral dose, folic acid malabsorption and deficiency is diagnosed.

Miscellaneous Laboratory Investigations

- ***Stool Examination***

a. ***Patients with Caeliac Disease***

NE—Stools are fluid/or semifluid, bulky, pale, frothy and offensive. These tend to float due to their high fat and gas content.

b. Suspected case of megaloblastic anaemia due to fish tapeworm (Diphyllbobothrium latum) worms produce B_{12} deficiency by eating up B_{12} from food.

Microscopic examination of stool demonstrate ova of the worm.

- ***Gastric Analysis***

A case of suspected pernicious anaemia ***shows histamine fast achlorhydria.***

- ***Serum Gastrin Level***

In 80% of patients of pernicious anaemia serum gastrin level is elevated. This test is not specific for pernicious anaemia.

- ***Other Biochemical Findings:***
  - ***Serum bilirubin:*** is usually at the upper limit of normal or it may be increased. Due to haemolysis of the peripheral cells and death of precursors in marrow.
  - ***Serum haptoglobin level:*** may be reduced.
  - ***Serum ferritin and serum Fe:*** are usually increased but decreases on proper treatment.
  - ***Serum lactate dehydrogenase (LDH):*** usually increased.
  - ***Serum gastrin level:*** In 80% cases in pernicious anaemia, serum gastrin level is increased.

- ***Demonstration of Parietal Cell Antibodies***

Perietal cell antibodies are IgG type and can be demonstrated by immunofluorescent techniques. The antibodies can be found in serum as well as in gastric juice.

Interpretations

- Serum antibodies to surface membrane and cytoplasmic antigens of gastric parietal cells are found in 85% patients of pernicious anaemia.
- Test is not specific as parietal cell antibodies are also found in 30 to 60% patients with chronic atrophic gastritis without pernicious anaemia and in sera of 35% patient's relatives. These antibodies can be found in some normal people, specially females over the age of 70 years.
- The antibodies are also found in sera of patients of other autoimmune diseases, viz. Hashimoto's thyroiditis, adult spontaneous myxoedema, Addison's disease, hyperthyrosidism, etc.

- ***Intrinsic Factor Antibodies***

Intrinsic factor antibodies are of ***two types:***

- Blocking antibodies
- Binding antibodies.

- ***Blocking antibodies:*** They react with vitamin B_{12} combining site of intrinsic factor and inhibit subsequent binding of B_{12}.
- ***Binding antibodies:*** They attach to a site distant from the B_{12} combining site and prevent linkage of the IF-B_{12} complex to bind to ileal receptor. They are usually found in patients who have blocking antibodies and titre is high.

Both antibodies are of serum IgG type. IF antibodies are also found in gastric juice. In gastric juice only blocking antibodies are found and they are of IgA type.

Interpretations

- Both types of IF antibodies are found in the sera of 20 to 30% patients with pernicious anaemia. Blocking antibodies are found in 50 to 70% patients.
- Blocking antibodies of IgA type are found in gastric juice in 50 to 70% patients of pernicious anaemia.
- Antibodies may be detected in a few cases of other autoimmune diseases, viz. spontaneous adult myxoedema, hyperthyroidism, Addison's disease, etc.

Note

Unlike parietal cell antibodies, IF antibodies are not found in chronic atrophic gastritis *not* associated with pernicious anaemia.

- ***Biopsies***

  - *Gastric biopsy:* In pernicious anaemia, chronic atrophic gastritis shows diffuse mucosal atrophy, most marked in body of the stomach. In 80 to 90% antral mucosa is spared.

Histologically atrophic mucosa shows heavy ***infiltration with lymphocytes*** and ***plasma cells.*** There is almost complete absence of chief and perietal cells, frequently with a change to intestinal type of epithelium.

- *Per oral jejunal biopsy:* In megaloblastic anaemia of folate deficiency due to ***caeliac disease*** peroral jejunal biopsy is recommended. The typical finding on jejunal biopsy is that of villous atrophy of the mucosa, with loss of normal villi, giving rise to appearance of a flat mucosa.

In tropical sprue: The biopsy shows a wide-spectrum of abnormalities. In severe cases, it may be similar to that seen in caeliac disease, but more frequently the abnormalities are much less.

Part Three

Miscellaneous

Chapter 25

Enzymes and Isoenzymes in Clinical Medicine

ENZYMES

Introduction

The investigation and interpretation of changes in serum enzymes in diseases is one of the most rapidly expanding fields in clinical biochemistry. ***Wröblewski*** and his coworkers in 1956 published their first papers on serum glutamate-oxaloacetate transaminase (S-GOT) and followed by serum lactate dehydrogenase (LDH) and brought the possibilities of these enzymes assays in general notice. Thus began the present efflorescence of clinical enzymology and large number of enzymes have been used for diagnosis and prognosis of various diseases.

A. GENERAL CONSIDERATIONS

1. Sources of Plasma Enzymes

They can be:
- plasma derived, and
- cell derived.

• *Plasma Derived Enzymes*

These act on substrates in plasma, and their activity is higher in plasma than in cells, e.g., coagulation enzymes. This group will not be further considered.

• *Cell Derived Enzymes*

These have a high activity in cells and overflow into the plasma. They are further subdivided into:

- *Secretory:* These are mainly derived from digestive glands and function in the extracellular space.
- *Metabolic:* These are concerned with intermediary metabolism and function in the cells and those enzymes found in the plasma are mainly derived from the soluble and microsomal fractions of the cells.

The cell derived enzymes enter the plasma in small amounts as a result of:
- continuous normal ageing of the cells; or
- owing to diffusion through undamaged cell membranes.

They leave the plasma through:
- inactivation;
- catabolism in general protein pool; and rarely,
- excretion in bile and urine.

2. Possible Mechanisms Responsible for Abnormal Levels

Serum level of a particular enzyme may be increased by diseases that provoke:

i. an increase in its rate of release, or
ii. a decrease in its rate of disposition or excretion.

Increased Serum Level

a. Increased release

- *Necrosis of cells:* Due to damage to cells of the tissue. The resultant pattern will depend on:

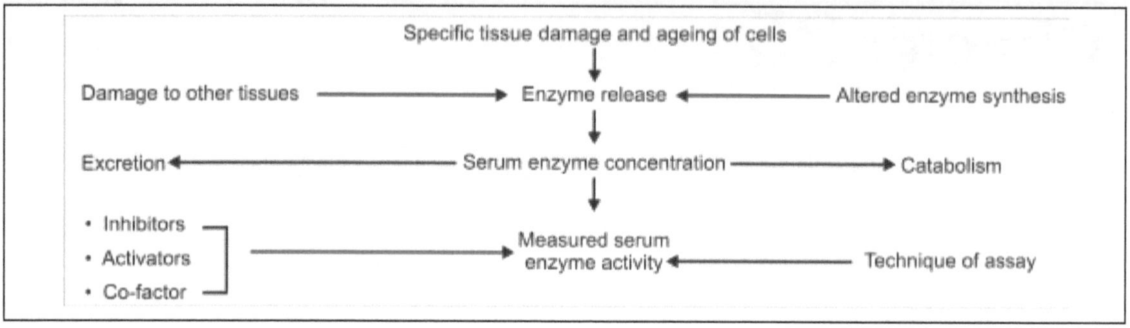

- Normal enzyme content of the tissue/organ.
- On the extent and type of necrosis.

- ***Increased permeability of cell membrane without necrosis of cells:*** Increased permeability without gross cellular damage/necrosis can increase the enzyme level, e.g.
  - In early stage of viral hepatitis, before jau-ndice appears, there is "ballooning" deg-eneration of liver cells, leading to elevated levels of transaminases (S-GPT).
  - Progressive muscular dystrophy—elevated levels of aldolase, GOT and CPK.
- ***Increased production of the enzyme within cell:*** Such a situation may be seen in treatment of patients with protein anabolic drugs, results in increased synthesis of liver cell ***transaminases*** and ***serum transaminases*** will increase by overflow.
- ***An increase in tissue source of enzymes:*** This is due to either increased rate of production in cells as mentioned above, or increase in the number of cells/and cell mass, as seen in malignancies, e.g. ***alkaline phosphatase*** increased in patients with osteoblastic bone lesions, or ***acid phosphatase*** increase in patients with carcinoma prostate.

b. Impaired disposition/excretion

As for example

- increased levels of serum LAP and ALP seen in patients with obstructive jaundice, and
- certain increased enzyme levels in cases of renal failure.

- ***Decreased Serum Levels***

a. ***Decreased Formation of the Enzyme*** Which may be:

(i) Genetic

Examples:

- Hypophosphatasia, with decreased ALP level in serum,
- Wilson's disease with decrease in serum caeruloplasmin.

(ii) Acquired

For example:

- In hepatitis decreased serum level of pseudocholinesterase due to decreased production.
- Decreased serum amylase in patients with chronic hepatic, or pancreatic diseases, or those who are severely malnourished.

b. ***Enzyme Inhibition***

For example, decreased serum pseudocholinesterase in insecticide poisoning.

c. ***Lack of Cofactors***

For example, decreased serum GOT level in pregnancy and cirrhosis.

3. Units of Serum Enzyme Activity

Various workers have used various units. It is better to have uniformity, the serum enzyme activity is expressed in '***international units***' (IU). ***Definition:*** One IU is defined as the activity of the enzyme which transforms one μ mole of substrate per minute under optimal conditions and at defined temperature, and expressed as IU/ml. When milli-micromole of the substrate is transformed/minute, it is IU/L or m-IU/ml.

4. Value of Serum Enzyme Assay in Clinical Practice

Single or serial assay of the serum activity of a selected enzyme or enzymes may provide information on the nature and extent of a disease process.

(a) Value in Diagnosis

As example, an enzyme assay of serum CK on the day of a suspected case of myocardial infarction will be helpful for diagnosis if ECG changes are doubtful.

(b) In Differential Diagnosis

When the differential diagnosis lies between a disease that is known to cause a particular pattern of serum enzyme change and one that does not, e.g. as an aid in differentiating myocardial infarction and pulmonary embolism both presenting with chest pain.

	Serum–GOT	*LDH*
• *Myocardial infarction*	↑	↑
• *Pulmonary embolism*	Normal	↑

(c) In Ascertaining Prognosis

Serial enzyme assay is required. When a disease regularly causes serum enzyme alterations and it is necessary to know the progress of the enzyme changing process in the tissue known to be diseased and how it may be altered by natural causes or in response to treatment, e.g.

- to ascertain progress in viral hepatitis, serial enzyme assays of S-GPT are of great help,
- response to endocrine therapy of carcinoma of prostate is shown by degree of reduction of the elevated serum acid phosphatase.

(d) Early Detection of a Disease

When damage to a tissue is suspected which is so slight that it cannot be detected otherwise. *For example:*

- Minimal hepatotoxic effects of antidepressant drugs can be detected by a raised serum ICD/or OCT before the patient is clinically ill.
- Increased S-GPT in early stage of viral hepatitis when jaundice has not appeared (subclinical stage).

B. CLINICAL SIGNIFICANCE OF ENZYME ASSAYS

Value of enzyme assays will be discussed organwise.

I. Serum Enzymes in Heart Diseases

Before the introduction of serum GOT assay for the investigation of myocardial infarction the heart had been a ***"biochemically inaccessible"*** organ. In cases of suspected myocardial infarction when clinical and ECG evidence was equivocal, there was no other means of specifically investigating possible injury to cardiac muscle.

Why Enzyme Diagnosis?

1. About 25 to 30% of myocardial infarctions are not diagnosed "antemortem" sometimes.
2. Clinical diagnosis and angiographic studies do not correlate in 25 to 33% of patients.
3. ECG findings may not be helpful if:
   - Prior left bundle branch block is present.
   - Old changes exist that may obscure current ECG interpretation.
   - Intramural infarctions may not change ECG pattern.
   - Diaphragmatic infarctions often missed on ECG.

Enzyme Assays Carried out in Myocardial Infarction

a. Commonly done

- *Creatine phosphokinase (CK)*
- *Aspartate transaminase (GOT) or (AST)*
- *Lactate dehydrogenase (LDH)*

b. Other enzymes which have been studied but not commonly done

- *γ-Glutamyl transpeptidase (GGTP)*
- *Histaminase*
- *Pseudocholinesterase*

1. Creatine Phosphokinase (CPK or CK)

This enzyme catalyzes the following reaction:

Creatine~ (P) + ADP → Creatine + ATP

This enzyme is also called as ***creatine kinase.*** It is found in high concentration in skeletal muscle, myocardium and brain but not found at all in liver and kidneys. Small amounts are found in lung, thyroid and adrenal gland. ***It is not found in RBCs and its level is not affected by haemolysis.*** It appears to be a sensitive measure of myocardial infarction and muscle diseases, but remains normal in patients with liver diseases.

Normal value: Serum activity varies from 4 to 60 IU/L (at 37°C)

Behaviour in acute myocardial infarction: After myocardial infarction, serum value is found to increase after about 6 hours, reaches a peak level in 24 to 30 hours, and returns to normal level in 2 to 4 days (usually in 72 hours).

Remarks

- Studies suggested that serum CK activity is a more sensitive indicator in early stage of myocardial ischaemia.
- Potentially ***more useful in subendocardial infarction.***
- No increase in activity noted in heart failure and coronary insufficiency.
- Magnitude of elevation was found to be greater than that observed with GOT or LDH.

Note

- ***Storage:*** There is 50% loss of serum CK activity after 6 hours at room temperature and 24 hours at refrigerated temperature. Hence, ***all determinations of serum CK activity should be done on fresh blood samples.***
- The above can be circumvented by adding to the reaction mixture cysteine or other compounds containing –SH group (cystein stimulated CPK assay).

2. Serum Glutamate Oxaloacetate Transaminase (S-GOT)

Also called as ***aspartate transaminase or aminotransferase*** (AST), the concentration of this enzyme is very high, in myocardium.

Normal value: Serum activity of S-GOT varies from 4 to 17 IU/L (25°C) (10-35 of original Karmen spectrophotometric units/ml).

Behaviour in acute myocardial infarction: In acute myocardial infarction, serum activity rises sharply within the first 12 hours, with a peak level at 24 hours or over and returns to normal within 3 to 5 days.

Remarks

- Level of serum enzyme has been correlated well with prognosis:
  - Levels > 350 IU/L usually fatal, (due to massive infarction).
  - Levels > 150 IU/L associated with high mortality.
  - Levels < 50 IU/L are associated with low mortality.
- Elevation has been noted in absence of any ECG change.
- ***Highest incidence of abnormal levels occurs on second day of infarction.***
- Rise depends on size of the infarction
- ***Extra cardiac factors:*** Elevation seen in other diseases, e.g. muscle disease and hepatic diseases. But these can be differentiated clinically and simultaneous determination of S-GPT. There is no rise of S-GPT in myocardial infarction.
- Re-infarction results in a secondary rise of S-GOT.

3. Lactate dehydrogenase (LDH)

LDH catalyzes the reversible conversion of pyruvic acid (PA) and lactic acid (LA).

Normal value: Normal serum LDH activity ranges from 60 to 250 IU/L (120-500 units/ml—original Karmen spectrophotometric method).

Behaviour in acute myocardial infarction: In acute myocardial infarction, serum activity rises within 12 to 24 hours, attains peak at 48 hours (2 to 4 days) reaching about 1000 IU/L and then return gradually to normal from 8th to 14th day.

Remarks

- The peak rises in S-LDH is roughly proportional to the extent of injury to the myocardial tissue.
- S-LDH elevation may persist for more than a week after CPK and S-GOT levels have returned to normal levels.
- S-LDH level > 1500 IU/L in acute myocardial infarction suggests a grave prognosis.

Disadvantage

The enzyme is ***relatively nonspecific for myocardial tissue.*** It is so widespread in body cells that coexistent disease processes in other organs may cause elevations.

Thus, S-LDH levels are raised in:

- Carcinomatosis
- Acute leukaemias
- Granulocytic leukaemia
- Pulmonary infarction
- Renal necrosis
- Muscle disease.

Less pronounced S-LDH increases are seen in inflammatory hepatic disorders.

Precaution:

Red blood cells are rich in LDH, hence avoid haemolysis. Haemolyzed samples should not be assayed.

4. *γ-Glutamyl Transpeptidase (G-GTP)*

Also called ***γ-glutamyl transferase (γ-GT),*** it catalyzes the transfer of the γ-glutamyl group from one peptide to another peptide or to an amino acid.

Highest tissue activity of this enzyme is found in kidneys, but activity is relatively high in liver, lungs, pancreas and prostate. Some activity is present in intestinal mucosa, thyroid gland and spleen. Normal heart contains very little γ-GT.

Normal value: Normal serum activity has been shown to be:

- ***Men*** : 10 to 47 IU/L
- ***Women*** : 7 to 30 IU/L

Behaviour in acute myocardial infarction: Several investigators recently have demonstrated increases in serum γ-GT in acute myocardial infarction. ***Increase serum activity is found to be late, peak activity between 7th and 11th day and lasts as long as a month.*** Hence, it has been proposed as a useful test for myocardial infarction in later stages. ***The enzyme does not come from heart muscle.*** They postulate that ***increased tissue levels develop with the repair process. Source of the enzyme is from vascular endothelium from angioblastic proliferation.***

Remarks

Elevated levels of serum activity are found in many other conditions also.

- ***In hepatobiliary disorders:*** It is useful in detecting obstructive jaundice, cholangitis and cholecystitis, with primary and secondary neoplasms of liver.
- Also found elevated ***in alcoholics and in alcoholic cirrhosis. γ-GT is the most sensitive indicator in alcoholics.***
- Increase serum activity seen with ***pancreatic diseases.***
- Elevated levels seen in epileptic patients with drug therapy with anticonvulsants, probably due to enzyme induction.
- Since serum γ-GT levels are not elevated in any form of bone disorders, it is ***a valuable parameter in differentiating between skeletal (bone) and hepatic dysfunction associated with increased serum-ALP.***

5. Histaminase

The enzyme histaminase occurs in different organs in various species. In man, however, normal plasma contains either very small amount of histaminase or none at all, but considerable amount of histaminase has been found in human heart muscle. Estimation of serum histaminase has been done by volumetric method of Kapeller-Adler.

Normal value: It ranges from 0.12 to 0.76 PU/ml (Mean 0.41 ± 0.17).

Interpretation:

- Raised histaminase found > 0.8 P.U/ml in 97.14% of ECG proved cases of myocardial infarction.

Pattern of Rise in Acute Myocardial Infarction:

Serum enzyme activity rises within 6 hours of myocardial infarction and persists for whole of first week.

Remarks

- It helps in early diagnosis of myocardial infarction even when ECG failed to reveal.
- It also has a prognostic value as higher serum histaminase levels were found to be associated with worse prognosis (mean value in fatal cases > 3.48 ± 0.97).

6. Cholinesterases

Cholinesterases are enzymes which hydrolyze esters of choline to give choline and acid.

There are **two types:**

- ***True cholinesterase:*** is responsible for destruction of acetyl choline at the neuromuscular junction and is found in nerve tissues and RB cells.
- ***Pseudocholinesterase:*** is found in various tissues such as liver, heart muscle and intestine and it is the type which is present in plasma.

Normal value: Normal value of serum pseudocholinesterase is 2.17 to 5.17 IU/ml (De la Huerga et al). By Michaelis method it is 1.05 to 2.45 units/ml (mean 1.5 ± 0.33).

Pattern in Acute Myocardial Infarction:

Elevation of plasma pseudocholinesterase was observed in 90.5% cases of acute myocardial infarction. Raised serum activity is found within 12 hours (or even as early as 3 hours found in some cases). ***Serum enzyme activity has been considered as a sensitive index for determination of cellular necrosis in myocardium.***

Serum enzyme activity in other conditions:

- Serum enzyme activity is decreased in acute hepatitis. Its regular low level in chronic hepatitis is more often found valuable (owing to diminished synthesis by hepatic cells).
- Cholinesterase is also ***inhibited by organophosphorous compound (insecticides)*** and serum cholinesterase assay is, therefore, useful to detect poisoning by these compounds in agriculture and industries ("Diazinon" poisoning).

II. Serum Enzymes in Liver Diseases

See the Chapter on Liver Function Tests.

III. Serum Enzymes in GI Tract Diseases

Assays in serum of proteolytic enzymes and their precursors or their inhibitors have not yet found a place in the normal investigation of diseases of GI tract. The only enzyme of GI origin which is regularly assayed is ***serum amylase.*** The other enzyme is ***serum lipase,*** but it is not routinely done in most of the laboratories.

I. Serum Amylase

There are problems in methodology and numerical, results of assay by one procedure cannot easily be converted by a factor to those obtained by another procedure and IU are difficult to apply.

Many laboratories use:

- A very quick and rapid ***"amyloclastic"*** method for rapid diagnosis.
- ***"Saccharogenic" method*** which is more accurate ***(Somogy's method).***

Normal value: By Somogy method—80 to 180 Somogy units/100 ml.

Interpretations

- ***Acute pancreatitis:*** Serum amylase assay is the investigation of choice in the diagnosis of acute pancreatitis. Serum enzyme activity > 1000 units seen within 24 hours and returns to normal within 3 days. Also urinary amylase increases and persists a little longer than serum activity.

- ***In other diseases:*** As amylase is secreted in the parotid glands, raised serum values not exceeding 1000 units, are usually found in ***mumps,*** and other forms of parotitis and also when there is salivary duct stone.

  This may be of value occasionally in differential diagnosis of:
  - Meningoencephalitis.
  - In facial swellings of other causes.
- A raised serum amylase though not usually exceeding 500 units is often found in other acute abdominal catastrophes like:
  - Perforated peptic ulcer.
  - Intestinal obstruction.
- After administration of opiates, raised values may be seen.

Macroamylasaemia

In some individuals, a form of amylase with a high molecular weight occurs in the circulation. It cannot pass the glomerular filter and consequently accumulates in the blood stream.

Macroamylasaemia should be suspected when there is

- an increase in serum amylase; and
- no increase in urinary amylase output.

Macroamylase can be formed by ***combination of ordinary serum amylase with an antibody.*** It can probably result from polymerization of the enzyme molecule.

2. Serum Lipase

Serum lipase assay is more specific in pancreatic disorders and remains raised for longer periods. But it is not valuable in practice because of the absence of quick assay methods.

The lipolytic activity of the serum may be determined by the amount of "olive-oil emulsion" hydrolyzed by a given quantity of serum in a given time at 37ºC. Values for lipase can be expressed as the amount of 0.05 N NaOH required to neutralize the FA produced by one ml of serum ***(Cherry-Crandall).*** A ***colorimetric assay*** has also been designed **(Seligman and Nachlas).**

Normal value:

a. ***By titrimetric method***—0.06 to 1.02 ml of 0.05N Sodium hydroxide.

b. ***By colorimetric assay***—9.0 to 20 m IU.

Remarks:

- Increase in serum lipase is a reflection of pancreatic disorders. In ***acute pancreatitis*** serum lipase activity increases promptly at the time of onset of symptoms, values as high as 2800 U/L having been reported. The subsequent fall is more gradual than in the case of amylase. Elevated levels persist in some cases 10 to 14 days or longer (less rapid removal from circulation).
- Elevated serum lipase levels also reported in perforated duodenal and peptic ulcers and in intestinal obstruction.
- Moderate increases of serum lipase were found in about 1/3 patients with cirrhosis.

"Provocative tests" with secretin and PZ, have been reported

- In ***normal*** cases duodenal juice amylase is increased and serum level is unaltered.
- In ***chronic pancreatitis*** duodenal juice value is unaltered but serum level increases.

IV. Serum Enzymes in Muscle Diseases

Enzyme assays used in muscle diseases are:

- *S-GOT/S-GPT*
- *Aldolase*
- *CPK.*

1. S-GOT/S-GPT

These are not used now.

2. Serum Aldolase

Aldolase was until recent years the enzyme of choice in the investigation of diseases of muscles being more sensitive than GOT. This enzyme catalyzes the interconversion of F-1-6di-(P) and triose (P). It has a wide tissue distribution specially found in high concentration in liver, skeletal muscle, brain. Also found abundant in neoplastic tissues.

Normal value: ranges from 2 to 6 m-IU

Remarks:

- Normal values of serum aldolase found in neurogenic muscular weakness e.g., in poliomyelitis, peripheral neuritis.
- Moderate increase in dermatomyositis, and muscular dystrophies.
- Highest values are seen in Duchenne type of muscular dystrophy.
- Increase in serum aldolase activity has also been reported in other conditions—liver diseases specially viral hepatitis, and myocardial infarction.

3. Serum CPK

Assay of serum aldolase has been replaced by serum CPK which is ***more sensitive*** and ***more specific.***

Remarks

- Serum CPK is slightly elevated occasionally in neurogenic muscular atrophy.
- Raised values are seen in most cases ***of muscular dystrophies*** and ***dermatomyositis,*** usually 1000 IU/L.
- ***Highest values are found in Duchenne type of muscular dystrophies*** (10,000 IU/L). The increase is most marked in acute phase, in early childhood; the actual value depend on both: (i) severity of the disease; or (ii) on mass of diseased muscle. The rise occurs before the clinical manifestations and serum enzyme levels are used to detect "carriers".
- Raised values are also found in hypothyroidism owing to secondary muscle disease.

V. Serum Enzymes in Bone Diseases

Serum ***alkaline phosphatase*** remains the only useful enzyme assay for investigation. ALP is a most valuable index of osteoblastic activity.

- Increases in serum ALP activity seen in rickets, osteomalacia, hyperparathyroidism and particularly in Paget's disease.
- In primary and secondary malignancies of bone, the level depends on the severity and degree of new bone formation. When the lesion is purely destructive as myelomatosis, the value is normal.
- In hypophosphatasia, where there is defective calcification, low tissue and serum ALP activity is observed.

VI. Value of Enzymes in Malignancies

Chief enzyme assays useful in malignancies are listed in Table 25.1.

1. Acid Phosphatase

There are ***two types*** depending on activity in different pH.

	Tissues found in
1. A type of acid phosphatase (pH = 6.0)	Erythrocytes
2. A type of acid phosphatase (pH = 5.0)	Prostate epithelium, spleen, kidney, plasma, liver, pancreas.

Table 25.1: Chief enzyme assays useful in malignancies

Enzymes assayed	*Diseases*
1. **Serum Acid phosphatase (AP)**	• Cancer of prostate with/without metastasis
2. **Serum alkaline phosphatase (ALP)**	• Metastasis in liver • Osteoblastic metastasis in bone. • Jaundice due to carcinoma of head of pancreas.
3. **Serum LDH, aldolase, phosphohexose isomerase**	• Widespread malignancies. • Advanced leukaemias.
4. **β-Glucuronidase in urine**	• Cancer of urinary bladder. • Cancer head of pancreas.
5. **LDH in effusion fluids**	• Local malignancies.
6. **LAP**	• Liver cell carcinoma. • Primary or secondary carcinoma superimposed on cirrhosis liver.

Normal value: Normal plasma contains small amount of acidphosphatase, 0.6 to 3.1 KA units/100 ml.

Precautions

1. It is an ***extremely labile enzyme*** so the enzyme assays should be done on fresh samples immediately.

- Avoid haemolysis due to presence of acid phosphatase in RB cells.

Remarks:

- Main value in relation to diagnosis of metastasizing prostate carcinoma. Enzyme is formed from mature prostatic epithelial cells. Not formed by immature prostatic epithelial cells.
- Highly anaplastic carcinoma may not produce the enzyme.
- Acid phosphatase of prostate is ***inhibited by L-tartarate. "Tartarate-liable" AP is more specific.***

  Normal value is 0.0 to 0.5 KA units %.
- ***Sullivan test'*** can be used in cases of highly anaplastic carcinoma to stimulate AP production.

  Injection of 25 mg of testosterone propionate is given daily for 5 days, may stimulate enzyme production by anaplastic cancer cells.
- ***Other conditions:*** Acid phosphatase activity in serum may also rise in certain other diseases:
  - Marked rise is seen in **Gaucher's disease** and it is characteristic of that disorder.
  - Occasional rise is seen in ***Paget's disease, hyperparathyroidism,*** and ***osteolytic metastasis*** from breast and other carcinomas.
  - Marked rise seen with thrombocytosis, chronic granulocytic leukaemia, myeloproliferative disorders, etc.

    Note: No rise occurs in lymphocytic leukaemias, or lymphomas.
  - A rise is seen in haemolytic anaemia.
  - Small elevations with thromboembolic disorders, e.g., pulmonary embolism.

2. β-Glucuronidase

Though it is not routinely done, it is useful in certain malignancies. β-Glucuronidase catalyzes ***glucuronotransferase*** reactions as well as the hydrolysis of β-D-glucopyranuranides by means of which its activity is usually estimated.

The enzyme is widespread in human tissues but is most abundant in liver, spleen, endometrium, breast and adrenals. Human RB cells contain little or no β-glucuronidase but leucocytes have a high enzyme content.

Normal value: Serum β-glucuronidase activity ranges from 210 to 550 m-IU for males, and 90 to 400 m-IU in females.

Remarks:

- Serum and urinary β-glucuronidase activity is ***increased markedly in cancer of urinary bladder.***
- Very high serum activity reported in ***carcinoma of head of pancreas*** and in 50% cases of ***cancer breast*** and ***cervix*** without liver metastasis.
- Serum β-glucuronidase activity increases in last trimester of pregnancy, and then falls to normal values by about the 5th of postpartum day.
- Assay of β-glucuronidase activity of vaginal fluid has been suggested as useful in diagnosis of malignancies of female genital tract.
- β-Glucuronidase activity in ascitic fluid has been found to increase twice in malignant diseases compared to ascitic fluid of nonmalignant origin.

ISOENZYMES

Definition:

Isoenzymes (or isozymes) are the physically distinct forms of the same enzyme but catalyze the same chemical reaction or reactions, and differ from each other structurally, electrophoretically and immunologically.

A. MULTIPLE FORMS PRESENTATION

There are a number of ways in which enzyme can be present in tissues in multiple forms.

1. The same enzymatic reactions are usually performed in different species by different proteins. **Example**—yeast ***alcohol dehydrogenase*** is chemically not the same protein as

any animal hepatic alcohol dehydrogenase. Such greatly differing forms of enzymes are often called as **"heteroenzymes"**.

2. Different tissues of a particular species often contain protein of very similar enzymatic activities which are chemically and physically distinct. **Examples** are:
   - ***"Acid phosphatase" of RBCs can easily be differentiated from that of prostate.*** Prostate acid phosphatase is extremely "heat-labile" even at 37°C and can be inhibited by ethanol and L (+) tartarate while acid phosphatase of RBCs are inactivated by 20% neutral formaldehyde.
   - ***Alkaline phosphatase*** isoenzyme of ***placental origin*** is extremely ***"heat-stable"***.
3. The term isoenzyme (isozyme) was originally used to describe multiple forms of an enzyme having the same biological enzymatic activity, which could be separated within the same cells of the same tissues. ***Example:*** using electrophoresis, most work has been done on LDH. There are five major isoenzymes of LDH, all of which are present in all tissues, but whose proportional distribution varies greatly from tissues to tissues.

- Very often cells fractionation by ultracentrifugation has shown that different subcellular fractions viz., soluble, microsomal, mitochondrial, nuclear have different isoenzymes distribution. It may become possible to correlate the intracellular location of these isoenzymes with their metabolic functions as has been done with isocitrate dehydrogenase (ICD) and malate dehydrogenase.

B. Value and Significance of Different Isoenzymes

1. LDH Isoenzymes

- LDH catalyzes the reversible oxidation of lactate to pyruvate.
- In blood serum as many as *5 (five) physically distinct isoenzymes* of this enzyme exist and are known as **LDH-1, LDH-2, LDH-3, LDH-4, and LDH-5.** All these isoenzymes though different physically they catalyze the same reaction of oxidation of LA to PA.

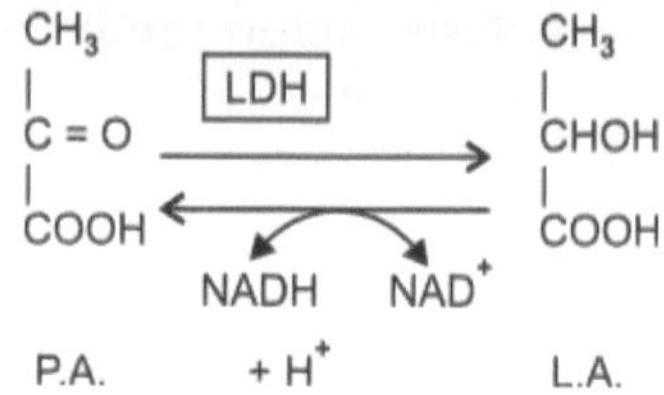

- The different forms can be separated by electrophoresis. The difference in electrophoretic mobilities is due to different electric charges on the isoenzymes due to difference in contents of acidic and basic amino acids. ***Examples are:***
  - **LDH-1** has the ***highest negative charge*** and hence moves fastest during electrophoresis. It contains a higher proportions of aspartate and glutamate than the other forms.
  - **LDH-5** is the slowest moving fraction.
- Though the same chemical reaction is catalyzed, the different isoenzymes may catalyze the same reaction at different rates. ***Example:*** rate of oxidation of –OH-butyrate is greater by LDH-1 and LDH-2, when compared with rate of oxidation of LDH-4 and LDH-5.
- The isoenzymes may have different physical properties also. ***Example:*** LDH-4 and LDH-5 are easily destroyed by heat, whereas LDH-1 and LDH-2 are not, if heated up to about 60°C ("Heat-resistant")
- The isoenzymes have different pH optima and K_m values. It has been shown that the existence of different isoenzymes is due to difference in the quarternary structure of the enzyme protein.

Structure of LDH Isoenzymes

- In man, there are **5 (five) principal isoenzymes** of LDH as mentioned above. A ***sixth, atypical isoenzyme*** LDH has been found in male genital tissues, called **LDHx.**
- Each isoenzyme protein is made up of four polypeptide subunits, thus, each is a ***"tetramer"***. Each subunit may be one of two types termed H and M and the different isoenzy-

Table 25.2: Possible combination of LDH

Type	*Polypeptide chains*	*Electrophoretic mobility*	*Tissue rich in isoenzyme type*
• **LDH-1**	(H_4) H H H H	Fast moving (fastest)	Found in myocardium
• **LDH-2**	(H_3M) H H H M		
• **LDH-3**	(H_2M_2) H H M M		
• **LDH-4**	(HM_3) H M M M		
• **LDH-5**	(M_4) M M M M	Slowest moving	Found in liver (hepatic)

mes contain H and M in different proportions.

Thus, five possible combinations occur as shown in Table 25.2.

Clinical significance

- After damage to either of these tissues viz., myocardium or liver, total serum LDH is increased and it may be useful to know the origin of this enzyme increase.
- ***In normal serum, LDH_2 (H_3M) is the most prominent*** isoenzyme and the slowest peak of LDH-5 is rarely seen.
- ***After myocardial infarction,*** the faster isoenzymes LDH-1 and LDH-2 predominate.
- ***In acute viral hepatitis,*** the slowest isoenzymes LDH-5 and LDH-4 (HM_3) predominate.

  However, differential diagnosis, by electrophoresis of a serum with a raised LDH of unknown origin though relatively simple, is not a method routinely adopted in all laboratories.

Chemical Differentiation of Isoenzymes of LDH: Attempts have been made at simpler chemical identification of these patterns by

i. ***heat stability,***
ii. ***inhibition with urea, and***
iii. ***reaction with changed "substrate".***

- ***Myocardial LDH (LDH-1)*** is found to be more **"heat stable"** than that of hepatic LDH (LDH-5).
- ***Hepatic*** **LDH (LDH-5)** is **inhibited by urea.** The above two properties have been utilised to differentiate these two isoenzymes by chemical methods.
- ***Reaction with changed substrate:*** *Cardiac LDH* (LDH-1 and 2) utilizes oxobutyrate preferentially to pyruvate as a substrate, whereas liver LDH (LDH-5 and 4) has relatively less activity with oxobutyrate.

LDH Isoenzymes in Malignancy

- Total serum LDH is frequently elevated in neoplastic diseases. In malignancies, isoenzyme pattern shifts towards slower migrating zone, there is increase usually LDH-3, LDH-4 and LDH-5.
- An increase in LDH-5 is seen ***in breast carcinoma, malignancies of CNS, prostatic carcinoma.***
- ***In leukaemias,*** rise is more in LDH-2, and LDH-3.
- ***Malignant tumours of testes and ovary*** show rise of LDH-2, LDH-3, and LDH-4.

2. Isoenzymes of CPK

In human tissues, CK isoenzymes occur in ***three distinct molecular forms.*** Each isoenzyme is a ***'dimer'*** consisting of two protomers 'M' (muscle) and 'B' (brain). Thus, three possible isoenzymes are shown in Table 25.3.

Table 25.3: Possible isoenzymes of CPK

Type	*Polypeptide chains*	*Electrophoretic mobility*	*Tissue type*
• **CK-1 (CPK-1)**	BB	Fast moving (more of -ve charge)	Brain type
• **CK-2**	MB	Intermediate	Hybrid type
• **CK-3**	MM	Slow moving	Muscle type

Atypical Isoenzymes

In addition to above three distinct forms, ***two atypical isoenzymes*** have been reported. They are:

- ***Macro-CK (CK-Macro)***
- ***Mitochondrial type (CK-Mi)***

Methods of Assay

Methods that are currently used for measurement of CK-isoenzymes are:

- Electrophoresis
- Ionexchange chromatography
- Radioimmuno assay (RIA)
- Immuno-inhibition.

Electrophoresis is a major method, and is the method of choice. It can be done routinely in laboratory.

Principle: The technique consists of performing electrophoresis on the sample using an overlay technique and then visualizing the bands under UV light.

1. The three major band separated as per their mobility are shown below.
2. The atypical bands can also be seen.
3. Sometimes a strongly fluorescent band appears which migrates in close proximity to CK-BB. The exact nature of this fluorescence is not known but it has been attributed to binding of fluorescent drugs or bilirubin by albumin.

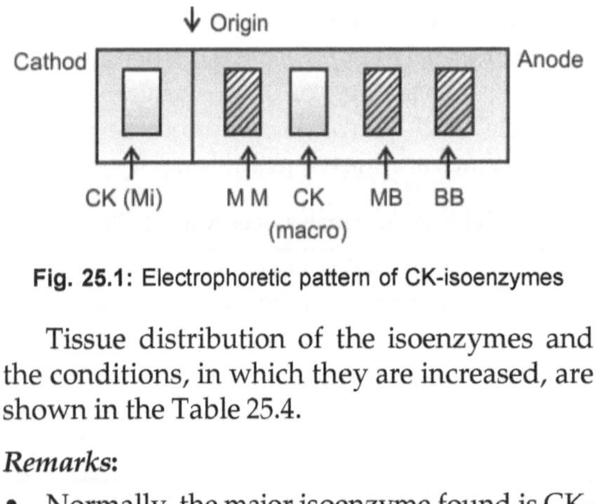

Fig. 25.1: Electrophoretic pattern of CK-isoenzymes

Tissue distribution of the isoenzymes and the conditions, in which they are increased, are shown in the Table 25.4.

Remarks:

- Normally, the major isoenzyme found is CK-MM. Values for MB isoenzyme varies from undetectable to trace amount, being less than 6% of total CK activity of plasma. It is claimed that CK-BB is also present in trace quantities in the sera of healthy persons (but most techniques employed cannot detect).

Note

CK-BB is not found in significant quantity in normal healthy person as its passage across the blood-brain barrier is hindered due to large molecular size, approximately 80,000. It is detectable in significant amount when extensive damage to brain tissue occurs and blood-brain barrier is disrupted.

- **CK-BB:**
  - Most common cause of elevation of CK-BB are:
    - Central nervous system damage.
    - Tumours (carcinomas).

    In these, it is usually more than 5 U/L and in the range of 10 to 50 U/l.
  - Other conditions listed in the Table 25.4, the activity is usually less 10 U/L.

    Note

    Presence of Macro-CK, an enzyme-immunoglobulin (Enz-Ig) complex is there. Recently, it has been reported that CK-BB is significantly increased in various carcinomas, viz, in adenocarcinomas, prostatic carcinomas. Thus, ***CK-BB may be useful as a "tumour-marker".***
- **CK-MB:**

  a. ***Cardiac diseases:*** Cardiac muscle contains significant amount of CK-MB isoenzyme (approximately 20% of all CK-MB). Hence, ***estimation of serum CK-MB is of immense value in diagnosis of acute myocardial infarction (AMI).***

  Demonstration of increased levels of CK-MB ≥ 6% of total CK is taken as most specific indicator of AMI. MB accounts for 4.5 to 20% of total CK activity of plasma of patients with recent AMI and total MB isoenzyme may be elevated 20 times above normal.

  In AMI, CK-MB levels begin to rise within 4 to 8 hours, peak at 12 to 24 hours, and return to normal levels within 48 to 72 hours.

  Note

  - Not specific as rise is observed in other cardiac disorders.

Table 25.4: CK isoenzymes in various tissues and their increase in diseases

Type of CK isoenzymes	*Tissues found*	*Conditions found elevated*
• CK-BB (CK-1)	Brain (principal tissue), Also found in bladder prostate, uterus, colon, stomach, lungs, thyroid	• Cerebrovascular accidents, • Anoxic encephalopathy • CNS shock • Placental or uterine trauma • Carcinomas • Carbon monoxide poisoning • Reye's syndrome • Acute and chronic renal failure.
• CK-MB (CK 2)	Heart (principal tissue) Skeletal muscle	• Myocardial infarction (principal cause) • Myocardial injury due to various causes, viz., ischaemia, angina, etc. • Duchenne muscular dystrophy • Polymyositis • Reye's syndrome • Carbon monoxide poisoning • Rocky mountain spotted fever
• CK-MM CK-3	Skeletal muscle Cardiac muscle	• Myocardial infarction • Muscular dystrophies • Polymyositis • Hypothyroidism • Severe strenous physical activity.

- CK-BB can be transformed to CK-MB which can account for unexplained CK-MB rise in lung cancer, acute cerebral disorders.

b. ***Non-cardiac diseases:*** CK-MB level may be increased in certain non-cardiac disorders as given in Table 25.4.

- **CK-MM**

CK-MM is the major isoenzyme found in striated muscle and normal healthy serum; skeletal muscle contains mainly CK-MM with a small amount of CK-MB. Hence, it is increased in AMI and in muscular dystrophies.

CK-MM elevation seen in hypothyroidism is probably due to:

- Involvement of muscle tissue (probably due to increased membrane permeability).
- Direct effect of thyroid hormones on enzyme activity.
- Probably slower clearance of CK as a result of hypometabolism.

Atypical CK Isoenzymes

1. **Macro-CK (CK-Macro)**

- ***Formation:*** Formed by aggregation of CK-BB with immunoglobulin, usually with IgG but sometimes IgA. and may also be formed by complexing CK-MM with lipoproteins.
- ***Electrophoresis:*** Electrophoretically migrates between CK-MB and CK-MM (Fig. 25.1).
- ***Incidence:*** It ranges from 0.8 to 1.6 %.
- ***Age and sex:*** Occurs most frequently in women above 50 years of age.
- ***Clinical significance:*** No specific disorder has been associated with this isoenzyme.

2. **CK-Mi (Mitochondrial CK-Isoenzyme)**

- ***Site and structure:*** It is present bound to the exterior surface of inner mitochondrial membrane of muscle, liver and brain. It can exist in dimeric form or as an oligomeric aggregates having high molecular weight of approximately 35,000.
- ***Electrophoresis:*** Electrophoretically, it migrates towards cathode and is behind CK-MM band.

- *Incidence:* It is not present in normal serum and incidence is from 0.8 to 1.7 %.
- *Clinical significance:* It is only present in serum when there is extensive tissue damage causing breakdown of mitochondria and cell wall. ***Thus, its presence in serum indicate severe illness.*** It is not related with any specific disease states, but it has been detected in cases of malignant tumours and cardiac abnormalities.

3. Isoenzymes of Alkaline Phosphatase (ALP)

ALP exists as a number of isoenzymes, the major isoenzymes found in serum are derived from liver, bone, intestine and placenta.

Assay: The techniques used most frequently for separating the isoenzymes are:

- Electrophoresis.
- Chemical inhibition.
- Heat inactivation.

Electrophoresis is considered the most useful single technique for ALP isoenzyme analysis. By starch gel electrophoresis at pH 8.6, at least ***six* isoenzyme bands** have been delineated.

- *Hepatic isoenzyme:* travels fastest towards the anode and occupies the same position as the fast α_2-globulin.
- *Bone isoenzyme*: the hepatic isoenzyme is closely followed by bone isoenzyme in β-globulin region.
- *Placental isoenzyme:* follows bone isoenzyme.
- *Intestinal isoenzyme.* Slow moving and follows the placental isoenzyme.

Remarks:

- The major ALP isoenzyme in normal serum of adult healthy person is derived from liver, and it shows main liver band. In growing child, bone isoenzyme predominates.

  The *presence* of *intestinal isoenzyme* in serum ***depends*** on ***blood group*** and ***secretor status.*** Individuals who have B or O blood group and are secretors are more likely to have intestinal isoenzyme.
- Nearly all tissues show a ***"subsidiary band"*** near the point of insertion, this approximates in position of serum β-lipoproteins.
- ***Liver isoenzyme*** can actually be ***divided into two fractions:***
  - The *major liver band.*
  - ***A subsidiary smaller fraction, called 'fast' liver or α_1-liver,*** which migrates anodal to the major band and corresponds to α_1-globulin.

  When total ALP levels are increased, it is the major liver fraction that is most frequently elevated.

Clinical significance

- The major liver band increased in many hepatobiliary diseases.
- 'Fast' liver band is found in many hepatobiliary diseases and in metastatic carcinoma of liver. The two subsidiary bands form a ***"doublet"*** which *is **of diagnostic significance in** extrahepatic obstructive jaundice.*
- ***Bone isoenzyme:*** increases due to osteoblastic activity and is normally elevated in children during periods of growth and in adults over the age of 50. In these cases, an elevated ALP level may cause difficulty in interpretation.
- ***In pregnancy:*** during last six weeks of pregnancy, placental isoenzyme of ALP increases. ***Placental isoenzyme*** is ***"heat stable"*** and resists heat denaturation at 65°C for ½ hour. It is inhibited by L-phenylalanine.
- Increases of intestinal isoenzyme occurs after consumption of fatty meal. It may increase in several disorders of GI tract and cirrhosis of liver. Increased levels are also found in patients undergoing chronic haemodialysis.

Characteristics of intestinal isoenzyme are given below:

- Slow moving in electrophoresis.
- Inhibited by L-phenylalanine.
- Resistant to neuraminidase.

Table 25.5: Increase/decrease of different enzymes in diseases

Serum enzymes	*Normal value*	*Concentrations increased in*	*Concentrations decreased in*
1. *Aspartate transaminase (AS-T) (S-GOT)*	4-17 IU/L	Myocardial infarction, elevation slight to moderate in muscle diseases, acute liver disease, toxic liver cells necrosis, haemolytic anaemia.	–
2. *Alanine transaminase (ALT) (S-GPT)*	3-15 IU/L	Marked increase in viral hepatitis. Slight to moderate in obstructive jaundice, cirrhosis liver, toxic liver cells necrosis, skeletal muscle disease	—
3. *Lactate dehydrogenase (LDH)*	60 to 250 IU/L	Acute myocardial infarction, acute hepatitis, also raised in muscle diseases, leukaemias, renal tubular necrosis, carcinomatosis, cerebral infarction, pernicious anaemia.	–
4. *Alkaline phosphatase (ALP)*	3 to 13 KA units% (23-92 IU/l) Infants and growing children 12-30 KA units per 100 ml	***Marked increase in obstructive jaundice (> 35 K.A. units %)***, bone diseases—rickets, Paget's disease, hyperparathyroidism. Slight to moderate increase in acute liver diseases, metastatic carcinoma, "space-occupying" lesions of liver, kidney disease, osteoblastic sarcoma.	–
5. *Creatine kinase (CK or CPK)*	4-60 IU/L	Marked increase in acute myocardial infarction, muscular dystrophies; mild to moderate rise in muscle injury, severe physical exertion, hypothyroidism.	–
6. *Aldolase*	2 to 6 m-IU	Muscular dystrophies, acute liver diseases, myocardial infarction, diabetes mellitus, leukaemias, etc.	—
7. *Amylase*	80 to 180 Somogyi units %	Acute pancreatitis, acute parotitis (mumps), perforated peptic ulcer, intestinal obstruction, macroamylasaemia, renal failure.	Acute liver diseases, D. mellitus
8. *Lipase*	1. Colorimetric assay 9.0 to 20 m-IU (Seligman and Nachlas) 2. Titrimetric method 0.06 to 1.02 ml of 0.05N NaOH. 3. Cherry-Krandal units. 1.0 to 1.5 units%	Acute pancreatitis, perforated peptic ulcer, cirrhosis liver, pancreatic carcinoma	Acute liver diseases, D. mellitus, vitamin A deficiency
9. *Cholinesterase*	2.17 to 5.17 IU/ml (130-310 units, de La Huerga)	Nephrotic syndrome, acute myocardial infarction	Acute liver diseases, Malnutrition, acute infectious diseases, organophosphorus poisoning (diazinon poisoning)

Contd...

Contd...

	Serum enzymes	Normal value	Concentrations increased in	Concentrations decreased in
10.	*Acid phosphatase (ACP)*	0.6 to 3.1 KA units/ 100 ml; Tartarate-labile ACP—0 to 0.8 KA units%	Metastasizing prostatic carcinoma, marked rise seen in Gaucher's disease, slight to moderate rise seen— Paget's disease, hyperparathyroidism, osteolytic lesions from breast carcinoma, thrombocytosis, slight increase after rectal examination (P.R.), chronic granulocytic leukaemia, myeloproliferative lesion	
11.	*Caeruloplasmin (Ferroxidase)*	3 to 58 mg%	Cirrhosis, bacterial infections, pregnancy	Wilson's disease (hepatolenticular degeneration)
12.	*Isocitrate dehydrogenase (I.C.D)*	0.9 to 4.0 IU/L	Marked increase seen in viral hepatitis, slight to moderate rise in cirrhosis liver,	
13.	*Ornithine carbamoyl transferase (OCT)*	8 to 20 m-IU	Marked elevation in viral hepatitis; slight elevation in cirrhosis liver, obstructive jaundice, metastatic carcinoma	—
14.	*Leucine amino-peptidase (LAP)*	15 to 56 m-IU	Moderate rise in viral hepatitis slight increase in cirrhosis liver, marked rise in superimposed hepatoma in cirrhosis liver, and in liver cell carcinoma	—
15.	*γ-Glutamyl transpeptidase* (γ-GT)	1 to 47 IU/L	Acute hepatobiliary diseases, alcohol abuse marked rise characteristic, alcoholic cirrhosis, slight to moderate increase seen in epileptic patients with drug therapy with anticonvulsants, pancreatic diseases	
16.	*5'-Nucleotidase*	2 to 17 IU/L	Acute liver diseases, obstructive jaundice, tumours	—

Atypical ALP-Isoenzymes—"Oncogenic Markers"

In addition to four major ALP isoenzymes, two more abnormal fractions are seen associated with tumours. They are:

- ***Regan isoenzyme.***
- ***Nagao isoenzyme.***

They have been called as *"carcino-placental ALP isoenzymes"* as they resemble placental isoenzyme. Frequency of occurrence in cancer patients is 3 to 15%.

Properties

- ***Regan isoenzyme:*** electrophoretically migrates to same position as bone fraction. It is extremely 'heat stable' and resists heat denaturation of 65°C for ½ hour. It is inhibited by L-phenylalanine.
- ***Nagao isoenzyme:*** may be considered as a variant of Regan isoenzyme. Other properties and electrophoretic mobility are similar to Regan isoenzyme. It can also be inhibited by L-leucine.

Clinical Significance

- ***Regan isoenzyme is produced by malignant tissues.*** It has been ***detected*** in ***various carcinomas of breast, lungs, colon*** and ***ovary.*** Highest incidence of positivity found in cancers of ovary and uterus.
- ***Nagao isoenzyme*** has been ***detected in metastatic carcinoma of pleural surfaces and adenocarcinoma of pancreas*** and ***bile duct.*** Both have prognostic significance. They disappear on successful treatment.

Chapter 26

Oncogenic Markers (Tumour Markers)

INTRODUCTION

- **What are Tumour Markers?**

Tumour "markers" are defined as a biochemical substance (e.g. hormones, enzymes, or proteins) synthesized and released by cancer cells or produced by the host in response to cancerous substance and are used to monitor or identify the presence of a cancerous growth. Tumour markers are different from substances produced by normal cells:

Sites: Tumour markers may be present: in blood circulation, in body cavity fluids, in cell membranes, in cell cytoplasm

- **Methods for Detection**

1. Immunohistological and immunocytological tests are used to dedect those tumour markers which are present only on cell-membranes and cytoplasm of cells and ***not in blood circulation.***

Examples:

- Immunofluorescence
- Immunoperoxidase
- Monoclonal antibody technology.

2. Biochemical methods are used for measuring tumour markers found in the blood circulation.

Examples:

- Radio-immuno assay (RIA)
- Enzymeimmune assay
- Immunochemical reactions.

- **Clinical Uses of Tumour Markers**

Ideally, tumour markers have following ***six potential uses*** in cancer patient care:

- **For screening** specially in asymptomatic population.
- **For diagnosis** in asymptomatic patients.
- As a ***prognostic predictor.***
- As an adjunct in clinical staging of the cancerous condition.
- For monitoring during treatment of the patients.
- For ***early detection for relapse/recurrence*** of the cancerous process.

Although it seems unlikely that an ideal tumour marker will be identified for every cancer, but several workable 'markers' are available and can be used.

Increasing our knowledge about the capabilities and limitations of existing tumour markers will enable the oncologist to use them judiciously in cancer patient care and treatment.

- **TYPES OF TUMOUR-MARKERS**

Two types of tumour antigens have been described:

- ***Tumour-specific antigens***
- ***Tumour-associated antigens***

1. Tumour-Specific Antigens

These are a direct product of oncogenesis induced by an oncogene (viral), radiation, chemical carcinogen or an unknown risk factor. Oncogenesis causes abnormalities of genetic information available to the cancer cells, which then subsequently synthesizes ***"neo-antigens"*** specific to cancer cells. They play an important role in clinical oncology.

2. Tumour-Associated Antigens

These are also called as ***"onco-foetal"*** proteins/antigens and shown to exist in both in embryo-foetal tissues and cancer cells. These are produced in large quantities in foetal life and released in foetal circulation. ***After birth,*** these onco-foetal antigens disappear from blood circulation and may be present in trace amounts in normal healthy adults. With the onset of malignancy in adult life, the synthesis of onco-foetal antigens in fetal life which was suppressed in adult life, is again reactivated with malignant transformation of cells and reappears in cancer cells and in blood circulation ***(retrogenetic expression theory).***

Examples of such onco-foetal antigens are:

- **CEA** (Carcinoembryonic antigen)
- **AFP** (Alpha-feto protein)

• CHARACTERISTICS OF AN IDEAL TUMOUR MARKER

An ideal tumour marker is yet to be found out. Ideal tumour marker must satisfy the following criteria:

1. Analytical Criteria

- The marker should have high ***sensitivity.*** The test method should be sensitive to measure very low concentrations. It should have high ***specificity.*** It should measure a particular tumour marker only and no other substances should interfere.
- The other analytical criteria should include high ***accuracy, and precision.***
- The method should be *simple* and easy to measure and should not be very *costly.*

2. Clinical Criteria

- The marker should be ***disease-sensitive*** and it must be positive in all patients with particular cancer. There should be no false-negative results. ***It should show increased level in presence of micro-metastasis*** and ***be able to detect relapse/ and recurrences.***
- The marker should have high ***disease-specificity*** and should not be detectable in normal healthy people. It should be associated only with a particular cancer and should not show increase with other tumours. It should not show rise in benign tumours, other diseases and should not show false positive results.
- It should be stable and should not show wide fluctuations.
- The marker should correlate well with cancerous process, i.e., its extent and the volume of the tumour.
- It should correlate well with cure rate and prognosticate the "high risk" cancer patients from "lower risk".
- It should be able to detect relapse/recurrence of the cancer.

CLASSIFICATION OF TUMOUR MARKERS

Quite a large number of "tumour markers" have been used in cancer. Their list is quite big and ***no universally accepted classification exists.*** Tumour markers which have been found clinically useful in cancer patients may be grouped as follows:

1. Tumour Associated Antigens (Onco-fetal Antigens)

a. • Carcinoembryonic antigen (CEA)
   • α-feto protein (AFP)

b. ***Other antigens:***
   • Tissue polypeptide antigen (TPA)
   • Pancreatic oncofetal antigen (POA)

- Colon-specific antigen
- Beta oncofetal antigen
- Tennessee antigen (TENAGEN)

2. Carbohydrate Antigens

Detected by monoclonal antibodies and are more organ and tumour-specific

a.
- CA-125
- CA-15-3
- CA-19-9
- CA 72-4 (TAG-72)
- CA 50

b. *Others:*
- Mammary serum antigen (MSA)
- MAM-6
- Mucin like carcinoma associated antigen (MCA)

3. Pregnancy Associated Antigens

a.
- Human chorionic gonadotropin-β sub-units (β-HCG).
- Placental like alkaline phosphatase (Regan isoenzyme-PLAP)

b. *Other antigens:*
- Pregnancy specific glycoprotein (SP-1).
- Human placental lactogen (HPL).
- α_2 pregnancy associated globulin (PAG).
- Other placental proteins.
- Sex hormone binding globulin (SHBG).
- Steroid binding β globulin (SBβG).

4. Hormones Used as Tumour Markers

a.
- Parathormone (PTH)
- Calcitonin
- Growth hormone (GH)
- ACTH

b. *Other hormones:*
- Insulin
- Glucagon
- Catecholamines
- Serotonin

5. Enzymes and Isoenzymes Used as Tumour Markers

a. *Enzymes synthesized by tumour tissue:*
- Prostatic acid phosphatase (PAP) and prostate specific antigen (PSA)
- Neuron specific enolase (NSE)
- LDH isoenzymes
- CK isoenzymes
- Glycosy l transferases II isoenzymes (GT II).

b. *Enzymes derived from organ tissues with metastatic carcinoma:*

1. *From bone:*
   - Bone isoenzymes of ALP (osteoblastic)
2. *From liver:*
   - Liver isoenzyme of ALP (from liver cells)
   - Gamma-glutamyl transferase (GGT)
   - 5'-Nucleotidase
3. *From prostate:*
   - Acid phosphatase (ACP)

6. Miscellaneous Tumour Markers

1. Sialic acid concentration in serum
2. Polyamines
3. Monoclonal immunoglobulins
4. Steroid receptors
   - Oestrogen receptors
   - Progesterone receptors
5. Cellular markers
   - T lymphocytes
   - B lymphocytes
6. α_1-antitrypsin (α_1-AT).

CLINICAL USEFULNESS OF DIFFERENT TUMOUR MARKERS

It is not possible to go into indepth discussion for all-tumour markers noted above. Discussion will be done on those biochemical tumour markers which are commonly done in hospitals, viz. CEA, AFP, and β-HCG. Other tumour markers will be discussed briefly.

A. COMMONLY USED TUMOUR MARKERS

1. Carcino Embryonic Antigen (CEA)

CEA is one of the onco-fetal antigens used most frequently and widely as a tumour marker in clinical oncology. It was originally described by **Gold** and **Freedman** as a tumour specific antigen present only in cancer cells, in the circulation of patients with gastrointestinal malignancy and in the normal epithelial cells of fetal GI tract, hence it was named as CEA ***because of its presence in both carcinoma and embryonic tissue.*** It was discovered in 1965 by raising antiserum against a colon cancer.

Properties of CEA and Chemical Composition

It is a **glycoprotein** with a molecular weight varying from 150,000 to 300,000 (average 185,000).

- *Protein Part*
  - A single polypeptide chain (monomeric unit) consisting of 30 amino acids with lysine at N-terminus.
  - By EM, it appears as a twisted rod.
  - Protein content is 46 to 75%
- *Carbohydrate Component*
  - Carbohydrates surround the protein and constitutes 45% to 57%.
  - On analysis of carbohydrates found to contain fucose, mannose and galactose.
  - N-acetyl galactosamine is low whereas large amount of N-acetyl glucosamine present.
  - Sialic acid varies significantly.

Physiology and Metabolism

- *Sites:* CEA is chiefly ***present in endodermally derived tissues,*** viz. GI mucosa, lungs and pancreas. It may also be present in non-endodermally derived tissues (?) —conclusive evidences lacking. It has been detected in GI tract of fetuses as early as three months of gestation and also found in embryonic liver, pancreas, and lungs. It has been detected in free brush border of normal mucosal cells and also in cytoplasm of colonic carcinoma cells.
- *Metabolism:* This is not known exactly. CEA is probably broken down in liver. It disappears from circulation in 3 to 4 weeks after removal of CEA-producing tumour.

Clinical Uses and Remarks

- CEA has been reported to be most useful as tumour marker in ***colorectal cancer.***
- It is elevated also in other malignancies. Found to be ***useful*** in ***breast cancer*** and ***Bronchogenic carcinoma of lung specially*** small cell carcinoma of lungs (SCLC).

  Other malignancies where the value is raised are:
  - Pancreatic carcinoma
  - Gastric carcinoma
  - Cancer of urinary bladder
  - Prostatic cancer, neuroblastomas, ovarian cancer and carcinoma of thyroids.
- *Value in colorectal cancer:*
  - Most valuable, has been ***used as an aid in diagnosis.*** Value of CEA as a tumour marker is greatest in colorectal cancer.
  - Has been ***useful in staging.*** Found to be elevated in 28% of patients with stage I colo-rectal cancer and in 45% of patients with stage II colorectal cancer.
  - Most important use of CEA has been monitoring the response of colorectal cancer to treatment.
  - Patients with colorectal cancer who initially had elevated CEA show return of CEA values to normal after complete and successful surgical removal. Values of CEA remain normal as long as remission persists (serial assays are helpful).
  - A rise again in post surgical patients is definite indication of relapse/recurrence.
  - ***Prognostic usefulness:*** patients of colorectal carcinoma with near normal pretreatment CEA levels had a lower incidence of metastasis. On the other hand, majority of patients having high CEA pretreatment levels developed metastasis.

Note:
CEA is considered as best available non invasive tumour marker for the postoperative monitoring of surgically treated patients with colorectal cancer.

- ***Value in other malignant tumours:***
  - Reports are conflicting. A role of CEA in monitoring the therapeutic response in patients with gastric carcinoma and lung carcinoma is not proven.
  - But in small cells lung cancer (SCLC) it is claimed that chemotherapy may show dramatic, short lived responses, monitoring the CEA level may be of value.

Limitations of CEA Assay

Though CEA is the most widely investigated and most frequently used tumour marker in clinical oncology, it has certain limitations.

- ***High false -ve results:*** A significant number of patients with adenocarcinoma of the GI tract will not have an elevated CEA level. ***Hence, a normal CEA value would not rule out the presence of cancer.***
- ***False +ve results:*** Abnormally elevated CEA values have been reported in certain benign diseases, viz. ulcerative colitis, in benign breast conditions, in emphysema, in rectal polyps and even in heavy smokers. In these cases increase in CEA levels is usually does not exceed 3 to 4 times of the upper limit of reference range.

2. Human Chorionic Gonadotropin (β-HCG)

HCG is a placental hormone. It is synthesized by the syncytiotrophoblastic cells of placental villi.

Normally, it is present in the serum of non pregnant women in very trace amounts or not at all. But it is markedly elevated in pregnancy. Maximum peak level is reached by 12 weeks of pregnancy, then it declines slowly, reaching 1/5th of peak by the end of 20th week and then continues at a very low level for a few days even after parturition. Measurement of elevated HCG in serum and urine has been used to diagnose pregnancy.

Chemistry

It is a **glycoprotein** with molecular weight averaging 45,000. Protein is present as a central core with branched carbohydrate side chains, which terminate with sialic acid. It is a dimer and has two dissimilar subunits:

- **α-sub unit,** and
- **β-sub unit**

- *α-subunit:*

Its molecular weight varies from 15,000 to 20,000 and consists of 92 amino acids. It is identical with α sub unit of FSH, LH and TSH

- *β-sub unit:*

The molecular weight varies from 25,000 to 30,000. β-sub unit or C-terminal part of the β-sub unit is specific immunologically.

Clinical Uses and Remarks for β-HCG

- The β-sub unit of HCG is typically measured because of its increased specificity and because some tumours secrete only β-sub unit.
- β-HCG is ***an ideal tumour marker for diagnosing and monitoring gestational trophoblastic tumours and germ cell tumours of testes and ovary.***
- Frequency of elevated β-HCG has been observed to be as follows:

• **Seminomas**	15%
• **Embryonal carcinomas**	50%
• **Terato carcinoma**	42%
• **Choriocarcinoma**	100%

  Specificity increases when AFP and LDH isoenzymes are done simultaneously. Both LDH and LDH-1 isoenzyme show increased levels in 50 to 80% of patients of testicular cancers.
- ***β-HCG in CS fluid:*** Recently, measurement of β-HCG in cerebrospinal fluid (CSF) has aided in diagnosis of brain metastases. *A*

serum/CSF ratio of less than 60 : 1 points to central nervous system (CNS) metastasis. The response of therapy in patients with CNS metastases can be monitored using HCG levels.

Limitations

Elevated β-HCG levels have also been reported in other tumours, viz. lung cancer, breast cancer, GI cancer, ovarian cancer, hypernephroma, etc.

Conclusion

In spite of limitations, ***serum β-HCG level is an ideal and superb "tumour marker" in patients with gestational trophoblastic tumours.*** Serial assays of β-HCG levels would be the best tool for monitoring the clinical course of those patients.

3. Alpha-Feto Protein (AFP)

Like CEA, α-feto protein (AFP) is another oncofetal antigen. AFP is synthesized in the liver, yolk sac and GI tract in fetal life and is released into the serum of fetus.

It is a normal component of serum protein in human fetus. The concentration is highest during embryonic and fetal life. At birth, the serum AFP declines to 1/100th of AFP value at the highest fetal concentration. At one year of life, the value decreases further and in normal adults it is negligible, less than 20 ng/ml.

Chemistry

It is a **glycoprotein** of molecular weight 61,000 to 70,000. Physically and chemically, it is related to albumin, pI is similar to albumin (4.8). It is a single polypeptide chain (monomeric unit) with regions in the interior being similar to human serum albumin. Protein constitutes 95% and carbohydrate moiety 5%.

Clinical Uses and Remarks

- AFP is the ***most specific and ideal tumour marker for primary carcinoma of the liver (hepatocellular carcinoma).*** Serum level of AFP level is elevated markedly. Hepatoma cells are analogous to fetal hepatocytes and are capable of synthesizing AFP.
- AFP assay has been used in case of hepatic mass:
  - in suspected hepatoma.
  - in patients with cirrhosis liver suspected to have superimposed hepatoma.
  - also serial assay in established case of hepatoma to follow the effect of therapy.
- AFP as tumour marker has been found to be also most useful in germ cell tumours of the testes and ovary. ***Serum AFP and β-HCG are the best available tumour markers for germ cell type of tumours.***

AFP is not elevated in seminomatous testicular tumours. It is found to be elevated in majority of the patients with non-seminomatous tumours, e.g. choriocarcinoma, embryonal carcinoma, yolk sac tumour, teratomas and teratocarcinomas.

Note:

- AFP is specifically elevated in embryonal carcinoma and yolk sac tumour.
- Combined use of AFP, β-HCG and LDH isoenzyme has proved clinically useful.

B. TUMOUR MARKERS NOT USED COMMONLY

A brief discussion with clinical usefulness of the other "tumour markers" will be done.

1. *Tissue Polypeptide Antigen (TPA)*

It was first evaluated as tumour marker in 1978 and is ***not tumour specific.*** Elevated levels are found in various malignancies, viz. in colonic cancer, breast cancer, prostatic cancer and metastatic cancer. It can be used in combination with other tumour markers which improves the sensitivity but diminishes the specificity of the other marker.

2. *Tennesee antigen (Tenagen)*

Though not in use routinely, its clinical usefulness has been shown in colo-rectal cancer, pancreatic cancer, lung cancer and stomach cancer.

3. CA 125

CA 125 is an antigenic determinant expressed by epithelial ovarian carcinomas that can be detected by a monoclonal antibody. ***It has been used for screening and diagnosis of ovarian carcinoma.***

CA 125 is ***not specific for ovarian carcinoma.*** It is also elevated in breast carcinoma and colo-rectal cancers. ***An elevated CA 125 level is observed in 80 to 90% patients with ovarian cancer.*** The elevation correlates well with tumour size and stage. Although an elevated CA 125 level is highly correlated with the presence of ovarian cancer, a normal value does not exclude the disease. **Combination of three markers CA 125, CA 15-3 and TAG 72 increased the specificity to 98.6%.**

4. CA 15-3

Has been found useful as tumour marker in breast carcinoma. CA 15-3 is an antigen that is detected by a monoclonal antibody generated against extracts of metastatic human breast cancer.

Most studies have shown that CA 15-3 level is a more sensitive marker than the CEA level. Elevated CA 15-3 levels are found in 70 to 80% of patients with metastatic or recurrent breast cancer. A more important role of CA 15-3 is early detection of recurrence.

Limitations

Though CA 15-3, is useful in breast cancer as a "marker", its specificity is low; because elevated levels have been observed in other malignancies and also in patients with benign breast lesions and liver diseases.

5. CA 19-9

It has been found useful as tumour marker in pancreatic cancer. It is an asialiated Lewis blood group antigen that is detected by monoclonal antibody. Like CEA, it was first detected in a colo-rectal carcinoma. It is found to be elevated markedly in patients with pancreatic cancer (80 to 100% cases). Sensitivity of CA 19-9 level in patients with pancreatic cancer is relatively high. Excellent correlations have been reported between CA 19-9 assay and relapse/recurrence in post-surgical resection cases.

Limitations:

CA 19-9 specificity is lowered as:
- It is found to be elevated in other malignancies also, viz. colorectal cancer (20%), hepatomas (20 to 50%) and gastric cancer.
- Elevated levels have also been found in benign disorders, e.g. pancreatitis, and liver diseases.

6. CA 72-4

It is a radioimmuno assay that detects a tumour-associated glycoprotein termed TAG 72, which has been found by immunohistochemistry in tissue sections from more than 90% of patients with ***colo-rectal, gastric*** and ***ovarian cancers*** and from 70% of patients with breast cancers. A correlation of TAG 72 level with disease stage has been shown in patients with ovarian cancer and gastrointestinal cancer.

7. CA 50

It is a carbohydrate antigen detected by monoclonal antibody found useful in ***lung cancer,*** gastrointestinal cancer including colorectal carcinoma. It is claimed that CA 50 level can be used to identify postoperative recurrences of colorectal cancer which are not identified by the CEA level.

8. Mammary Antigens

Several new antigens have been recognized by monoclonal antibodies being identified in patients with breast cancer. They have been proposed as "tumour markers".

- ***MCA (Mucin-like carcinoma associated antigen):*** is a mucin glycoprotein that is deteced by monoclonal antibody against human breast cancer cell lines. The antigen is not sensitive in early stage of breast cancer.

- *MAM 6:* an epithelial membrane antigen present on ductal and alveolar epithelial cells that is detected by monoclonal antibody raised against human milk-fat globule membranes.
- *MSA (Mammary serum antigen):* it is detected by an antibody raised against a whole cell suspension of intraductal breast cancer. ***Studies have shown MSA to be superior than CA 15-3 as a tumour marker in breast cancer.*** It has ***better sensitivity and specificity.*** Incidence of elevated level in patients with stage I and stage II breast cancer has been observed to vary from 68 to 90% and specificity from 82 to 95%.

Recent Advances: Excerpt—A New Breast Cancer Markers

- **MAP (Mitogen Activated Protein) Kinase**

Recently a new breast cancer "marker" found. It is called as "mitogen activated protein (MAP) kinase". Normally this enzyme helps cells to divide. But breast cancer cells were found to contain up to 20 times of the enzyme level found in normal. This enzyme in excess appears to be the "trigger" for breast cells to proliferate wildly, a hallmark of cancer.

Researchers claim to be hopeful to use the ***"MAP-kinase marker" to distinguish cancerous breast lumps from harmless benign one.*** The test is performed on biopsy tissues taken after a woman has had a suspicious looking mamogram. MAP-kinase levels were found to be 5 to 20 times higher in Breast Cancer as compared to normal breast tissue. More studies are needed to repeat the results and to determine if inhibiting MAP-kinase can influence the growth of breast cancer.

9. Prostatic Acid Phosphatase (PAP) and Prostate Specific Antigen (PSA)

PAP has been recognized as a tumour marker for prostatic cancer since 1938. But it is not an ideal marker. Its use has been hampered by poor sensitivity and specificity.

PSA is an organ-specific, localized to prostatic ductal cells. As a tumour marker it is nearly an ideal marker and better than PAP. Levels are undetectable in women, in normal men (below < 2.0 ng/ml), but it is elevated in benign or malignant prostatic disease.

The clinical recurrence/relapse of prostate cancer is associated with raised serum PSA levels in 90 to 100% of patients. PSA has been found to be very sensitive in detecting disease recurrence.

10. Neuron-specific Enolase (NSE)

Recently the use of NSE as a specific tumour marker has been advocated ***for tumours of neuro-endocrine origin.*** Although NSE has been detected with various tumours, studies of NSE as serum tumour marker have been found to be extremely useful in ***neuroblastomas,*** and ***lung cancer.***

Immunoreactive NSE is found in the tumours of most patients with "small-cell carcinoma of lung" (SCLC). NSE level is found to be elevated in serum in 80 to 87% of cases of SCLC.

Limitations

Specificity is rather low. In 10% patients of non-SCLC and non-malignant lung diseases elevations are seen.

11. Other Tumour Markers and Their Clinical Uses

Other tumour markers with their clinical uses are tabulated below.

Tumour markers	Tumour types and associated abnormalities
A. Hormones	
• ACTH	Lung cancer, carcinoids, pancreatic carcinoma, medullary carcinoma of thyroid
• Catecholamines	Pheochromocytoma
• Insulin	Insulinoma
• Glucagon	Glucagonoma

• Gastrin	Gastrinoma
• Serotonin	Carcinoids
• Calcitonin	Medullary carcinoma of thyroid, lung cancer

B. Enzymes

• Total LDH	Lymphomas, leukaemia, germ cell tumours, breast and lung cancer and others
• LDH 1	Germ cell tumours, ovarian carcinoma, osteosarcoma
	Other abnormalities
	Acute myocardial infarction, Renal infarct Haemolytic disease
• LDH 2,3,4	Leukaemias Lymphomas
• LDH 5	Hepatoma, breast cancer, prostatic cancer, colorectal cancer
	Other abnormalities:
	Hepatitis and other benign liver diseases Skeletal muscle injury

• Alkaline Phosphatase (ALP)

• Fast liver isoenzyme	Metastatic liver cancer
• Bone isoenzyme	Metastatic bone disease Benign bone disease
• Regan isoenzyme	Lung cancer, ovarian Cancer, breast cancer, colonic cancer, uterine cancer
• Nagao isoenzyme	Metastatic carcinoma of pleural surfaces, Adenocarcinoma of pancreas and bile duct

• Prostatic acid phosphatase (ACP)	Prostatic cancer

• Creatine kinase (CK/CPK)

• Isoenzyme CK-BB useful as a "tumour marker"	Adenocarcinomas, prostatic carcinoma
• α_1-antitrypsin (α_1-AT)	Germ cell tumours of testes and ovary

CONCLUSION

During the past two decades, there has been remarkable efflorescence in search of "tumour-markers". Since the introduction of CEA, numerous tumour-markers have been identified and have been used by oncologists in cancer patient care. As seen from above discussion, as diagnostic tools, tumour markers have certain limitations. Quite a number of them lack in specificity. Most of the markers can be elevated in benign disorders also. A few markers are not elevated in early stages of malignancy. Also, the lack of tumour markers does exist in patients with tumours, and hence, ***a negative result does not exclude the diagnosis of cancer.***

Further research for more specific and more sensitive tumour markers is in progress. Monoclonal antibody technology has opened a new era and has sparked the search for tumour markers that are more organ and tumour specific.

Part Four

Inborn Metabolic Diseases (Inborn Errors of Metabolism)

Chapter 27

Inborn Metabolic Diseases (Inborn Errors of Metabolism)*

INTRODUCTION

Inborn Metabolic Diseases (IMDs), previously known as Inborn Errors of Metabolism (IEM) constitute a heterogenic group of disorders with an underlying genetic aetiology affecting one or many of the metabolic pathways. With rapid advancement in the molecular techniques and related diagnostic methodologies, the list of the malfunctioning/mutant genes that form the foundation of metabolic imbalance leading to these disorders is consistently increasing. ***All of the IMDs are extremely rare*** in their occurrence, the ***individual prevalence not more than 1 in 5000 live births,*** but as a group with overlapping clinical presentation like mental retardation, spasticity, hepatosplenomegaly, ataxia, cardiomyopathy; they contribute consideraly to the childhood morbidity and mortality all over the world. Many of these IMD cases go unreported and unattended in the absence of a confirmed diagnosis inspite of a strong clinical suspicion. In most cases of IMDs such as phenylketonuria, galactosaemia, urea cycle disorders, organic acidemias present with nonspecific symptoms like an acute episode of infection, loss of consciousness with or without seizures or vomiting, the retardation of mental development is always lurking behind these symptoms. Brain, at the time of birth, is probably the most immature organ in the body and is due to undergo a long and complex series of developmental changes over many years during which it is susceptible to chemical derangement at many stages during this development. Nearly every metabolic disease has several forms that vary in the age of onset, clinical severity and quite often, the mode of inheritance.

Most of the inherited disorders are transmitted in an autosomal recessive fashion but autosomal dominance and X-linked inheritance is also known in number or IMDs. Single gene defects, commonly associated with an enzyme or a transport protein thus compromising a metabolic pathway, result in abnormalities in the synthesis or catabolism of proteins, carbohydrates, fats, amino acids or other body metabolites. The clinical signs and symptoms are due to the toxic accumulations of substrates before the block, intermediates from alternate metabolic pathways, and/or defects in energy production and utilisation caused by the deficiency of products beyond the block.

Lysosomes are the catabolic factories of biological systems and thus the warehouses of a large battery of enzymes involved in the regular turnover/catabolism of specific biomolecules. Single point or multiple mutations in the gene(s) for a number of lysosomal enzymes result in

Contributed by Professor R Chawla, MSc, DMRIT, PhD, Professor of Biochemistry , Faculty of Medicine, Addis-Ababa University, Ethiopia, ex-Professor of Biochemistry, Christian Medical College, Ludhiana (Punjab)

unnatural accumulations of these metabolites leading to a group of IMDs known as *lysosomal disorders.* These storage disorders are catalogued according to the target biomolecules stored in excess, e.g. glycogen storage diseases, mucopoly-saccharidosis, sphingolipidosis, mucolipi-dosis and polysaccharidosis.

Another group of inherited disorders ***involves the defective function of one or more of the circulating plasma proteins,*** viz. oxygen carrying proteins, clotting factors and metal transport proteins. These disorders then precip-itate the symptoms like deficient oxygen trans-port function (anaemias and thalassemias), compromised blood clotting (hemophilias, thro-mbophilia, afibrinogenemia), accumulation of abnormal haemoglobin or catabolic products (bilirubinaemias, porphyrias) or excess/de-ficiency of essential micronutriants (Wilson's disease, Zellweger's syndrome, Menke's disease, haemochromatosis).

Defective connective tissue and neuro-muscular disorders also form an important category of IMDs. The victims of these disorders would present with a wide range of disabilities depending upon the tissue or the organ affected most by the disorder. The symptoms could include changes in the facial features, heart and blood vessel problems, irritability during infancy, dental and kidney abnormalities, hyperacusis (sensitive hearing), musculoskeletal problems and premature aging. Impaired vision and deafness are quite common features of this group of IMDs. Some examples of these disorders are Duchenne's muscular dystrophy, Williams syndrome, Alport's syndrome and Werner's syndrome, etc.

A number of central nervous system dis-orders are also now known to have an under-lying inherited biochemical basis. The genetic basis of a number of common diseases, hitherto known as acquired disorders, is now becoming clearer day-by-day. At least twelve forms of epilepsy have been demonstrated to possess some genetic basis. For example, LaFora Disease (Progressive myoclonic, type 2), a particularly aggressive epilepsy, is characterised in part by the presence of glycogen-like LaFora bodies in the brain. Alphasynuclein fragments are implicated in both Parkinson's and Alzheimer's diseases; therefore, there might be a shared pathogenic mechanisms between the two, Parkinson's disease is long known to be due to the deficiency of defective synthesis of neuro-transmitter DOPamine. In Alzheimer's disease, formation of lesions made of fragmented brain cells surrounded by amyloid-family proteins, are characteristic and an enzyme that may be res-ponsible for the increase in amyloid production characteristic of Alzheimer's disease is under study.

Classification of the Major Metabolic Disorders

According to the metabolic pathway or the tissue function affected, the IMDs may be grouped as follows:

1. Disorders of carbohydrate metabolism
2. Disorders of protein amino acid metabolism
3. Disorders of fat metabolism
4. Errors in nucleotide metabolism
5. Disorders with defective protein functions
6. Disorders of oxygen carrier proteins and their metabolism
7. Disorders of metal transport and metabolism
8. Peroxisomal disorders
9. Errors of DNA repair

It is not possible to discuss all the metabolic disorders. The following inborn metabolic diseases will be discussed.

A. Disorders of carbohydrate metabolism
B. Disorders of amino acid metabolism
C. Disorders of lipid metabolism
D. Inborn errors of Defective DNA repair and Purine and Pyrimidine metabolism

A. Disorders of Carbohydrate Metabolism

A.1. Galactosaemias

A group of inherited enzyme deficiencies that feature ***elevation in the levels of blood galactose*** are referred to as galactosaemia. The ***birth incidence*** of classical galactosaemia has been estimated to be 1 per 47,000 in the white population.

Biochemical: The classical form of galactosaemia is ***caused by "galactose-1-phosphate uridyltransferase"*** (GALT) gena defect and presents in infancy with failure to thrive, vomiting and intracranial hypertension. Other clinical symptoms may include **mental retardation, jaundice, hepatosplenomegaly and cataracts.**

The gene has been mapped to chromosome 9 at the locus 9p13.

The first detailed description of galactosaemia was given by **Goppert (1917).** The patient presented with **large liver, icterus, failure to thrive, and urinary excretion of albumin and sugar.** After exclusion of galactose from the diet these signs and symptoms normalised. He was mentally retarded (developmental quotient of 14 months at 36 months of age). He tolerated sucrose, maltose, glucose, and fructose at doses of 2 g/kg, but after lactose or galactose administration, there was dose-dependent galactosuria. Two of his siblings had died within 6 weeks of birth probably due to the same enzyme defect as the autopsy showed hepatomegaly in both the siblings.

Three kinds of enzymes of the galactose metabolism viz. **UDP-Hexose-1-Phosphate Uridy1 Transferases, Galactokinase and 4-Epimerases (Fig. 27.1)** have been implicated in these disorders characterised by galactosaemia with slight variations in the signs and symptoms.

Jaundice or intrinsic liver disease may be accentuated by the severe haemolysis occurring in some patients. There appears to be a high frequency of neonatal deaths due to *E. coli* sepsis, with a fulminant course. Ovarian failure in many affected girls may indicate *in utero* damage from galactosaemia. Pregnancy is rare in women with

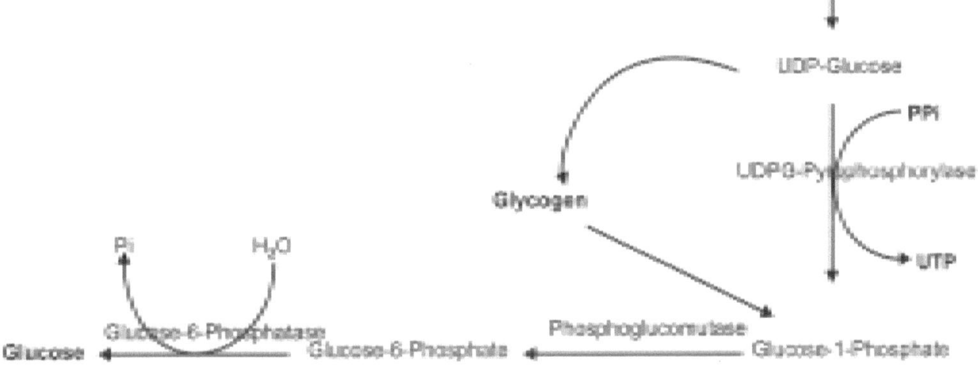

Fig. 27.1: Metabolism of Galactose (Deficiency of Enzymes in Red → Galactosaemias)

galactosaemia because of the high frequency of hypergonadotropic hypogonadism with ovarian atrophy.

Molecular genetics: With the several mutations that have been identified at the GALT locus, the tendency for clinical complications to develop varies from apparent clinical normality in the relatively common ***Duarte type*** to perhaps mild symptoms in the ***S135L variant*** and to the ***severe galactosaemia syndrome*** in the ***'classic', Indiana, and Rennes variants. Beutler et al. (1965)*** suggested that some persons with intermediate levels of the enzyme are not heterozygotes for the usual galactosaemia but rather are homozygotes for what they termed the 'Duarte' variant. Heterozygotes for this variant have about 75% normal activity.

- Using G for the allele causing classic galactosaemia and D for the Duarte allele (N314D), **Elsas et al. (1994)** proposed that the **D/N, D/D, and D/G genotypes** show approximately 75%, 50%, and 25% of normal GALT activity, respectively. The Duarte allele is associated with an isoform of the enzyme that has more acidic pI than normal. This variant, with decreased activity of GALT, is know ***as D2*** (Holton et al. 2001).
- Another biochemical variant has been called the ***'Los Angeles (LA) varient', or 'D1' by Ng et al. (1973)*** and others. The LA variant occurs when the N314D allele is in *cis* configuration with L218L.
- Another type of galactosaemia is associated with the S135L mutation, previously called the 'Negro' variant. The difference in behaviour of the metabolism of galactose in these patients may be due to the development of an alternative pathway.

Diagnosis: ***Biochemical and urinary findings:***

- Increase blood galactose level ↑, Blood sugar level decreases ↓ (Hypoglycaemia), ***Inorganic P decreases ↓, due to utilisation of PO_4 for gal-1-p.***

Urine:

- Increased excretion of galactose in urine↑, (galactosuria)
- Albuminuria, and amino aciduria: amino acids excreted usually are *serine, alanine* and *glycine.*

Biochemical and urinary findings:

- Increase blood galactose level ↑
- Decrease blood sugar level (hypoglycaemia)
- Inorganic phosphate decreases ↓, due to utilisation of Po_4 for gal—I—P.

Urine:

- Increased excretion of galactose in urine ↑ (galactosuria)
- Albuminuria and amino aciduria, amino acids excreted usually are ***serine, alanine*** and ***glycine***
- Ophthalmoscopic examination shows presence of cataract galactosaemia deficiency at present chiefly indetified
- ***By assaying for the enzyme in red cells or cultured skin fibroblasts.*** Because the enzyme is expressed in cultured cells, prenatal diagnosis is feasible.
- Mass screening for galactosemia in newborns is feasible and is routinely used where filter paper placed in diaper, then air dried and part stain for galactose with aniline phthalate and heated for 5'at 105°C. If galactose is present brown colour appears on stain.

On the basis of a screening of newborns in Massachusetts, **Shih et al. (1971)** found only 2 cases of galactosaemia among 374, 341 births. Noth infants died with *Escherichia coli* sepsis in the neonatal period. Since *E. coli* sepsis can be a presenting manifestation of galactosemia, results of the neonatal screening must be reported promptly to the clinician.

CLINICAL MANAGEMENT

Long-term results of treatment have been disappointing; IQ is low in many despite early and seemingly adequate therapy. For example, the retrospective study by **Schweitzer et al. (1993)** of 134 galactosaemic patients born between 1955 and 1989 in the Federal Republic of Germany. The cause of the unsatisfactory outcome of seemingly good control of galactose intake and the disturbances in long-term development despite treatment are unclear. Possibilities include chronic intoxication by galactose metabolites or deficiency of galactose-containing glycoproteins and/or glycolipids as a result of an overrestrictive galactose-free diet.

A.2. Fructosuria

Alternative titles: Hepatic Fructokinase Deficiency, Ketohexokinase Deficiency Fructosuria is a benign, asymptomatic defect of intermediary metabolism characterised by the presence of large amounts of fructose in urine sufficient to give a positive reducing sugar test. Small amounts of fructose occur in the urine of normal individuals ingesting a regular diet but amounts sufficient to give a positive test for reducing sugar in the routine examination occur only in essential fructosuria, familial fructose intolerance, and advanced liver disease.

Prevalence: Fructosuria appears to be more common in the Jew population, is inherited in ***autosomal recessive*** fashion and is often ***found to co-exist with other disorders like Diabetes Mellitus and Sickle Cell disease Thallassaemia.*** This disorder was first described independently by **Czapek (1876)** and **Zimmer (1876)** in a man who also suffered from diabetes mellitus.

The enzyme involved is hepatic fructokinase, also known as ketohexokinase (KHK; EC 2. 7.1.3). This enzyme catalyses the first step of metabolism of dietary fructose, conversion of fructose to fructose-1-phosphate. Ketohexokinase, or fructokinase, like gluco-kinase (GCK) and glucokinae regulator (GCKR), is present in both liver and pancreatic islets. ***KHK is the first enzyme with a specialised pathway that catabolises dietary fructose*** ***(Fig. 27.2).***

Alternative mRNA species and alternative KHK isozymes are produced by alternative polyadenylation and splicing of the KHK gene (Gene map locus 2p23.3-p23.2). In a well characterised family in which 3 of 8 sibs had fructosuria, all affected individuals were found to be compound heterozygotes for **2 *mutations: gly40-to-arg and ala43-to-thr. Both mutations resulted from a G-to-A transition,*** and each altered the same conserved region of the KHK protein. KHK and GCKR genes are present together in close proximity on the same chromosomal locus and the co-localisation of these metabolically connected genes has implications for the interpretation of linkage or allele association studies in type 2 diabetes. It also raises the possibility of coordinate regulation of GCKR and KHK by common regulatory elements.

Khachadurian (1963) described **non-alimentary fructosuria** in an 18-month-old Arab boy **who suffered from sickle-cell thalassaemia.**

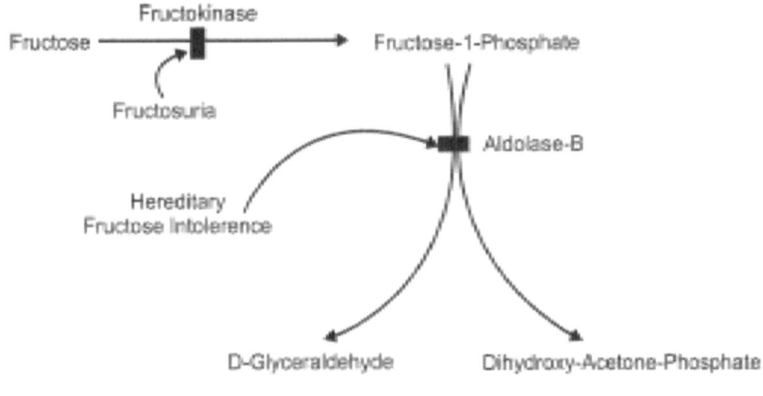

Fig. 27.2: Metabolic defects in Fructosuria and Hereditary Fructose Intolerence

The fructose tolerance test was normal and fructosuria persisted after fructose was entirely excluded from the diet, but had decreased markedly when the patient was seen 2 years later. Both the spleen and the liver were enlarged. The patient's parents were first cousins. Urine samples from both parents were negative for a reducing substance. Urine samples from the brother and 2 sisters showed intermittent fructosuria.

Clinical management: Fructosuria is essentially a benign condition but occasional hepatosplenomegaly has been documented. Dietary restriction of fructose reduces the urinary excretion.

A 3. Hereditary Fructose Intolerance

Alternative titles: Fructosaemia, fructose-1-phosphate aldolase deficiency, fructose-1, 6-bisphosphate aldolase B-deficiency.

Most of the cases of fructose intolerance are severely ill infants with recurrent hypoglycaemia and vomiting, occurring at the time of weaning when fructose or sucrose is added to the diet and resulting in marked malnutrition. ***Hyperuricaemia and hyperuricosuria are commonly associated features. Hepatomegaly*** may be present and a test dose of fructose often precipitates hypoglycaemic shock. There is a marked aversion to sweets and fruits in the adult patients.

Biochemical: The defect resides in aldolase B (EC 4.1.2.13), which catalyses the cleavage of fructose-1-phosphate to form dihydroxyacetone phosphate and D-glyceraldehyde. Both structural and controller mutations may exist, as well as more than one type of structural mutation. Two of the reported cases had a near normal ratio of fructose-1-phosphate aldolase to fructose diphosphate aldolase, suggesting a controller mutation.

In aldolase 'B'-deficient tissues, cytoplasmic accumulation of fructose-1-phosphate leads to sequestration of inorganic phosphate with resulting activation of AMP deaminase that catalyses the irreversible deamination of AMP to IMP (inosine monophosphate), a precursor of uric acid. In the cytoplasm, AMP, ADP, and ATP are maintained in a state approaching equilibrium. Depletion of tissue ATP occurs through massive degradation to uric acid and impairment of regeneration by oxidative phosphorylation in the mitochondria because of inorganic phosphate depletion. In the cell, ATP exists largely as a 1:1 complex with magnesium. Depletion of ATP in tissues leads to deletion of magnesium concentration also.

MOLECULAR GENETICS

The ***aldolase B gene consists of 9 exons,*** the first of which is untranslated. The cognate mRNA encodes 364 amino acids. ***The gene has been found to be located on chromosome 9 at a gene map locus 9q22.3.***

The ***molecular genetic defects*** in fructose intolerance have been found to be quite ***heterogeneous caused by single base substitutions*** resulting in amino acid replacements, non-sense codons or caused by small (4 bp) or large (up to 1.65 kb) deletions. Recurrent mutations have been observed in exons 5 and 9. Haplotype analysis suggested that the A149P and A174D mutations originated from a single founder and achieved a relatively high frequency through genetic drift.

The ***mutant aldolases are mis-sense variants*** and could be classified into **2 principal groups:**

- ***Catalytic mutants,*** with retained tetrameric structure but altered kinetic properties (W147R, R303W, and A337V), and
- **Structural mutants,** in which the homotetramers readily dissociate into subunits with greatly impaired enzymatic activity, e.g., A174D and N334K. It appears that the integrity of the quaternary sturcture of aldolase B is critical for maintaining its full catalytic function.

DIAGNOSIS

Most, if not all, patients with fructose intolerance have ***neonatal hypoglycaemia, lactic acidosis, and an abnormal fructose or glycerol loading*** test.

Hypoglycaemic attacks occur later in life and are associated with severe ***hyperuricaemia and metabolic acidosis.*** Hypoglycaemia and hypophosphataemia may be demonstrated within 1 hour after an oral dose of fructose in these subjects. ***Since aldolase B is normally present in kideney*** and ***intestinal mucosa*** as well as in liver, the ***enzyme deficiency can only be demonstrated in the biopsy samples of any of these tissues.***

Oberhaensli et al. (1987) used ^{31}P magnetic resonance spectroscopy to study the effect of fructose on liver metabolism in patients with this disorder. In heterozygotes, the method could be used to diagnose fructose intolerance and to monitor patient compliance with a restricted diet. Ingestion of small amounts of fructose was followed by an increase in sugar phosphates and decrease in inorganic phosphate in the liver. Fructose also induced a larger increase in plasma urate in heterozygotes than in control subjects. Heterozygosity for this disorder may predispose to hyperuricaemia.

Paolella et al (1987) described a ***Restriction Fragment Length Polymorphism (RFLP) within the ALDOB gene*** useful in the study of hereditary fructose intolerance.

Cross et al. (1988) reported the ***first identification of a molecular lesion in the ALDOB gene*** in this disorder. A ***G-to-C transversion in exon 5*** created a new recognition site for the ***restriction enzyme AhaII*** and ***resulted in a substitution of proline for alanine at position 149*** of the protein within a region critical for substrate binding. Utilising this novel restriction site and the polymerase chain reaction (PCR) they were able to demonstrate the existence of this mutation in a large number of European fructose intolerance patients.

CLINICAL MANAGEMENT

Therapeutic measures include **restriction of fructose intake** and avoidance of prolonged fasting, particularly during febrile episodes. Stringent limitation of fructose intake normally results in accelerated growth.

Clinical case report: ***Marks et al*** (1989) described the obstetrical management of a woman with fructose intolerance. Her first child had failure to thrive and died at 6 months; autopsy showed cirrhosis and pulmonary oedema, with a clinical diagnosis of *E. coli* sepsis. Her second child also had fructose intolerance and died at age 5 years from acquired immunodeficiency syndrome contracted from a neonatal blood transfusion. On a strict fructose-free diet, her third pregnancy proceeded well; the child, who was also found to have fructose intolerance, did well on a fructose-free diet. Diagnosis of fructose intolerance was said to have been verified in the mother by biopsy of the liver.

A 4. Hyperglycerolaemia

(***Alternative title:*** Glycerol Kinase Deficiency)
Types: There are ***3 clinically distinct forms of glycerol kinase deficiency*** that affects the male children of the carrier mothers: infantile, juvenile, and adult.

- The infantile form is characterised by adrenal hypoplasia, psychomotor retardation, growth delay, osteoporosis, and in some patients myopathy histologically similar to that of Duchenne muscular dystrophy.
- The juvenile GKD reported at the age of more than 2 years presents with episodic vomiting, gastroenteritis, metabolic acidosis, stupor, and coma.
- Patients with the **adult form** of glycerol kinase deficiency are usually identified through hyperlipidaemia testing. They have **pseudotriglyceridaemia** because the large amount of glycerol in their serum is falsely identified as triglyceride. These adults have no apparent clinical problems. The pedigrees in all reported cases are consistent with **X-linked inheritance.** There is no adrenal hypoplasia wit the adult form of X-linked glycerol kinase deficiency.

Gaudet et al (2000) undertook a study of fasting plasma glycerol levels in a cohort of 1.056 unrelated men and women of French-Canadian descent. Family screening in the initial cohort identified 18 men from 5 families with severe hyperglycerolaemia (values above 2.0 mmol/l and demonstrated an X-linked pattern of inheritance. Linkage analysis of the data from 12 microsatellite markers surrounding the Xp21.3 GK gene resulted in a peak load score of 3.46, centred around marker DXS8039.

Biochemical and Molecular Genetics

The locus for glycerol kinase and that for X-linked adrenal hypoplasia are in the segment Xp21-p11.2 on the X-chromosome. The deletion with breakpoints at p11.2 and p21 has been documented as the cause. Linkage of primary adrenal hypoplasia and glycerol kinase deficiency is supported by description of coincidence of the 2 disorders in a number of studies. The deletion at the same locus has also been documented in the patients with a combination of Duchenne muscular dystrophy (DMD), adrenal hypoplasia (AH), and glycerol kinase deficiency (GK).

Investigations of glycerol kinase deficiency by **Seltzer et al (1985)** suggested that primary adrenal hypoplasia seen in association with glycerol kinase deficiency in cases of Xp deletion is not due to the loss of a separate (closely linked) locus but rather is a pleiotropic effect of the glycerol kinase deficiency. In the infantile form of GK deficiency, adrenocortical hypoplasia with insufficiency is a consistent feature (observed in 12 patients in 6 families). The deficiency of outer mitochondrial membrane-bound GK restricts glycerophospholipid synthesis and hence the activation of steroidogenesis.

Some authors suggest that the syndrome is likely due to deletion of several closely linked genes, comparable to the cause of the **WAGR syndrome** on 11p and perhaps the **Langer-Giedion syndrome** on chromosome 8 and other "contiguous gene" syndromes; whereas others favour separate loci for AHX, GK, and DMD. The latter point out that congenital adrenal hypoplasia has been reported with DMD and with GKD without muscle disease. **Patients with progressive muscular dystrophy tend to have larger deletions** that included markers known to derive from the DMD locus. The findings in the patients with isolated GK deficiency **suggested that the AH and GK loci are separate and distinct.** DMD, GK and AHC are located in that order from centromere. The conclusion is based on the finding of patients who suffered from DMD and GK deficiency without AHC and other patients who suffered from all 3 disorders.

A gene responsible for gonadotropin deficiency (GTD) is located in the Xp21 region.

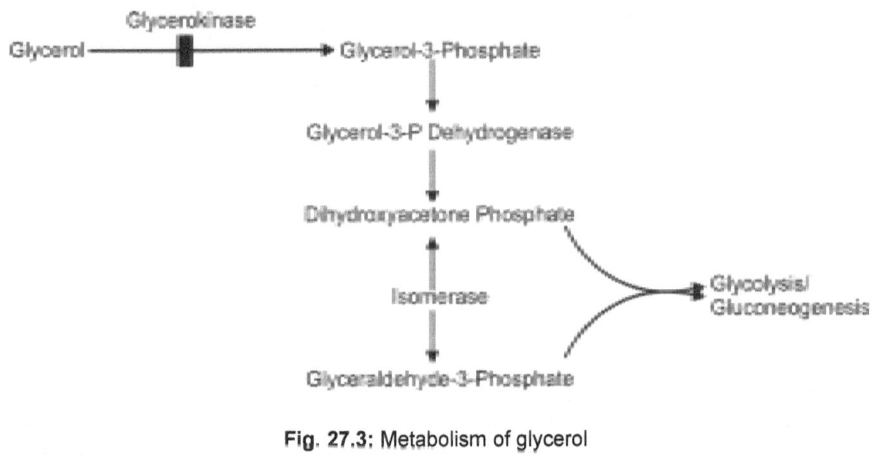

Fig. 27.3: Metabolism of glycerol

Kallmann's syndrome is determined by a **mutation on Xp,** and gonadal dysgenesis of the XY female type appears to be determined by a gene in the Xp22-p21 region.

Diagnosis

Demonstration of hyperglycerolaemia in the clinically relevant individuals calls for the ***estimation of glycerokinase activity in the leucocytes.*** GK deficiency can be demonstrated by evaluating plasma triglycerides by a routine clinical method that measures glycerol released after lipolysis. With the help of chromosomal and genetic mapping the deletion of the Xp21 band can often be noticed. High resolution cytogenetic investigation of blood cells for an interstitial deletion within Xp21 can be tried in the patients and their mother or maternal females. DNA isolated from leucocytes can be studied by using multiple probes. Molecular genetic studies with conventional Southern blot and PCR analyses may show the evidence of deletion in some of the patients.

Adrenal function tests should be performed to rule in/out the coexistent adrenal hypoplasis. Patients with muscular weakness may be probed with the entire cDNA for the dystrophin protein to find out the deletions extending through the 3-prime end of the dystrophin gene.

In pregnant women, who have earlier given birth to the children with GK deficiency, deficient activity of the enzyme in the cultured amniocytes can help in the decision-making regarding termination of the pregnancy. The amniotic fluid generally shows high amounts of glycerol.

Management: A low-fat diet often results in dramatic clinical and developmental improvement.

A 5. Lactose Intolerance

Alternative names: Lactase deficiency; Milk intolerance; Disaccharidase deficiency; Dairy product intolerance.

Lactose intolerance is the inability to digest lactose, a type of sugar, a disaccharide found in milk and other dairy products. It is ***caused by a deficiency of the enzyme lactase.***

Causes, Incidence and Risk Factors

Lactose intolerance occurs ***when the small intestine does not produce enough of the enzyme lactase.*** Infant intestine produces this enzyme so they can digest milk, including breast milk. Before humans became dairy farmers, most people did not continue to drink milk, so their bodies did not produce lactase after early childhood.

People from cultures in which adult consumption of milk and milk products occurred earliest are less likely to suffer from lactose intolerance than those from areas where dairy farming began more recently. As a result, *lactose intolerance is more common in Asian, African, African-American, Native American, and Mediterranean populations than it is among northern and western Europeans.*

Lactose intolerance can begin at various times in life. In Caucasians, it usually starts to affect children older than 5 years of age. In African-Americans, lactose intolerance often occurs as early as 2 to 3 years of age.

Lactase deficiency may also ***occur as a result of intestinal diseases*** such as caeliac disease, sprue and gastroenteritis, or it may follow gastroduodenal surgery. Temporary lactase deficiency can result from viral and bacterial enteritis, especially in children, when the mucosal cells of the intestine are injured.

When ***people with lactose intolerance consume milk products,*** they may have symptoms such as

- abdominal bloating,
- excessive intestinal gas,
- nausea, diarrhoea, and
- abdominal cramping.

Lactose intolerance is very common in adults and is not dangerous. Many adults have some degree of lactose intolerance by age 20 (approximately 30 million Americans).

Lactose intolerance is sometimes **seen in premature babies.** Full-term babies generally do not show signs of lactose intolerance until they are at least 3 years old.

Biochemical: Lactose cannot be completely digested and absorbed in the small intestine and passes into the large intestine, where bacteria convert it to toxic products that cause ***abdominal cramps and diarrhoea. The problem is further complicated because undigested lactose and its metabolites increase the osmolarity of the intestinal contents, favouring the retention of water in the intestine.*** In most parts of the world where lactose intolerance is prevalent, milk is not used as a food by adults, although milk products predigested with lactase are commercially available in some countries. In certain human disorders, several or all of the intestinal disaccharidases are missing. In these cases, the digestive disturbances triggered by dietary disaccharides can sometimes be minimised by a controlled diet.

Clinical management: Eliminating milk from the diet can result in a deficiency of calcium, vitamin D, riboflavin, and protein. Therefore, a milk substitute is a necessity. For infants younger than two years old, Soy formulas are adequate substitute. Good alternatives for toddlers are soy or rice milk. Older children may also use lactase-treated cow's milk.

A 6. Glucose-6-Phosphate Dehydrogenase Deficiency

Glucose-6-phosphate dehydrogenase (G6PD) deficiency increases the vulnerability of erythrocytes to oxidative stress. Clinical presentations include ***acute hemolytic anemia, chronic hemolytic anaemia, neonatel hyperbilirubinaemia,*** and an absence of clinical symptoms. The disease is rarely fatal.

G6PD deficiency occurs with increased frequency throughout Africa, Asia, the Mediterranean, and the Middle East. In the United States, black males are most commonly affected, with a prevalence of approximately 10 percent. Prevalence of the deficiency is correlated with the geographic distribution of malaria, which has led to the theory that ***carriers of G6PD deficiency may incur partial protection against malarial infection.*** Cases of sporadic gene mutation occur in all populations.

Biochemical

G6PD catalyses nicotinamide adenine dinucleotide phosphate (NADP) to its reduced form, NADPH, in the pentose phosphate pathway (Fig. 27.4). ***NADPH protects cells from oxidative damage.*** Because erythrocytes do not generate NADPH in any other way, they are more susceptible than other cells to destruction from oxidative stress. The level of G6PD activity in affected erythrocytes generally is lower than in other cells, Normal red blood cells that are not under oxidative stress generally exhibit G6PD activity at approximately 2 percent of total capacity. Even with enzyme activity that is substantially reduced, there may be few or no clinical symptoms.

A total deficiency of G6PD is incompatible with life. The G6PD-deficient variants are grouped into different classes corresponding with disease severity (Table 27.1).

Neonatal Hyperbilirubinaemia

The ***prevalence of neonatal hyperbilirubinaemia is twice*** that of the general population in males who carry the general population in males who carry the defective G6PD gene and in

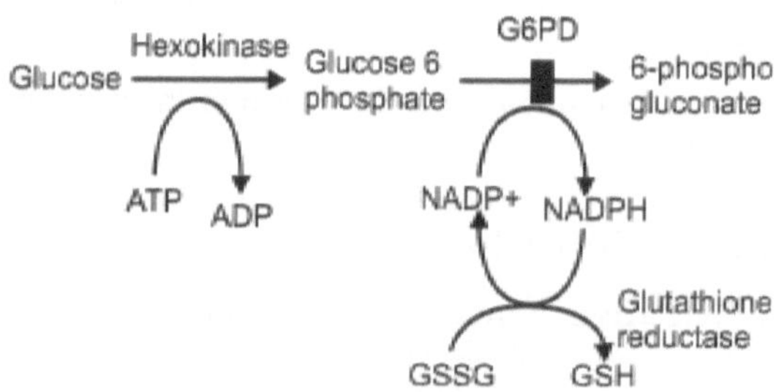

Fig. 27.4: Pentose phosphate pathway and block in G6PD deficiency

Table 27.1: Classes of G6PD enzyme variants

Class	*Level of deficiency*	*Enzyme activity*	*Prevalence*
I.	**Severe**	Chronic nonspherocytic haemolytic anaemia in the presence of normal erythrocyte function	Uncommon; occurs across populations
II.	**Severe**	Less than 10 percent of normal	Varies; more common in Asian and Mediterranean populations
III.	**Moderate**	10 to 60 percent of normal	10 percent of black males in the United States
IV.	**Mild to none**	60 to 150 percent of normal	Rare
V.	**None**	Greater than 150 percent of normal	Rare

G6PD = glucose-6-phosphate dehydrogenase.
Information from references 1 and 7

homozygous females. ***It rarely occurs in heterozygous females.*** The mechanism by which G6PD deficiency causes neonatal hyperbilirubinaemia is not completely understood. Although haemolysis may be observed in neonates who have G6PD deficiency and are jaundiced, other mechanisms appear to play a more important role in the development of hyperbilirubinaemia. Hyperbilirubinaemia is likely secondary to impairment of bilirubin conjugation and clearance by the liver leading to indirect hyperbilirubinaemia. ***Infants with G6PD deficiency and a mutation of uridine diphosphoglucuronate glucuronosyl-transferase-1 gene promoter (UDPGT-1) are particularly susceptible to hyperbilirubinaemia*** secondary to decreased liver clearance of bilirubin. UDPGT-1 is the enzyme affected in Gilbert disease. ***G6PD deficiency should be considered in neonates who develop hyperbilirubinaemia within the first 24 hours of life,*** a history of jaundice in a sibling, bilirubin levels greater than the 95th percentile, and in Asian males. G6PD deficiency can lead to an increased risk and earlier onset of hyperbilirubinaemia, which may require phototherapy or exchange transfusion. In certain populations, hyperbilirubinaemia secondary to G6PD deficiency results in an increased rate of kernicterus and death, whereas in other populations this has not been observed. This may reflect genetic mutations specific to different ethnic groups.

Acute Haemolysis

Acute haemolysis is caused by infection, ingestion of fava beans, or exposure to an oxidative drug. Medications that should be avoided in patients with G6PD deficiency are listed in Table 27.2. Haemolysis occurs after exposure to the stressor but does not continue despite continued infection or ingestion. ***This is thought to be a result of older erythrocytes having the greatest enzyme deficiency and undergoing haemolysis first.*** Once the population of deficient erythrocytes has been hemolyzed, younger erythrocytes and reticulocytes that typically have higher levels of enzyme activity are able to sustain the oxidative damage without haemolysis.

Clinically, acute haemolysis can cause ***back or abdominal pain and jaundice*** secondary to a ***rise in unconjugated bilirubin.*** Jaundice, in the setting of normal liver function, typically does not occur until greater than 50 percent of the erythrocytes have been haemolysed. Drugs that cause haemolysis in G6PD deficient persons inflict oxidative damage to erythrocytes leading to erythrocyte destruction. ***Haemolysis typically occurs 24 to 72 hours after ingestion,*** with resolution within four to 7 days. Oxidative drugs ingested by a woman who is breastfeeding may be transmitted in breast milk and can cause acute haemolysis in a G6PD deficient child.

Table 27.2: Medications that should be avoided by persons with G6PD deficiency*

Drug name	*Use*
• Primaquine	Antimalaria agent
• Dapsone	Antimicrobial for treatment of leprosy
• Flutamide (Eulexin)	Antiandrogen for treatment of prostate cancer
• Mafenide ceam (Sulfamylon)	Topical antimicrobial
• Methylene blue (Urolene Blue)	Antidote for drug-induced methemoglubinaemia
• Nalidixic acid (NegGram)	Antibiotic used primarily for urinary tract infections
• Nitrofurantoin (Macrodantin)	Antibiotic used primarily for urinary tract infections
• Phenazopyridine (Pyridium)	Analgesic for treatment of dysuria
• Rasburicase (Elitek)	Adjunct to antineoplastic agents
• Sulfacetamide (Klaron)	Antibiotic (ophthalmic and topical preparations)
• Sulfamethoxazole (Gantanol)	Antibiotic used in combination preparations (i.e. trimethoprim-sulfamethoxazole (TMP-SMX; Bactrim, septra)
• Sulfanilamide (AVC)	Antifungal agent for treatment of vulvovaginal *Candida albicans* infection

Diagnosis

The diagnosis of G6PD deficiency is made by a ***quantitative spectrophotometric analysis or, more commonly, by a rapid fluorescent spot test detecting*** the generation of NADPH from NADP. The test is positive if the blood spot fails to fluoresce under ultraviolet light. In field research, where quick screening of a large number of patients is needed, other tests have been used; however, they require definitive testing to confirm an abnormal result.

Tests based on polymerase chain reaction detect specific mutations and are used for population screening, family studies, or prenatal diagnosis. In patients with acute haemolysis, testing for G6PD deficiency may be falsely negative because older erythrocytes with a higher enzyme deficiency have been haemolysed. Young erythrocytes and reticulocytes have normal or near-normal enzyme activity. Female heterozygotes may be hard to diagnose because of X-chromosome mosaicism leading to a partial deficiency that will not be detected reliably with screening tests.

G6PD deficiency is one of a group of congenital haemolytic anaemias, and its diagnosis should be considered in children with a family history of jaundice, anaemia, splenomegaly, or cholelithiasis, especially in those of Mediterranean or African ancestry. Testing should be considered in children and adults (especially males of African, Mediterranean, or Asian descent) with an acute haemolytic reaction caused by infection, exposure to a known oxidative drug, or ingestion of fava beans. Although rare, G6PD deficiency should be considered as a cause of chronic non spherocytic haemolytic anaemia across all population groups. Newborn screening for G6PD deficiency is not performed routinely in the United States, although it is done in countries with high disease prevalence. The World Health Organisation recommends screening all newborns in populations with a prevalence of 3 to 5 percent.

Screening Test Based on Dye Decolourisation

The Screening test based on dye decolourisation procedure where haemolysates are incubated in the presence of excess glucose-6-phosphate as substrate and NADP as coenzyme together with brilliant cresyl blue dye. Dehydrogenation of glucose-6-phosphate as the result of the presence of glucose-6-phosphate dehydrogenase (G6PD) in the reaction mixture leads to reduction of NADP to NADPH. The added dye is reduced to a colourless compound in proportion to the amount of NADPH formed. Absence or deficiency of the enzyme thus results in a significantly prolonged dye-decolourisation time. This is one of the routinely used screening test available in a laboratory.

A 7. Glycogen Storage Diseases (GSD)

Introduction

The first clinical description of a patient with glycogen storage disease was reported by van Creveld (1928), a 7-year-old boy who presented with a ***markedly enlarged liver, obesity,*** and ***small genitalia.*** The initial diagnosis of adiposogenital dystrophy had to be abandoned because of the further clinical and metabolic findings, the results of which were ingeniously interpreted as reflecting increased combustion of fat resulting from 'insufficient mobilisation of glycogen'. This was the first reported patient with GSD III, as proved later enzymatically. The description of GSD I by ***von Gierke (1929)*** came next. ***Pompe (1932)*** described a case of 'idiopathic hypertrophy of the heart,' now known to be GSD II. (Pompe was a close friend of van Creveld and was killed by the Nazi Germans very shortly before the liberation of The Netherlands in 1944).

These are a ***group of inherited disorders associated with glycogen metabolism, familial in incidence and characterised by deposition of normal and abnormal type and quantities of glycogen in the tissues.*** The effects of glycerol administered by mouth on levels of glucose and of lactate, together with the response to epinephrine or glucagons, permitted differentiation of the several types of hepatic glycogenosis (I, II, III, and IV). The glycogen storage diseases are notable examples of genetic heterogeneity. Glycogenosis I in particular illustrates pleiotropism with simulation of primary gout and xanthomatosis. Liver adenomas are often present and may undergo malignant transformation. The metabolic basis of GSDs is represented in the Figure 27.5. A number of types and variants have been reported, the major ones are discussed in Figure 27.6.

1 GSD TYPE 1: vON GIERKE DISEASE

Aetiology and Biochemical Features

The **von Gierke** disease is ***characterised by the deficiency of Glucose-6-phosphatase*** (EC 3.1.3.9) in the liver cells and in the intestinal mucosa. The liver and kidney are involved, and hypoglycaemia

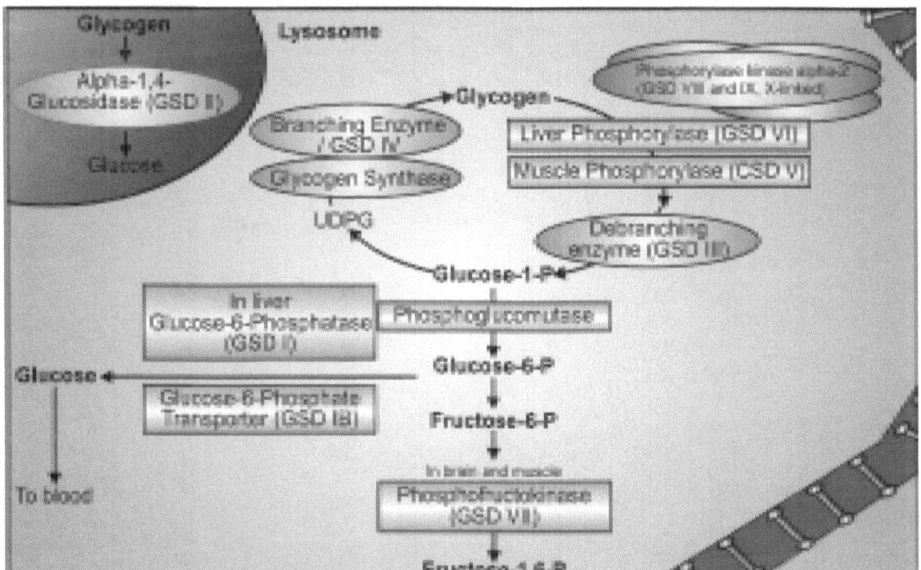

Fig. 27.5: Metabolic blocks causing glycogen storage diseases

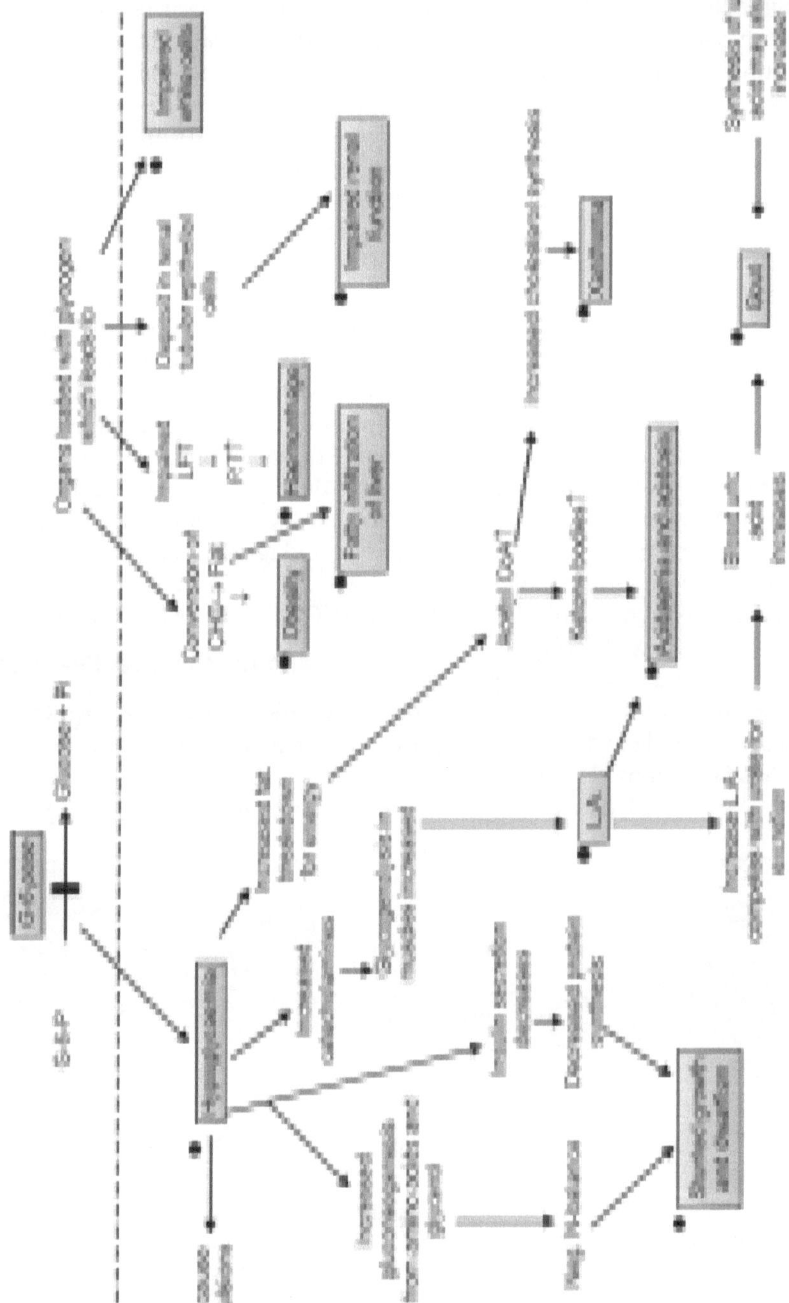

Fig. 27.6: Showing biochemical changes and correlation of clinical finding in Type-I

is a major problem. Lipidaemia also occurs and may lead to xanthoma formation. Survival to adulthood, previously rare, is now the usual situation. Hyperuricaemia has been observed in a considerable number of patients and in some, clinical gout has occurred. Inhibited tubular secretion of uric acid due to hyperlactic acidaemia and ketonaemia, and overproduction of uric acid have been postulated. The patients with partial GSDI have low or absent blood-glucose response to glucagons. Their hypoglycaemic symptoms occur with exercise, suggesting that they are unable to respond by increasing their hepatic glucose production above a certain level. Pancreatitis in association with hypertriglyceridaemia or severe metabolic acidosis has been reported in isolated cases.

Adult patients may have chronic renal disease. Gout, nephropathy, and renal stones are not the only complicatios; after a period of 'silent' hyperfiltration, renal damage develops with proteinuria, hypertension and renal dysfunction. Biopsies of such patients show focal glomerulosclerosis

GSDI subtypes: A second type of von Gierke disease has been proposed in which, although glucose-6-phosphatase activity is present on *in vitro* assay, glucose is not liberated from glucose-6-phosphate *in vivo.* They referred to this as 'functional deficiency of glu-6-phoshatase and the subtype is labelled as GSD1b against the classical GSDIa. It was noticed that G6Pase activity requires 2 components of the microsomal membrane:

1. A glucose-6-phosphate specific transport system that shuttles G6P, pyrophosphate, glucose and inorganic phosphate in and out of the endoplasmic reticulum cytoplasm (a G6P translocase), and
2. An enzyme, glucose-6-phosphate phosphohydrolase, bound to the luminal surface of the membrane. The deficiency of either of the two components can lead to the development of von Gierke disease.
3. Transport proteins, termed T1, T2, and T3, which allow the substrates and products glucose-6-phosphate, phosphate (and pyrophosphate), and glucose to cross the endoplasmic reticulum membrane. Defects in the three transport proteins are referred to as types Ib, Ic, and Id glycogen storage disease, respectively.

Molecular Genetics

The ***human D-glucose-6-phosphatase cDNA, its gene, and the expressed protein, have been characterised.*** Several mutations in the G6PC gene have been detected that completely inactivate the enzyme in persons with type Ia glycogen storage disease.

The gene contains 5 exons and spans approximately 12.5 kb. ***The gene has been mapped to the locus 17q21.*** A number of mutations have been reported from the same gene. Most of these mutations are G ◊ A or G ◊ C transitions causing the amino acid substitutions at functionally important positions of the enzyme.

Clinical Management

Symptoms usually resolve after the introduction of frequent meals high in cornstarch. Dietary manipulation with raw cornstarch diet as a measure to counteract hypoglycaemia, the common denominator in the pathogenesis of the main manifestations of the disorder, has been found to give beneficial results. The indicators of proximal renal tubular dysfunction improve in patients who were given dietary therapy such as total parenteral nutrition, nocturnal nasogastric infusion of glucose, or frequent oral administration of uncooked cornstarch.

2. GLYCOGEN STORAGE DISEASE II

Alternative titles: Acid Alpha-1, 4-Glucosidase Deficiency, GAA Deficiency, **Pompe Disease,** Acid Maltase Deficiency.

DESCRIPTION

Glycogen storage disease II, an ***autosomal recessive disorder,*** is the prototypic lysosomal storage disease. In the ***classic infantile form (Pompe disease), cardiomyopathy and muscular hypotonia are the cardinal features;*** in the ***juvenile and adult forms, involvement of skeletal muscles dominates*** the clinical picture. The expected number of individuals born with GSD II has been estimated to be 1 in 40,000 births.

Glycogen storage disease II (GSD II) is caused by mutation in the gene encoding acid alpha-1, 4-glucosidase (GAA), which has been mapped to chromosome 17.

CLINICAL FEATURES

Infantile Onset (Pompe Disease)

In classic cases of Pompe disease, affected children are prostrate and ***markedly hypotonic with large hearts. The tongue may be enlarged.*** Although the enzyme is deficient in all tissues, muscle weakness and heart involvement are the most common features. The liver is rarely enlarged, except as a result of heart failure, and hypoglycaemia and acidosis do not occur as they do in GSD I. ***Death usually occurs in the first year of life*** in the classic form of the disorder and cardiac involvement is sriking. Indeed, Pompe (1932) reported this condition as 'idiopathic hypertrophy of the heart, 'and ' cardiomegalia glycogenica' is a synonym.

Aetiopathology and Biochemistry

The ***defect*** in type II glycogen storage disease ***involves acid alpha-1, 4-glucosidase (acid maltase),*** a lysosomal, enzyme. Whereas the glycogen is distributed rather uniformly in the cytoplasm in the other glycogen storage diseases, it is enclosed in lysosomal membranes in this form of the disease.

In a case of infantile acid alpha-glucosidase deficiency, the ***defect was a structural mutation causing synthesis of a catalytically inactive, cross-reacting material (CRM)-positive, enzyme protein. On the other hand, the mutation in the adult form causes a reduction in the amount of enzyme protein.*** An inverse correlation was found between the severity of clinical manifestations and the level of residual enzyme activity in fibroblasts. The kinetic and electrophoretic properties of residual enzyme in fibroblasts from adult patients were identical to those from controls. The mutation may, therefore, affect the production or degradation of enzyme rather than its structure of catalytic funcation.

Deficiency of catalytically active mature enzyme in lysosomes was common to all clinical phenotypes but, in most cases, was more profound in early-onset than in late-onset forms of the disease.

MOLECULAR GENETICS

Glycogen storage disease type II is ***inherited as an autosomal recessive trait.*** The gene for the alpha-1, 4-glucosidase enzyme (GAA) has been ***mapped to*** the locus 17q25.2-q25.3.

Multiple mutations in the acid maltase gene have been shown to cause glycogen storage disease II, e.g. a single basepair substitution of G to A at position 271 and a single mutation in intron 1 of the acid maltase. Compound heterozygosity for mutations within a family have also been detected.

DIAGNOSIS

The adult form of the disease can be diagnosed ***in cultured skin fibroblasts.*** Morphologically and biochemically, the newly grown fibres of cultured muscle showed the same changes as did biopsied muscle.

Creatine kinase (CK) elevation is a sensitive market of GSD II. In patients presenting with a slowly progressive proximal muscle weakness or with respiratory insufficiency, measurement of serum levels of CK is recommended, followed by ***measurement of acid alpha-glucosidase activity in leukocytes,*** using glycogen as a substrate. To rule out the pseudodeficiency state seen in carriers of the GAA2 allele, patients with depressed leucocyte activity should have a repeat assay in cultured fibroblasts using artificial substrate.

CLINICAL MANAGEMENT

A ***high-protein, low-carbohydrate diet is an effective therapy*** in adults with acid maltase deficiency. Striking improvement in respiratory function has been observed.

Amalfitano et al. (2001) reported the results of a phase I/II open-label single-dose study of recombinant human alpha-glucosidase infused intravenously twice weekly in 3 infants with infantile GSD II. The results of more than 250 infusions showed that recombinant human GAA was generally well toterated. Steady decreases in heart size and maintenance of normal cardiac function for more than 1 year were observed in all 3 infants. These infants lived well past the critical age of 1 year (16, 18, and 22 months old at the time of this study) and continued to have normal cardiac function. Improvements of skeletal muscle functions were also noted; 1 patient showed marked improvement and had normal muscle tone and strength as well as normal neurologic and developmental evaluations.

3. GLYCOGEN STORAGE DISEASE III

Alternative titles: **Forbes Disease,** Cori Disease, Limit Dextrinosis, Amylo-1, 6- Glucosidase Deficiency, Glycogen Debranching Deficiency, Amylo-1, 6-Glucosidase, 4-Alpha-Glucanotransferase

Clinical Features

The clinical features in Glycogen Storage Disease III are ***milder than those of type I,*** and ***involvement of heart and skeletal muscle adds other features.*** Patients have liver involvement manifested by ***hepatomegaly and hypoglycaemia;*** a few patients have muscle weakness and wasting but no clinically apparent liver disease; and many patients have both liver and muscle problems, subclinical evidence of cardiac involvement in the form of ventricular hypertrophy is also observed in ECG and echocardiography. **Momoi et al. (1992)** divided the GSDIII patients into 4 groups:

a. with childhood onset of both muscle weakness and hepatic disorders;
b. with onset of muscular symptoms in adulthood while liver symptoms started in childhood;
c. with muscle weakness starting in adulthood long after liver symptoms in childhood had disappeared; and
d. with only muscle symptoms as adults without any sign or history of liver dysfunction after childhood.

The overall incidence of type III GSD in the United States is about 1 in 100,000 live births, it is unusually frequent among North African Jews in Israel (Prevalence 1 in 5,400; carrier prevalence 1 in 35).

Enzyme Defect

The ***deficiency in this disorder*** concerns glycogen debranching enzyme, a large monomeric protein with a molecular weight of 160,000 to 170,000. The ***2 catalytic activities*** of debranching enzyme are amyo-1, 6-glucosidase (*EC 3.2.1.33*) and oligo-1, 4-1, 4-glucanotransferase (*EC 2.4.1.25*). The 2 activities are determined at separate catalytic sites on the polypeptide chain and can function independently of each other. The structure of stored glycogen is abnormal "Limit Dextrin Type" with short and missing outer chains.

Biochemical Changes

Activities of serum aspartate and alanine transaminases, lactate dehydrogenase, creatine kinase and alkaline phosphatase are markedly elevated during infancy. The serum enzyme activities decline around puberty concomitantly with a decrease in liver size. Although ***periportal fibrosis and micronodular cirrhosis*** indicate the presence of hepatocellular damage during childhood, the decline in serum enzyme activities with age and the absence of overt hepatic dysfunction suggest that the fibrotic process may not always progress.

Patients with both myopathy and liver involvement have an enzyme defect in both tissues, whereas patients with only liver involvement lack enzyme activity in liver and have normal activity in muscle. The debranching enzymes in liver and muscle are immunochemically similar and in the patients studies, the absence of debrancher protein is responsible for the disorder.

Remarkable variability, both clinically and enzymatically, is a feature of glycogen debranching enzyme deficiency. Most patients have disease involving both liver and muscle (type IIIa); however, approximately 15% of all GSD III patients have only liver involvement without apparent muscle disease (type IIIb). AGL glucosidase and AGL transferase activities are selectively absent in types IIIc and IIId. During infancy and childhood, the disease may be indistinguishable from type I glycogen storage disease; hepatomegaly, hypoglycaemia, hyperlipidaema, and growth retardation are predominant features of both.

MOLECULAR GENETICS

The gene for the debranching enzyme has been mapped to chromosome number one at a locus 1p21. Although the glycogen debranching enzyme in liver and muscle appears to be encoded by a single gene, its expression in these tissues is under separate genetic control. This is corroborated by the fact that type IIIb. Patients have absent enzyme activity in the liver but retain enzyme activity in muscle. A full-length cDNA of the liver enzyme contains 7072 bp with a 4596-bp coding region. The liver mRNA sequence is identical to the muscle sequence for most of the length, except for the 5-prime end in which the liver sequence diverges completely from the muscle sequences beginning with the putative transcription initiation site to the ninth nucleotide upstream of the translation initiation codon. Thus, the muscle and liver isoforms are generated via differential RNA transcription, with an alternative first exon usage, from a single debrancher gene. It has been suggested that the human AGL gene contains at least 2 promoter regions that confer differential expression of isoform mRNAs in a tissue-specific manner.

The mutations causing the non-functionig enzyme are heterogeneous and ***a number of different mutations*** have been reported from different GSDIII patients. **In Japan,** 7 mutations, including 1 splicing mutation was identified from seven families. Two mutations have been found to be more frequent. Each of which was found in the homozygous state in multiple patients, and each of which was associated with a subset of clinical phenotype in those patients with that mutation. One mutation was indetified in homozygosity in a confirmed GSD IIIa **Caucasian patient** who presented with mild clinical symptoms. The IVS32-12A-G mutation had an allele frequency of around 5.5% in GSD III patients tested. The other common mutation, the novel mutation 3964delT, was identified in an **African-American patient** who had a severe phenotype and early onset of clinical symptoms. The mutation was later identified in several other patients and was observed at a frequency of around 6.7%. Together, these 2 mutations can account for more than 12% of the molecular defects in GSD III patients.

Diagnosis: The ***two enzyme activities*** of the debranching enzyme viz. amylo-1, 6-glucosidase (*EC 3.21.33*) and oligo-1, 4-1, 4-glucanotransferase (*EC 2.4.1.25*), can be ***demonstrated in the leucocytes*** as well as in liver and ***muscle biopsy*** samples.

Prognosis: Mostly patients survive well into the adulthood with progressive muscular weekness.

4. GLYCOGEN STORAGE DISEASE IV

Alternative titles: Glycogen Branching Enzyme Deficiency, GBEI Deficiency, Andersen's Disease, Brancher Deficiency, Glycogenosis IV, Amylopectinosis

The first case of GSD IV was reported by Andersen (1956) as 'familial cirrhosis of the liver with storage of abnormal glycogen.' Ten years later, the biochemical defect was identified to be the deficiency of the ***alpha-1, 4-glucan branching enzyme also known as Glycogen Branching Enzyme (GBE1).*** Mutation in the same gene causes an allelic disorder, adult polyglucosan body disease (APED). The ***enzyme deficiency results in tissue accumulation of abnormal glycogen with fewer branching points and longer outer branches, resembling an amylopectin-like structure, also known as polyglucosan (Fig. 27.7).***

CLINICAL FEATURES

Glycogen storage disease type IV is a clinically heterogeneous disorder. The typical 'classic' hepatic presentation is liver disease of childhood, progressing to lethal cirrhosis. The most common form of GSD IV presents in the first 18 months of life with failure to thrive, hepatosplenomegaly, and liver cirrhosis. There is progression to portal hypertension, ascites, and liver failure, leading to death by age 5 years.

Types of GSD IV

On the basis of the age of onset GSD IV can be classified into ***4 categories:***

a. **Perinatal:** The infants present with fetal akinesia deformation sequence (FADS), generalised oedema, serve hypotonia, and arthrogryposis of the lower limbs at birth. The condition is fatal within days of birth.

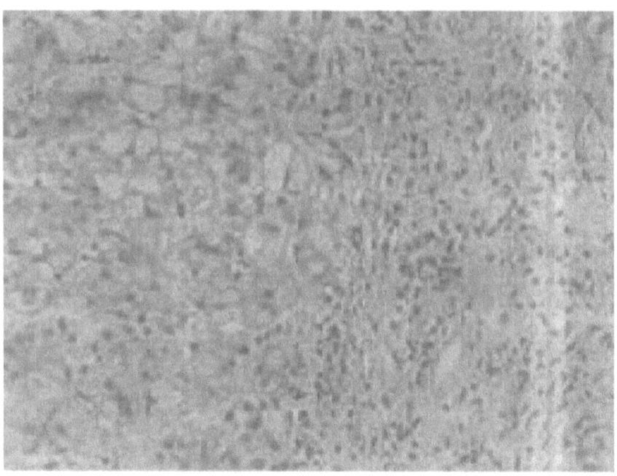

Fig. 27.7: Liver histology of a GSD IV patient showing accumulation of polyglucosan

b. **Congenital:** Infants present with ***hypotonia, neuronal involvement, and death*** in early infancy. The classic clinical manifestation of liver cirrhosis may not be present, although amylopectin-like inclusions can be found in hepatocytes.

c. **Childhood:** Diagnosed in early childhood, this form of GSDIV presents with ***severe myopathy, dilated cardiomyopathy, heart failure, dysmorphic features,*** and subclinical neuropathy and the patients die before puberty.

d. **Adult:** ***Rarely, GSD IV may present in the adult life.*** The clinical features are generally restricted to muscular dysfunction. Symptoms begin with progressive difficulty in climbing the upstairs. Hyperlordotic posture, wadding gait and proximal limb weakness are associated features.

MOLECULAR GENETICS

The ***gene for GBE1 enzyme has been mapped to locus 3p12.*** All forms of GSD IV are caused by mutations in the same gene and significant retention of GBE activity may be the reason for mild or non-progressive forms of the disease. ***Two mis-sense mutations and one nonsense mutation in the GBE gene have been identified*** in the classic hepatic form of GSD IV. Transient expression experiments showed that these mutation inactivated glycogen branching enzyme activity. In a patient with the non-progressive hepatic form of GSD IV, a compound heterozygosity for 2 GBE1 mutations was identified; one of these resulted in complete loss of GBE activity, whereas the other resulted in loss of approximately 50% of GBE activity. Large deletion or insertions have also been reported in some cases.

Diagnosis

A **simple iodine test** shows ***formation of a blue coloured complex*** of glycogen and iodine. The liver shows the main imvolvement, resulting from a defect of amylo (1, 4 to 1, 6) transglucosidase (brancher enzyme). Liver enzymes in all the patients of GSD IV are raised.

Enzymatic assay of GBE1 shows deficient branching enzyme in liver, skeletal muscle, and skin fibroblasts. This enzyme activity may be normal in circulating erythrocytes and leucocytes. The diagnosis of both homozygotes and heterozygotes can be made on the basis of the study of branching enzyme activity in erythrocytes. Brown and Brown (1989).

Management

Liver transplantation seems to be the ***only successful treatment.*** The longest survival reported is 73 months in a patient who received a transplant at the age of 31 months. Although it might appear that the liver failure would be reversed by successful transplantation but the progressive and probably fatal myopathy, cardiomyopathy, or encephalopathy would be inevitable. However, the patients appear to remain healthy and the accumulations of glycogen in the heart and muscle at the time of liver transplantation seems to diminish. The systemic microchimersim occurs after liver allotransplantation and can ameliorate pancellular enzyme deficiencies.

5. GLYCOGEN STORAGE DISEASE V

Alternative titles: **McArdle's Disease,** Myophosphorylase Deficiency, Muscle Glycogen Phosphorylase Deficiency, PYGM Deficiency.

McArdle disease is a ***relatively benign disorder*** of glycogen metabolism, except the patients are at risk of renal failure as a complication of myoglobinuria McArdle's disease, or glycogen storage disease type V (GSDV), is caused by ***mutation in the gene encoding muscle glycogen phosphorylase (PYGM).*** The ***inheritance*** appears to be ***autosomal recessive*** although some reports of dominant characteristics have been published.

The original patient, first reported by McArdle (1951), was a 30-year-old man who experienced first muscle pain and the weakness and stiffness with exercise of any muscle. Symptoms disappeared promptly with rest. Blood lactate did not increase after exercise, suggesting that the patient was unable to convert muscle glycogen into lactate. The cause of the disorder was identified by Schmid and Mahler (1959) as a glycogenolytic defect in the muscle with the absence of myscle phosphorylase.

CLINICAL FEATURES

The clinical symptoms of McArdle' disease ***usually begin in young adulthood*** with ***exercise intolerance*** and ***muscle cramps. Transient myoglobinuria*** may occur after exercise but this may ***precipitate acute renal failure.*** Patients may report muscle weakness, myalgia, and lack of endurance since childhood or adolescence. Later in adult life, there is persistent and progressive muscle weakness and atrophy with fatty replacement. The muscle cramps are 'electrically silent,' showing no activity on electromyography, which may lead to interpretation of psychoneurosis. The patients might be able to continue exercise without difficulty ('second wind' phase) after an initial fatigue which recovers very fast.

As for the other GSDs, clinical heterogeneity is also observed in McArdle's disease with the presentation of characteristic clinical features in various age groups. The range of the onset of clinical features is as wide as 4 weeks to 60 years.

MOLECULAR AND BIOCHEMICAL FEATURES

The ***gene*** for the ***muscle glycogen phosphorylase*** has been mapped to the locus 11q13. ***A number of point mutations in the PYGM gene*** have been reported in patients with McArdle's disease. The most common is a nonsense mutation, arg 49-to-ter (R49X) that has been reported to be the cause of GSD V in more than 75% of the patients. The mutation (s) can be identified by RELP analysis.

Glycogen phosphorylase is the major protein (~5% of total protein) in myocytes. By immunodiffusion and gel electrophoresis, various workers have demonstrated the presence of the myophosphorylase protein in patients who had no myophosphorylase activity. The studies using Western, Southern a well as Northern blot techniques have indicated a wide range of defects at the molecular levels that can result in GSD V. Some of the patients show total or partial lack of PYGM protein while others show the normal transcription of mRNA and its translation into the phosphorylase protein. The causative factor of the disease could be as wide as the phosphorylation defect of the protein to the intramuscular deficiency of pyridoxal phosphate that is a covalently linked factor of muscle phosphorylase enzyme.

Diagnosis

All the subjects with clinical features can be tested for McArdle's disease based on the development of brief painful cramps during exercise.

- The ***ischaemic forearm exercise test*** for McArdle's disease invariably causes muscle cramps and pain in patients with this glycolytic defect.
- ***Low post exercise plasma lactate levels*** also indicate McArdle's disease.
- ***Post-exercise peak lactate-to-ammonia ratios*** clearly separated patients from the healthy individuals.
- Myoglobin should be estimated in urine after exercise to assess the risk of developing renal failure.
- Ross et al. (1981) ***used ^{31}P nuclear magnetic resonance to*** study McArdle's disease. The inorganic phosphate resonance gives a direct measurement of intracellular cytoplasmic pH in muscle. During exercise, the pH fell relatively little, while phosphocreatine was shown to fall during aerobic exercise and was rapidly exhausted during minimal ischaemic exercise.

6. GLYCOGEN STORAGE DISEASE VI

Alternative titles: Hers disease, Phosphorylase Deficiency, Glycogen-Storage Disease of Liver, Glycogen Phosphorylase (Liver) Deficiency, PYGL deficiency.

Glycogen Storage Disease VI (Hers disease) is also a ***relatively benign disorder*** caused by the ***partial or total lack of liver glycogen phosphorylase*** (EC 2.4.1.1) activity. The disease appears to be ***inherited through autosomal recessive traits.*** It may be noted that there is confusion in the numerology of the glycogen storage diseases: hepatic phosphorylase deficiency, here designated GSD VI, is labelled GSD VIII by some of the workers.

BIOCHEMICAL AETIOLOGY AND CLINICAL FEATURES

Liver glycogen phosphorylase enzyme brings about glycogenolysis in liver to contribute to the blood glucose. The inability of the patients to utilise liver glycogen for maintenance of blood glucose results in moderate hypoglycaemia, which may then trigger the oxidiation of fatty acids causing ketosis. The clinical picture is one of ***mild to moderate hypoglycaemia, mild ketosis, growth retardation, and prominent hepatomegaly.*** Heart and skeletal muscle are not affected. The prognosis seems to be excellent.

The liver phosphorylase cDNA appeared to represent an evolutionary mosaic; the segment encoding the N-terminal 80 amina acids contained more than 90% G+C at the third codon position. The high G+C content in the N-terminal region of the liver message indicates that this segment was spliced onto the liver gene from the muscle gene long after the divergence of liver and muscle tissues. Possibly skeletal muscle, which undergoes a fall in pH and a rise in temperature during exercise, represents a stressful environment that selectively maintains high G+C content in expressed genes.

The gene for the liver phosphorylase has been located at chromosome number 14 at locus 14q21-q22. Two splice site mutations and two mis-sense mutations have been attributed to Hers disease. The pedigree analysis has shown that all the seventeen affected individuals in

Mennonite family could be traced back to a single couple living in Pennsylvania in the 1830s. A splice site abnormality of the intron 13 splice donor was estimated to be present on 3% of Mennonite chromosomes and the frequency of the disease was estimated to be 1 in 1,000 in that population. A number of other insertion, substitution or deletion mutations have been reported in the PYGL gene by different workers in different populations across the world.

Diagnosis

- Hepatomegaly, linear growth retardation and fasting hypoglycaemia are the characteristic features that suggest a GSD.
- ***Liver biopsy*** histology shows enlarged hepatocytes with a granular substance consistent with glycogen.
- The ***enzyme may be estimated*** in the liver biopsy samples.
- Like in all the other GSDs, liver function enzymes like alanine transaminase and pyruvate transaminase would be elevated in a major proportion of the patients.
- DNA sequencing of the PYGL gene to look for specific mutations on intron #13 or intron #14 can be helpful in detecting the carriers as well as prenatal identification of the affected child.

Clinical management: The management of the patients of GSD VI is primarily directed at stabilising the blood glucose levels to avoid ketoacidosis. The patient is advised frequent small meals. The prognosis is good.

Six classical types of GSDS are shown in the Table 27.3.

A 8. MUCOPOLYSACCHARIDOSIS

Introduction

Mucopolysaccharides (MPS) are the heteropolysaccharides with complex structures, primarly composed of amino sugars and uronic acid. They are also rich in sulphates, which give them an

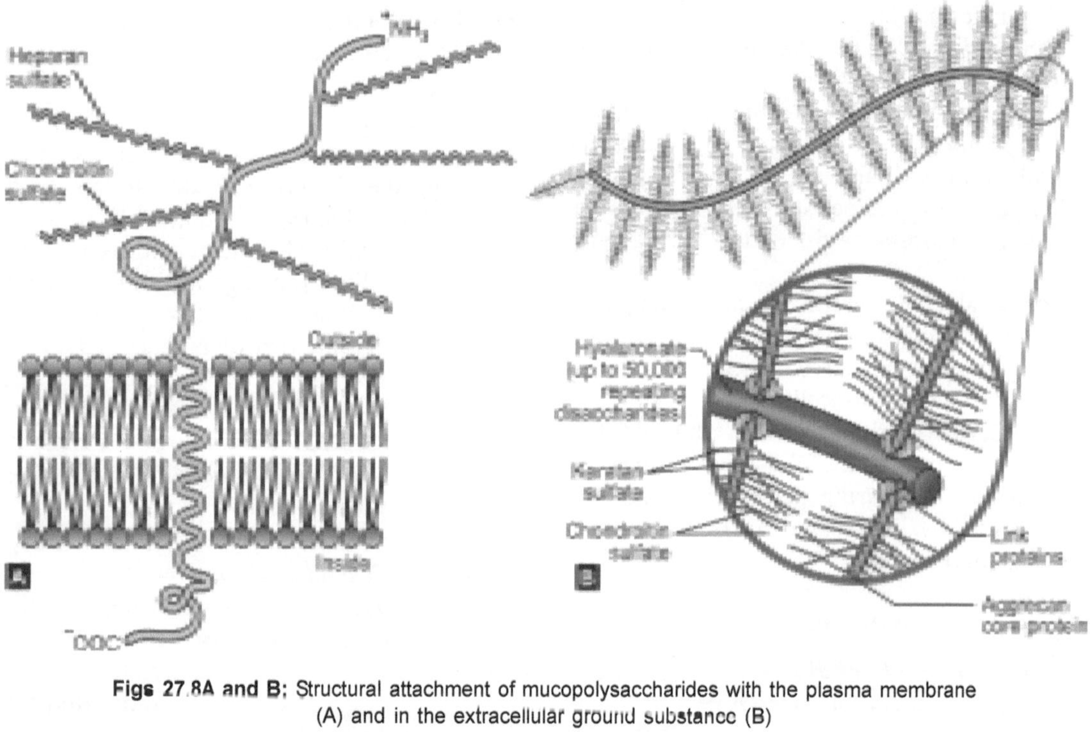

Figs 27.8A and B: Structural attachment of mucopolysaccharides with the plasma membrane (A) and in the extracellular ground substance (B)

Table 27.3: Glycogen storage diseases (GSDs)

Type	*Name*	*Deficient Enzyme*	*Inheritance*	*Structure of Glycogen*	*Organs Affected*	*Clinical Features*
I.	**von Gierke Disease**	*G-6-pase*	Autosomal recessive	Normal (Metabolically NOT available	Liver, Kidney, Intestine	Hypoglycaemia, Ketosis and Acidosis L.A. ↑, Uric Acid ↑ Failure to thrive, Hepatomegaly
II.	**Pompe's Disease**	*Acid Maltase* (Present in Lysosomes. Catalyses breakdown of oligosaccharides)	Autosomal recessive	Normal	Liver, Heart, Smooth and Striated muscles	Cardiomegaly, Muscle hypotonia, No Hypoglycaemia
Note: Infants die of cardiac failure and Bronchopneumonia. Death usually before 9 months. A few survive 2½ years.						
III.	**Limit Dextrinosis (Forbe's Disease)**	*Debranching enzyme*	Autosomal recessive	***Abnormal,*** 'Limit Dextrin' type Short missing Outer branches	Liver (18%), Heart and Muscle (6%)	Moderate Hypoglycaemia, Acidosis, Progressive myopathy, Hepatomegaly
Note: Patients survive well to adult life.						
IV.	**Amylopectinosis (Andersen's Disease)**	*Branching enzyme*	Not known	• ***Abnormal*** ("Amylopectin" type) • Very long inner and outer unbranched chains, very few branch point	Liver, Heart, Muscle, RE System	Moderate hypoglycaemia Hepato-splenomegaly, Ascites, Nodular Cirrhosis of liver, Hepatic failure
Note: Prognosis Fatal, Longest survival reported as 4 years.						
V.	**MacArdle's Disease**	*Muscle Phosphorylase*	Autosomal recessive	Normal	Skeletal muscle (Excess normal glycogen muscles)	Muscle cramps on exercise, Pain in muscle, weakness and stiffness of muscle
Note: Affects children and adults, Muscle recovers with rest—Due to utilisation of FA for energy, after inj. epinephrine/glucagon → Blood sugar ↑ (shows Liver Phosphorylase not affected)						
VI.	**Her's Disease**	*Liver Phosphorylase*	Autosomal Dominant	Normal	Liver, Leucocytes	Hypoglycaemia, Mild to moderate acidosis, Hepatomegaly
Note: Presents like a mild case of Type-I, the condition has also been reported to occur in association with Fanconi syndrome.						

acidic character. They are also called as 'glycosamino glycans'. MPS are important structural components of many tissues, especially the cartilage, tendons, cornea, connective tissue and ground substance. The diverse functions associated with MPS include cellular osmotic potential; lubrication of joints; cell migration and differentiation in the embroyonic tissues; cell adhesion and cell-cell interaction; blood group substances and anticoagulants; and transparency of the cornea.

The MPS are dynamic molecules, i.e. they are regularly synthesised and broken down. ***The breakdown is mainly carried out by the hydrolytic enzymes present in lysosomes. Deficiency*** of the lysosomal hydrolytic enzyme(s) can lead to a series of genetic disorders characterised by accumulation and excretion of intermediates of polysaccharide catabolism. The un-natural accumulation of these MPS in tissues interferes with the cellular function causing a number of ***clinical features*** such as ***mental retardation, characteristic facial appearance, corneal clouding and hearing loss.***

1. MPS TYPE I: ALPHA-L-IDURONIDASE DEFICIENCY

Alternative titles: Hurler's Syndrome (Fig. 27.9)

The first to be identified among the mucopolysaccharidosis, hence titled as mucopolysaccharidosis type I (MPS I), the Hurler's syndrome is an ***autosomal recessive*** disorder ***characterised*** by • severe mental retardation, • hepatosplenomegaly, • ***progressive corneal clouding,* • *conductive hearing loss*** and ***skeletal deformity with characteristic facial features.*** The disease traces a very severe course, particularly after the first year of life. ***Cardiac involvement*** becomes ***prominent with valvular dysfunction*** and progressively frequent coronary events. Lung tissue gets affected leading to impaired ventilation.

Biochemical Defect

The ***biochemical defect*** lies in the ***deficiency of α-L-iduronidase (IDUA; EC 3.2.1.76), the lysosomal enzyme*** that hydrolyses the terminal alpha-L-iduronic acid residues of the glycosamino-

Table 27.4: Types of mucopolysaccharidosis and their characteristics

Type	*Name*	*Enzyme Defect*	*Inheritance*	*Urinary MPS*
MPS-I	Hurler's syndrome	*α-L-Iduronidase*	Autosomal Recessive	Dermatan SO_4 Heparan SO_4
MPS-II	Hunter's syndrome	*Iduronate sulphatase*	X-Linked recessive	Chondriotin SO_4 B Heparan SO_4
MPS-III	San-Filipo's syndrome (A,B,C)	A: *Sulphaminidase* B: *α-N-acetyl glucosaminidase* C: *Acetyl transferase*	Autosomal Recessive	Heparan SO_4
MPS-IV	Morquio syndrome	*N-acetylgalactosamine -6-sulphatase*	Autosomal Recessive	Keratan SO_4
MPS-V	Scheie syndrome	*α-L-Iduronidase*	Autosomal Recessive	Dermatan SO_4
MPS-VI	Maroteaux-Lamy syndrome	*N-acetylgalactosamine —4-sulphatase*	Autosomal Recessive	Dermatan SO_4

Salient features of each one of the mucopolysaccharidosis are discussed below.

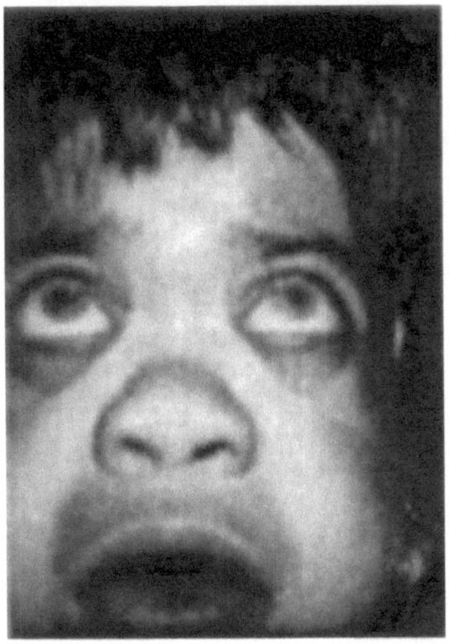

Fig. 27.9: Hurler's syndrome facial features with corneal clouding

glycans dermatan sulfate and of heparin sulfate. The enzyme was originally defined as the 'Hurler's corrective factor'. Normal mucopolysaccharides are synthesised, but they cannot be completely broken down, leading to the accumulation and ***urinary excretion of dermatan sulphate and heparan sulphate.***

The IDUA enzyme was purified from human liver and consists of a ***single polypeptide-74 kD protein*** with a ***26-amino acid signal peptide*** that is cleaved immediately before the amino terminus. The gene for the enzyme has been assigned to ***chromosome number 4 at the locus 4p16.3.*** Alternative splicing of the mRNA gives rise to closely related proteins in fibroblasts, liver, kidney, and placental RNA.

Nature of Mutation

The most common mutation, responsible for Hurler's syndrome in a number of (43%) MPS I patients, is a ***single base substitution that introduces a stop codon at position 402 (W402X) of the alpha-L-iduronidase protein.*** The mutation is associated with an extremely severe clinical phenotype in homozygotes. Patients who are compound heterozygotes having one allele carrying the W401X mutation have a wide range of clinical phenotypes. ***Two additional mutations, one that introduces a stop codon at position 70 (Q70X)*** and the other that ***alters the proline at position 533 to an arginine (P533R) in the 653 amino acid*** alpha-L-iduronidase protein, have also been detected in a number of families carrying Hurler's syndrome.

2. MPS TYPE II: IDURONATE 2-SULFATASE DEFICIENCY

Alternative titles: Hunter's Syndrome

The proteoglycan or glycosaminoglycans (Fig. 27.10) are present on the cell surface where they perform a number of functions including cell-cell interaction and molecular recognition. The proteoglycans containing chondroitin sulphate B and heparin sulphate require iduronate

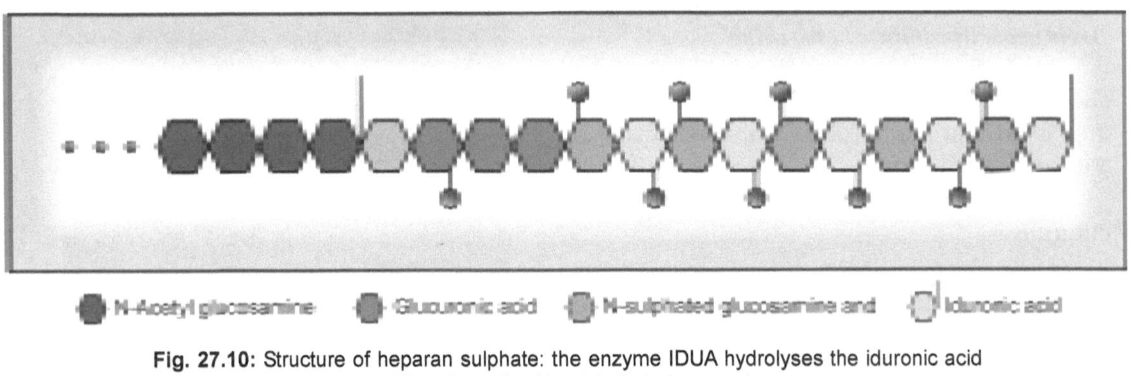

Fig. 27.10: Structure of heparan sulphate: the enzyme IDUA hydrolyses the iduronic acid residues from the N-sulphated glucosamine

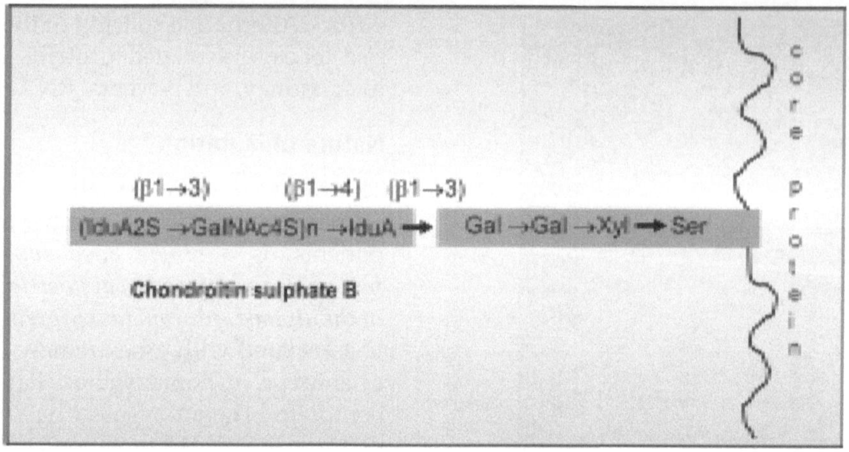

Fig. 27.11: A Proteoglycan containing chondroitin sulphate B

sulfatase enzyme for their regular turnover. Mucopolysaccharidosis II arises from ***iduronate sulfatase deficiency,*** which ***results*** in ***tissue deposits of mucopolysaccharides and urinary excretion of large amounts of chondroitin sulfate B and heparitin sulfate.***

CLINICAL FEATURES

Sex-linked mucopolysaccharidosis differs from the autosomal type (MPS I) in being on the average less severe and in not showing clouding of the cornea. Features are dysostosis with dwarfism, grotesque faces (Fig. 27.12) ***hepatosplenomegaly*** from mucopolysaccharide deposits, ***cardiovascular disorders*** from mucopolysaccharide deposits in the intima, ***deafness, and excretion of large amounts of chondriotin sulfate B and heparitin sulfate in the urine.***

The fibroblasts from patients with this disorder show metachromatic cytoplasmic inclusions and about half the fibroblasts of heterozygotes show such inclusions.

Two forms of MPS II are distinguishable clinically.

- ***(A) Severe form (MPS IIA):*** These patients have ***progressive mental retardation*** and ***physical*** disability and death occurs before the age of 15 years in most cases.
- ***(B) Mild form (MPS IIB):*** The disorder is milder in progression and is compatible with survival to adulthood, and reproduction is known to have occurred. Intellect is impaired

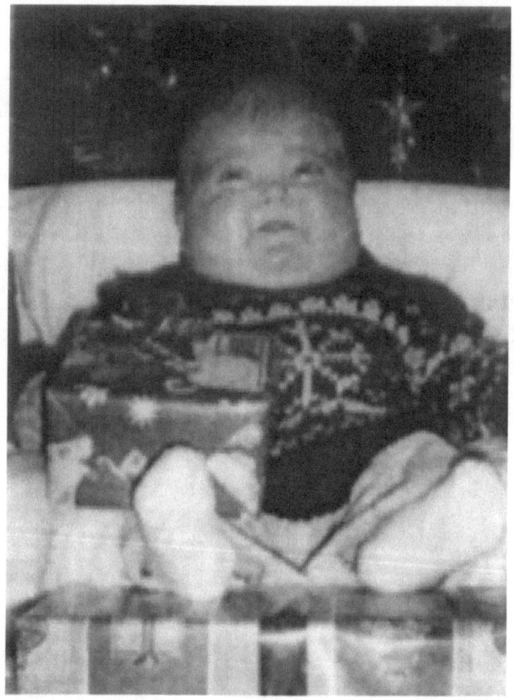

Fig. 27.12: Hunter's syndrome: gross features and dwarfism

minimally, if at all. Hobolth and Pedersen (1978) described a kindred with 6 cases of mild Hunter's syndrome remarkable for survival to ages 65 and 87 in 2 of the cases and for progeny from 3 affected males.

Hyper-pigmentation spots (Mongolian spots) are a long-lasting symptom in Hunter's disease. Although initially thought to be independent of the primary disorder, the spots are now recognises as essential features that may lead to early diagnosis in patients with mild forms of Hunter's syndrome.

- ***Electron microscopic findings*** show that pigment-bearing dermal melanocytes contained many free melanosomes in stage IV. These were surrounded by extracellular sheaths and encircled by elastic fibres.

Incidence: In United Kingdom, the estimated frequency of Hunter's syndrome is about 1 in 1,32,000 male births. ***The severe form was found to be 3.38 times more frequent than the mild form. The highest incidence*** of Hunter's syndrome has been reported from Israel, i.e. 1 in 34, 000 male live births. It is suggested that the high frequency of Hunter's disease in Israeli Jews is compatible with genetic drift. An incidence of approximately 1 in 3,20,000 live births (1 in 165,000 male live births) was obtained for Hunter's syndrome in ***Australia.***

Inheritance: Hunter's syndrome is the ***only polysaccharidosis disorder with X-linked inheritance.*** There has been a long controversy regarding autosomal/X-linked inheritance because a number of patients were found to be having a normal karyotype. Now it is recognised that the **gene** for the enzyme induronate sulphatase is present on X-chromosome at locus Xq28. In case of normal karyotypes, the non-random X-inactivation has been found to be the defect behind Hunter's syndrome. X/autosome translocation could also be responsible for the apparent normal karyotype in the patients or the heterozygous carriers.

Molecular characterisation of the DNA extracted from the Hunter's syndrome patients has demonstrated the ***presence of short or large deletion of several Xq27.3-Xq28 loci.*** Gene rearrangement of IDU sulphatase gene has also been observed in some of the patients. In the affected families, segregation in favour of selection of Hunter's gene has been observed.

Diagnosis

Detection of the Carriers

- **Tonnesen et al (1983)** found intercellular uptake of lysosomal enzymes in cultured fibroblasts, which is prevented by addition of either mannose-6-phosphate or fructose-I-phosphate to the culture medium. They ***developed a technique that uses the incorporation of 35_S-sulphate in the hair-follicle fibroblasts in the presence and absence of fructose 1-phosphate.*** The technique has been successfully tested by studying various mixtures of normal and Hunter's cells in culture as well as obligatory carriers.
- **Schroder et al (1993)** used ***different carrier detection tests, i.e. IDS activity in serum, sulfate incorporation in cultured skin fibroblasts, and RFLP*** analysis in 13 unrelated families with 16 patients and 36 females at risk for MPS II. Twenty-nine females were confirmed as carriers, and in 5 women, the heterozygous state was exclu-ded. The use of the intragenic IDS cDNA probes and flanking probes provided accurancy in carrier detection that was equal to or better than that in biochemical methods.
- **Timms et al (1998)** described carrier testing using direct dye primer sequencing of PCR products to identify mixed bases in an obligate carrier.
- ***Prenatal diagnosis*:** The prenatal diagnosis of Hunter's syndrome may be possible ***by measurement*** of iduronate sulfatase in the mother's serum. The level of IDS consistently rises in the serum of pregnant women. In pregnancies with Hunter-affected male fetuses, serum enzyme levels did not change. The normal increase occurs usually by the 6th to 12th weeks.

Clinical Management

- ***Bone marrow transplant:*** A number of bone marrow transplant attempts have been made with limited success. Out of the ten patients reported till 1999, only three survived for more than seven years. In 2 who had survived long-term, there had been a steady progression of physical disability and mental handicap. One patient had maintained normal intellectual development, with only mild physical disability.
- ***Gene therapy: Braun et al (1993)*** tested *in vitro* the correction of the enxyme defect in the Hunter's syndrome, ***using an amphotropic retroviral vector*** containing the humen IDS coding sequence. Lymphoblastoid cell lines from patients with Hunter's syndrome were transduced with the vector and expressed high levels of IDS enzyme activity, 10-to 70-fold higher than normal human peripheral blood leucocyted or lymphoblastoid cell lines. The transduced cells failed to show accumulation of $^{35}SO_4$ into glycosaminoglycan, indicating that recombinant IDS enzyme participated in glycosaminoglycan metabolism.

3. MUCOPOLYSACCHARIDOSIS TYPE III

(Sanfilippo Syndrome)

The Sanfilippo syndrome, or mucopolysaccharidosis III, is a lysosomal storage disease due to impaired degradation of heparan sulfate. The syndrome is characterised by severe central nervous system degeneration, but only mild somatic disease. Onset of clinical features usually occurs between 2 and 6 years; severe neurologic degeneration occurs in most patients between 6 and 10 years of age, and death occurs typically during the second or third decade of life.

Types:
MPS III ***can be due*** to deficiency of four different enzymes concerned with the metabolism of heparan sulphate (Fig. 27.10) and hence have been classified accordingly.

- **Type A:** *Hepara N-sulfatase deficiency*
- **Type B:** *α-N-acetylgucosaminidase*
- **Type C:** *Acetly CoA: alpha-glucosaminide acetyltransferase*
- **Type D:** *N-acetylglucosamine 6-sulfatase*

Type A has been reported to be most severe, with earlier onset and rapid progression of symptoms and shorter survival.

3 A. MPS Type IIIA (Sanfilippo Syndrome A)

Alternative tiles: Heparan Sulfate Sulfatase Deficiency, Sulfamidase Deficiency

CLINICAL FEATURES

In the Sanfilippo syndrome, of which 4 enzymatically distinct forms are recognised, only heparan sulfate is excreted in the urine. The ***clinical features*** are ***severe mental defect*** with relatively mild somatic features (Moderately severe claw hand and visceromegaly, little or no corneal clouding or skeletal, e.g. vertebral change). The ***rediologic findings*** in the skeleton are relatively mild and include ***persistent biconvexity of the vertebral bodies*** and ***very thick calvaria.*** The presenting problem may be marked over-activity, destructive tendencies and other behavioural aberrations in a child of 4 to 6 years of age.

Incidence

In British Columbia, between 1952 and 1986, only 4 cases of MPS IIIA were observed, giving a frequency of 1 in 324,617 live births. Using multiple ascertainment sources, **Nelson et al (2003)** obtained an incidence rate for Sanfilippo syndrome (all forms combined) in Western Australia for the period 1969 to 1996 of approximately 1 in 58,000 live births.

Diagnosis

- **Prenatal diagnosis:** The conventional method for the prenatal diagnosis was based on ^{35}S-radiolabelled heparin incorporation into the cells from chorionic villus sampling or aminiotic fluid. **Kleijer et al (1996)** used an artificial substrate and a 2-step salfamidase assay. Unequivocal assignment of the fetal status in 5 affected pregnancies and 7 pregnancies with a normal outcome confirmed the reliability of the test.

- **Carrier testing:** Enzymatic methods to identify heterozygotes by studying leukocytes or fibroblasts have been described and are reasonably reliable.

CLINICAL MANAGEMENT

Severe behavioural disturbance is a very common feature of Sanfilippo syndrome, and one of the more difficult aspects of the disorder to manage. Many patients require hospitalisation in a closed psychiatric ward.

Robertson et al (1998) described a series of 6 patients with MPS III who had cerebrospinal shunts inserted in an attempt to ameliorate behaviour that had proved refractory to conventional treatment. Symptoms improved significantly in all the patients.

3 B. MPS Type III B (Sanfilippo Syndrome B)

Alternative titles: N-Acetyl-Alpha-D Glucosaminidase Deficiency, NAGlu Deficiency

Sanfilippo syndrome B is an ***autosomal recessive*** lysosomal storage disorder ***characterised by the accumulation of heparan sulfate.*** Sanfilippo syndrome B, or mucopolysaccharidosis type IIIB, is csused by mutation in the gene encoding N-alpha-acetylglucosaminidase (NAGLU).

Clinically, patients have progressive neurodegenertion, behavioural problems, mild skeletal changes, and shortened lifespan. The clinical severity ranges from mild to severe **(Chinen et al 2005).**

BIOCHEMICAL FEATURES

The ***biochemical defect*** in Sanfilippo syndrome B is the ***absence or decreased activity of alpha-N-acetylglucosaminidase enzyme.*** The ***gene*** for the enzyme has been mapped to the ***chromosome number 17 at locus 17q21.***

Although the enzyme deficiency can be demonstrated in the patients, there is a lot of heterogeneity among the heterozygous carriers. In fact, a so-called 'hyperactive' allele has been documented in which case the carriers might have an abnormally high activity of the enzyme. The findings suggest that normal levels of the NAGLU enzyme can be found in obligate heterozygotes due to heterozygocity of a 'hyperactive' gene with a 'deficient' gene.

DIAGNOSIS

- Abnormal excretion of heparan sulfate in the urine is the primary indicative test for the disorder.
- ***The deficiency of the enzyme glucosaminidase*** can be detected in the plasma and leukocytes.
- **Prenatal diagnosis:** The prenatal diagnosis of Sanfilippo syndrome B has been successfully achieved by ***chorionic villus sampling. Elevated heparan sulfate in the amniotic fluid complemented the enzyme assay.***

CLINICAL MANAGEMENT

Bone marrow transplant: Vellodi et al (1992) performed bone marrow transplantation in twin sisters with Sanfilippo syndrome B. The diagnosis was made at the age of 18 months and the transplant was first done from the haploidentical father. There was no engraftment in either, so a second transplant was carried out with success from the haploidentical mother. Follow-up for 9 years post-transplant showed that neither twin was as handicapped as the untreated brother at the same age; other evidence of beneficial effect was also recorded.

3C. MPS Type IIIC (Sanfilippo Syndrome C)

Alternative titles: Acetyl-CoA Alpha-Glucosaminide N-Acetyltransferase Deficiency

Mucopolysaccharidosis type IIIC, also known as Sanfilippo syndrome C, is caused by a deficiency of alpha-glucosaminide N-acetyltransferase (EC 2.3.1.3), an enzyme with properties of a lysosomal membrane transporter **(Ausseil et al 2004).** The syndrome comprises several forms of lysosomal storage disease due to impaired degradation o heparan sulfate. The deficient, an acetyltransferase, catalyses the conversion of alpha-glucosaminide residues to N-acetylglucosaminide in the presence of actyl-CoA.

CLINICAL FEATURES

The dysmorphic signs reported in some of the patients include ***coarse facies, hypertelorism, low-set ears, depressed nasal bridge, and coarse hair. Mild hepatosplenomegaly and high lumbar vertebral bodies*** are observed radiographically. They demonstrate delayed motor development. Urinary heparan sulfate excretion is increased.

BIOCHEMICAL FEATURES

The lysosomal-membrane enzyme deficient in MPS IIIC ***catalyses the transfer of an acetyl group*** from cytoplasmic acetyl-CoA to ***terminal alpha-glucosamine residues of heparan sulfate*** with lysosomes. ***It was the first non-hydrolytic acivity identified as occurring in lysosomes.*** The enzyme appears to carry out a ***transmembrane acetylation of glucosamine*** via a ping-pong mechanism.

Acetylation of terminal alpha-linked glucosamine residues inside the lysosome is a required step in the degradation of heparan sulfate. Although acetyl-CoA is the acetyl donor in this reaction. It is unlikely that this cofactor could exist stably in the acidic and hydrolytic ambience of the lysosome. N-acetyltransferase provides a means for cells to use cytoplasmically derived acetyl-CoA in heparan sulfate degradation without transporting the intact molecule across the lysosomal membrane. Vectorial transport of the acetyl group across the lysosomal membrane appears to be a unique solution to a complex enzymatic and compartmental problem.

DIAGNOSIS

Klein et al (1981) described ***an assay for the detection in leukocytes*** of homozygous and heterozygous carriers of Sanfilippo syndrome type C. Affected individuals had no residual activity of acetyl-CoA: alpha-glucosaminide N-acetyltransferase. It was also noted that the enzyme was strongly membrane-bound.

Prenatal diagnosis: MPS IIIC in a fetus has been ***diagnosed by enzymatic studies of chorionic villus biopsy material*** obtained at 10 weeks' gestation.

3D. MPS Type IIID (Sanfilippo Syndrome D)

Alternative titles: N-Acetylgucosamine-6-Sulfatase Deficiency

Mucopolysaccharidosis type IIID is ***caused by mutation in the gene encoding N-acetylglucosamine-6-sulfatase (GNS)*** and hence the deficiency of the corresponding enzyme. MPS IIID cannot be distinguished clinically from the other forms of Sanfilippo syndrome. The patients show coarse facies, mild mental retardation and 'characteristic behavioural disturbances'. The girls might show hirsutism. ***All patients excrete excessive heparan sulfate in the urine.*** Severe deficiency of N-acetylglucosamine-6-sulfate sulfatase can be demonstrated in cultured skin fibroblasts. Northern blot analyses in some patients show apparently normal mRNA for N-acetylgucosamine 6-sulfatase; thus, abnormal translation or premature degradation may be responsible for the enzyme defect.

Siciliano et al (1991) reported the cases of 2 adolescent sisters, the daughters of first-cousin Italian parents. The elder child was 19 years old. Her early milestones were mildly delayed: she was able to stand at 1 year and to walk by herself at 2 years. Speech began at the age of 2.5 years and was limited to a few words. At the age of 4, the patient started to show progressive speech loss and aggressive behavior. By age 10, she showed complete loss of contact with her environment and was unable to walk unaided.

The younger sister was somewhat less retarded and attended elementary school for 5 years. Although with little advance.

BIOCHEMICAL FEATURES

The cultured skin fibroblasts are unable to release sulfate from N-acetylglucosamine-6-sulfate linkages in heparan sulfate-derived oligosaccharides. Keratan sulfate-derived oligosaccharides bearing the same residue at the nonreducing end are normally degraded. The activity directed against heparan sulfate is deficient in this form of Sanfilippo syndrome, designated type D by **Kresse et al (1980).**

From genomic DNA of a patient with MPS IIID, **Mok et al (2003)** amplified and sequenced the promoter and 14 exons of GNS. ***They found a homozygous non-sense mutation in exon 9*** which predicted a premature termination mutation, arg 355 to ter (R355X). They also found 2 common synonymous coding SNPs and genotyped these in samples from 4 ethnic groups.

Independently, **Beesley et al (2003)** reported the molecular diagnosis of Sanfilippo disease type D, They identified a l-bp deletion in the GNS gene in an affected patient.

4. MPS TYPE IV (MORQUIO SYNDROME)

Alternative titles: Galactosamine-6-Sulfatase Deficiency; Galns Deficiency

4A. MPS IVA (MORQUIO SYNDROME A)

The condition described simultaneously and independently by Morquio (1929) in Montevideo, Uruguay, and Brailsford (1929) in Birmingham, England, was the entity in which we now recognise the occurrence of corneal clouding, aortic valve disease, and ***urinary excretion of keratosulfate.*** A miscellany of ***skeletal disorders*** are included in the Morquio category. These ***include*** various ***types of spondylo-epiphyseal dysplasia*** and ***multiple epiphyseal dysplasia.*** This and some other forms of spondylo-epiphyseal dysplasia are prone to the dangerous complications of ***atlantoaxial dislocation, due to hypoplasia of the odontoid. The classic oral abnormalities*** have been described as: ***maxillary anterior teeth being widely spaced snad flared.*** The posterior teeth are tapered and have pointed cusp tips. The enamel in some patients is pitted and in roentgenograms was less than one-fourth of its normal thickness. The hard palate was broad and flat.

The ***enzyme deficiency*** involves ***6 sulfatase,*** which works on both keratin sulfate and chondroitin sulfate, the defect concerns galactosamine-6-sulfate sulfatase. The fibroblasts from some cases of MPS IVA show deficiency of glycoprotein neuraminidase (sialidase; acylneuraminyl hydrolase; (EC 3.2.1.18) activity in addition to the expected deficiency of N-acetylgalactosamine-6-sulfate sulfatase (EC 3.1.6.4). Residual neuraminidase activity is low or low normal.

There are severe, intermediate, and mild forms of N-acetylgalactosamine-6-sulfate (GalNAc-6-S) sulfatase deficiency.

In British Columbia, between 1952 and 1986, 6 cases of MPS IVA were observed, giving a frequency of 1 in 216, 412 live births.

Using Multiple ascertainment sources, **Nelson et al (2003)** obtained an incidence rate for MPS IVA in Western Australia for the period 1969 to 1996 of approximately 1 in 6,40, 000 live births.

Diagnosis: ***Excretion of keratin sulfate is increases 2 to 3 times over normal. Examination of urinary glycosaminoglycans by two-dimensional (2D) electrophoresis technique*** proved to be reliable and efficient with no false-negative results.

Beck et al (1992) made the diagnosis of MPS IVA at 23 weeks of gestation. A previously born child was affected. Ultrasound showed moderate ascites, and keratin sulfate was found in the amniotic fluid. The diagnosis was confirmed after pregnancy termination.

4B. MPS TYPE IV (MORQUIO SYNDROME B) (Alternative Titles: β-Galactosidase Deficiency)

Arbisser et al (1977) reported a 14-year-old girl with mild dysostosis multiplex, odontoid hypoplasia, short stature, cloudy cornease, and keratinsulfaturia, but no detectable central nervous systems abnormalities. ***Betagalactosidase activity was deficient in cultured fibroblasts,*** but galactosamine-6-sulfate sulfatase activity (deficient in classic MPS IV A) was normal.

The ***enzyme system concerned in cleavage of galactose from complex carbohydrates*** and other substances involves a number of different beta-galactosidase activities such as:

- Gm(1)-beta-galactosidase isozymes A and B,
- A neutral beta-galactosidase
- A galactocerebroside-beta galactosidase. Therefore, some patients show the coexistence of GM1-gangliosidosis. Cell hybridization studies demonstrated that MPS IVB and the infantile and adult forms of GMI-gangliosidosis belong to the same complementation group.

4.6 MPS TYPE VI (MAROTEAUX-LAMY SYNDROME)

Alternative titles: Arylsulfatase B Deficiency; N-Acetylgalactosamine-4-Sulfatase Deficiency

The ***clinical characteristics*** of the Maroteaux-Lamy syndrome are ***striking osseous and corneal changes*** (like those of MPS I) ***without intellectual impairment*** until late, if at all. Only (or predominantly) ***chondroitin sulfate B is excreted in the urine.*** Of all the mucopolysaccharidoses, MPS VI usually shows the most striking ***inclusions in circulating white blood cells.***

Types

As in other mucopolysaccharidoses, as well as in other lysosomal diseases, mild and severe forms are observed.

- The ***classic form*** has severe physical changes, including hydrocephalus due to meningeal involvement, leading to death in the teens as a rule.
- The ***mildest form*** of the disease is characterised by short stature, corneal clouding, Legg-Perthes-like disease of the hips and aortic stenosis. Cases of intermedi-ate severity have also been observed.
- Glaucoma develops in a number of patients. It has been suggested that the initial mechanism is secondary angle closure due to thickening of the cornea. Obstruction of the trabecular meshworks by mucopolysaccharides, causing secondary open-angle glaucoma, is an alternative mechanism.

Diagnosis

In all forms of the disease, striking ***leukocyte inclusions*** and ***deficiency of arylsulfatase B*** (N-acetylgalactosamine 4-sulfatase) are found. ***Azurophilic cytoplasmic inclusions in the polymorphonuclear leukocytes,*** so-called ***Alder granules*** are more striking in MPS VI than in any of the other mucopolysaccharidoses, with the possible exception of MPS VII.

- With an ***immunochemical technique coupled with enzyme kinetic analysis, Brooks et al. (1990)*** described a monoclonal-based system for immunoquantification of the enzyme deficient in this disorder, which is normally present at low levels.

4.7 MPS TYPE VII (SLY SYNDROME) (Alternative titles: Beta-glucuronidase deficiency)

Sly et al. (1973) described a patient with skeletal changes consistent with a mucopolysaccharidosis, hepatosplenomegaly and granular inclusions in granulocytes. Fibroblasts demonstrated ***deficiency of beta-glucuronidase*** (EC 3.2.1.31). Both parents and several sibs of the mother showed an intermediate level of the enzyme. Later the syndrome came to be known as 'Sly Syndrome'. ***Asymptomatic thoracic kyphosis and mild scoliosis*** are the main clinical

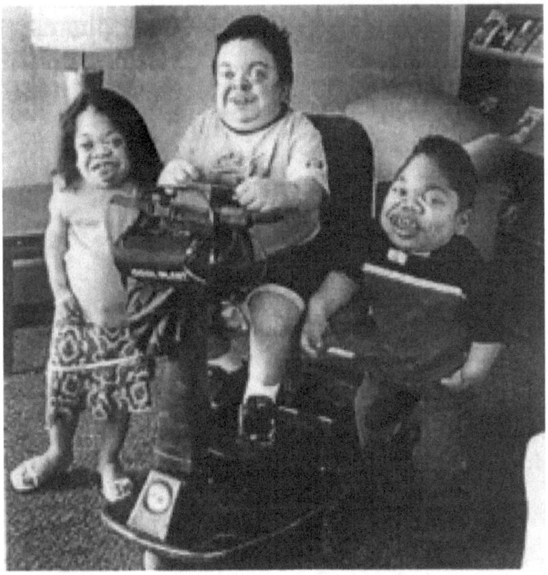

features. ***Hernia, hepatosplenomegaly, corneal clouding and dwarfing wear absent.***

MPA VII was the first ***autosomal*** mucopolysaccharidosis for which chromosomal assignment was achieved. Several laboratories confirmed the assignment of beta-glucuronidase to ***chromosome 7*** and refined it to the locus 7q21.1-q22.1

Prenatal diagnosis: The fact that beta-glucuronidase deficiency is the cause of non-immune hydrops fetalis and can be diagnosed by enzymatic assay of chorionic villi was demonstrated by van Eyndhoven et al (1998). ***Chorionic villus sampling was performed*** in the eleventh week and beta-glucuronidase deficiency in chorionic villi indicated that the foetus was affected. After termination in the twelfth week, signs of early hydrops fetalis were observed. The authors emphasised the significance to morphologic examination of the foetus and placenta for the diagnosis of MPS VII. ***Oedema of the neck and back*** makes a presumptive diagnosis of MPS VII, which can be confirmed by the finding of very low enzyme activity in chorionic villus cells.

Therapeutic enzymes: In enzyme replacement therapy for lysosomal storage diseases, infused therapeutic enzymes are targeted to lysosomes of affected cells by interactions with cell surface receptors that recognise carbohydrate moieties, scuch as mannose and mannose 6-phosphate, on the enzymes.

LeBowitz et al. (2004) ***tested an alternative, peptide-based targeting system for delivery of enzymes to lysosomes*** in a murine MPS VII model. This strategy depended on the interaction of a fragment of insulin-like growth factor II (IGF2), with the IGF II binding site on the bifunctional, IGF II cation-independent mannose 6-phosphate receptor. A chimeric protein containing a portion of mature human IGF II fused to the C terminus of human beta-glucuronidase was taken up by MPS VII firoblasts in a mannose 6-phosphate-independent manner, and its uptake was inhibited by the addition of IGF II. Furthermore, the tagged enzyme was delivered effectively to clinically significant tissues in MPS VII mice and was effective in reversing the storage pathology. Hopefully, the therapeutic enzymes would be developed further for all types of mucopolysaccharidosis and the future for these unfortunate group of patients could be brightened (Table 27.5).

Table 27.5: Types of mucopolysaccharidoses

Types	*Inheritance*	*Enzyme defect*	*Somatic skeletal changes*	*Mental retardation*	*Cardio-pulmonary*	*Hepato-splenomegaly*	*Corneal clouding*	*Hearing loss*	*Urinary MPS*
MPS-I (Hurler's syndrome)	Autosomal recessive	α-L-Iduronidase (A-Lysosomal hydrolase)	+++	Severe after one year	Valvular and coronary disease, Impaired ventilation	+++	Progressive	Present *(Conductive)*	Dermatan SO_4 *Heparan SO_4*
MPS-II (Hunter's syndrome)	Sex linked recessive	Iduronate sulfatase	++ to +++	Severe but gradual in onset	Valvular disease, pulmonary hypertension, impaired ventilation	+++	Rare	Present (early onset) *Perceptive*	—Do—
MPS-III SAN Filipos syndrome A, B & C	Autosomal recessive	A-sulfamidase B-α-N-acetyl Glucosaminidase C-Acetyl transferase	Mild	+++	Not described	++ (Moderate)	Absent	Present	Heparan SO_4
MPS-IV (Morquio syndrome)	" "	N-Acetyl galactosamine 6-sulfatase	+++	Absent or slight	Aortic regurgitation	Slight	Present, Late onset	Present, not severe	Keratan SO_4
MPS-V (Scheie syndrome)	Autosomal recessive	α-L-Iduro-nidase	Mild	Essentially absent	Aortic valvular disease	Variable	+++	Variable	Dermatan SO_4
MPS-VI (Maroteaux-Lamy syndrome)	" "	N-acetyl galactosamine 4-sulfatase *(Aryl sulfatase B)*	+++	Absent	Cardiac murmurs	Moderate ++	Present	"	Dermatan SO_4

B. Amino Acid Metabolic Disorders

B. 1 PHENYLKETONURIA

Alternative titles: Phenylalanine Hydroxylase Deficiency, Pah Deficiency, Oligophrenia, Phenylpyruvica Folling Disease, Hyperphenylalaninemia, Phenylalaninemia Phenylketonuria is an inborn error of metabolism resulting from a deficient activity of phenylalanine hydroxylase (EC 1. 14.16.1) and is characterized by hyperphenylalaninemia and mental retardation. The ***clinical features*** include a 'mousy' odor in urine; light pigmentation; peculiarities of gait, stance, and sitting posture; eczema; and epilepsy. Normal mental functionality is very rare among untreated patients with phenylketonuria. Barat et al. (2002) suggested that serum phenylalanine variations may contribute to osteopenia in patients with classic PKU.

The **incidence of PKU** varies in different populations across the world. Probably the hghest incidence has been reported from Ireland i.e. 1 per 4,500 in Ireland and the lowest among the Ashkenazi Jews. In Europe, PKU is found in about 1 per 12,000; while an average incidence of about 1 per 8, 000 has been reported in the US Caucasians. The data from Asian population is lacking.

Classical PKU is ***inherited*** in a strictly ***autosomal recessive*** manner and is the ***result of mutations in the structural gene for phenylalanine hydroxylase.*** Most variation in classical PKU is due to heterogeneity in the mutant alleles with many patients being compound heterozygotes rather than homozygotes for one particular mutant allele.

Early diagnosis of phenylketonuria (PKU), a cause of mental retardation, is important because it is treatable by dietary means. The basic defect in PKU is phenylalanine hydroxylase deficiency.

Widespread screening of neonates for phenylketonuria brought to light a class of patients with a disorder of phenylalanine metabolism milder than that in PKU. These patients show serum phenylalanine concentrations well below those in PKU, but still several times the normal values. These patients grouped as ***non-PKU hyperphenylalaninemia (HPA)*** have levels of phenylalanine hydroxylase about 5% of normal, although PAH activity lower than 20% of normal or plasma phenylalanine concentration above 600 micromol/1 is classified as phenylketonuria.

Intelligence quotient (IQ) is low in almost all the PKU subjects and has been correlated to the phenylalanine concentrations. Although early and continuous treatment (low phenylalanine diet) did not necessarily lead to normalization of overall IQ, brain phenylalanine concentration (determined by NMR spectroscopy) correlate very well with clinical phenotype. White-matter alterations are also observed in all patients.

Meternal Phenylketonuria

The occurrence of mental retardation in the offspring of homozygous mothers is an example of a genetic disease based on the genotype of the mother. Spontaneous first trimester abortions, intrauterine and postnatal growth retardation are common in PKU pregnancies; while ***microcephaly*** and even ***cardiac malformations*** may be present in the newborns. The frequency of congenital abnormalities increases with increasing maternal phenylalanine levels.

Biochemical Defect and Pathogenesis

The basic biochemical abnormality in PKU, as stated above, is the ***block at the conversion of phenylalanine to tyrosine by the enzyme phenylalanine hydroxylase. The resultant accumulation of phenylalanine and its alternate metabolic products viz. phenyl pyruvic acid, phenyl lactic acid and phenyl acetic acid*** along with the resultant deticiency of tyrosine contributes to most of the clinical features. ***Phenylpyruvic acid inhibits pyruvate decarbo-***

xylase in brain but not in liver and it has been suggested that this ***accounts for the defect in formation of myelin and mental retardation in this disease.*** It has been postulated that the significant incidence of learning disabilities even in treated patients with PKU may be due, in part, ***to reduced production of serotonin*** as a result of deficient tryptophan transport across the neuronal cell membrane. Tryptophan transport might be reduced owing to the competition from phenylalanine for the transporter. Children with phenylketonuria tend to have ***fair skin*** and ***fair hair*** which might be due to the impaired melanin synthesis.

The hydroxylation of phenylalanine is highly complex (Fig. 27.13). At least three enzymes are known to be involved and mutation at any one of the genes can affect the pace of the reaction. Furthermore, multiple alleles probably exist at the locus (or loci) determining the phenylalanine hydroxylase apoenzyme. Thus, there is much opportunity for many varieties of hyperphenylalaninemia. The phenylalanine hydroxylase in a patient with PKU could be a structurally altered form of the normal molecule that results form different allelic mutations in the structural gene. A total absence of PAH protein has also been reported even in the presence of normally active mRNA for PAH, which means that the mutations in the PAH gene might affect the translation or even stability of the protein.

Hyperphenylalaninemia may also result from a deficiency of Dihydropteridine Reducatse (DHPR) or from a defect in the synthesis of biopterin. These defects do not result in classic PKU but instead show defects in PAH and other enzymes dependent on the biopterin as cofactor. In contrast to classical PKU, the clinical syndromes resulting form defects in biopterin metabolism are not treatable with simple dietary phenylalanine restriction.

Classification

The PKU accordingly may be classified into the following types (Table 27.6) :

Table 27.6: Classification of phenylketonurias and their biochemical defects

Type	*Condition*	*Bilchemical Defect*
I	Classical PKU	Absent PAH activity
II	Presistent Hyperphenylalaninemia	Low PAH activity
III	Transient Mild Hyperphenylalaninemia	Maturational delay of PAH
IV	Dihydropteridine Reductase (DHPR) Deficiency	Deficient or Absent DHPR
V	Abnormal Dihydropteridine Function	Dihydropteridine synthesis defect

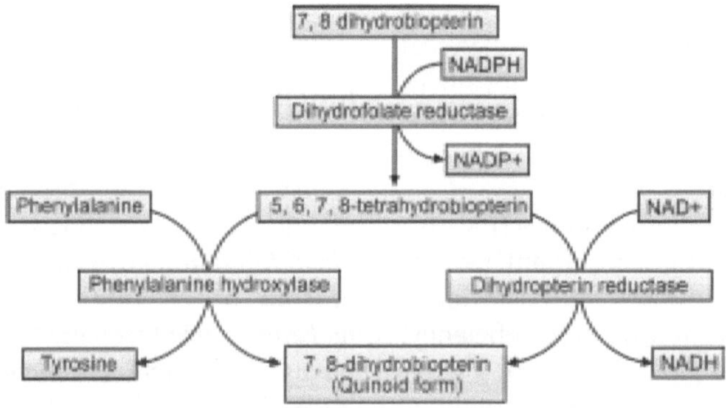

Fig. 27.13: Hydroxylation of phenylalanine and possible enzymes (red) responsible for phenylketonuria

Most PAH mis-sense mutation impair enzyme activity by causing increased protein instability and aggregation. The phenylalanine binding domains of PAH appear to reside on its N-terminal ***(46-48 and 65-69)*** and some N-terminal PAH mutation might be responsible for PKU due to impaired phenylalanine-mediated activation of PAH. With the help of *in vivo* NMR spectroscopic measurement of brain phenylalanine transport, Weglage et al. (2002) suggested that the transport of phenylalanine may vary from individual to individual. The blood-brain barrier transport characteristics and the resultant brain phenylalanine levels are causative factors for the individual clinical outcome in PKU patients.

By *in situ* hybridization, the PAH gene locus has been mapped to the chromosome #12 at locus 12q22-q24.1.

DIGNOSIS

1. *Blood and Urinary Phenylalanine levels:* Normal blood phenylalanine levels are 58+/-15μM/I in adults, 60+/-13 μM/1 in teenagers, and 62+/-18μM/1 (mean +/-SD) in childhood. In the newborn, the upper limit of normal is 120 μM/1 (2 mg/dl). In untreated classical PKU, blood levels as high as 2.4 mM/1 can be found.
2. *Ferric Chloride Screening Test:* Add a few drops of 10% ferric chloride solution to a small sample of urine of the patient in a test tube. Phenylpyruvic acid present in the urine acids a green of blue colour for one to two minutes; it then gradually fades. **Note:** The test must be carried out on ***fresh urine***
   - Phenylpyruvic acid may disappear quite rapidly in alkaline urine by oxidation
   - Ferric chloride Screening Test: $FeCl_3$ test is routinely used to screen for the PKU neonates.
3. *Guthrie's Test:* **Screening test** based on the Guthrie bacterial inhibition assay which based on the principle that the growth of bacteria on agar containing B-2 thienylalanine, a competitive inhibitor of phenylalanine, is a function of the phenylalanine added to the medium, makes use of the high serum phenylalanine (about 30 times normal). The inhibition is prevented by phenylalanine, phenylpyruvic acid and phenyllactic acid, an activity specific to these compounds. When a punched out disc of a paper is placed on the surface of the medium and incubated, these substances diffuse out and neutralize tha inhibitor. The spores then germinate and zone of growth appears around the disc, the diameter of which is related to their concentration in the blood, similar discs prepared form phenylalanine standards used for quantitative measurement. A droplet of blood obtained by heel-prick and dried on filter paper is obtained a few days after birth and assayed.
4. *Paper Chromatography:* Execssive urinary excretion of phenylalanine can easily be detected with the help of paper chromatography. The ***urine of the PKU patients have a 'mousy odor' due to excretion of phenyl acetic and phenyl lactic acids conjugated to glutamine.***
5. *RFLP and Prenatal Diagnosis:* Restriction Fragment Length Polymorphism (RFLP) has been used for the confirmation of mutations in the PAH gene. Many of these mutations have been shown to create/disrupt the restriction sites that could show up on the RFLP pattern of PCR amplified DNA. *Lidsky et al. (1985)* first reported the use of RFLP to achieve prenatal diagnosis of a PKU homozygote as well as heterozygote. Taking advantage of the 'illegitimate' transcription of the PAH gene in circulating lymphocytes, *Kalaydjieva et al. (1991)* identified 3 silent mutations in the PAH gene, in codons 232, 245, and 385, linked to specific RFLP haplotypes in several Caucasian populations. All 3 mutations created a new restriction site and were easily detected on PCR-amplified DNA. The combined analysis of these markers and 1 or 2 PKU mutations formed a simple panel of diagnostic tests that could be used for the prenatal diagnosis in

the progeny of PKU families. *Forrest et al. (1991)* used a modification of the chemical cleavage of mismatch (CCM) method to identify mutations in PAH in PKU. They stated that 'judicious choice of probes gives the CCM method the potential to detect close to 100% of single-base mutations'.

CLINICAL MANAGEMENT

Phenylketonuria is ***treatable by a low phenylalanine diet.*** In treated patients, severve white matter abnormalities are predominantly associated with blood phenylalanine levels above 15 mg/dl. A study of well controlled PKU (blood phenylalanine levels <10 mg/dl) has shown that ***the brain damage visible on MRI can be eliminated/minimized by the low phenylalanine diet.*** The IQ of the affected children can also be brought to near normal provided the therapy is started within two weeks of birth. Earlier view of the scientists that the dietary restriction may be lifted after 8 years of age, have now been challenged and it has suggested that the continuation of diet restriction would be beneficial for the patients.

The fetal damage from maternal PKU can also be largely and perhaps entirely prevented by dietary therapy, but that therapy must begin before conception for the best chance of a normal infant. *Fisch et al. (1993)* suggested that surrogate motherhood should be recommended as alternative management of PKU in women who wish to have children.

- **Hoskins *et al.* (1980)** showed that the ***plant enzyme phenylalanine ammonia lyase*** (PAL; EC 4.3.1.5) ***will survive in the gut long enough to deplete the phenylalanine derived from food protein*** and so ***reduce the rise in blood phenylalanine*** that otherwise occurs after a protein meal. **Sarkissian et al (1999)** described ***usage of ancillary PAL to degrade phenylalanine.*** PAL, a robust enzyme without need for a cofactor, ***converts phenylalanine to trans-cinnamic acic,*** a harmless metabolite. They concluded that the ***appropriate dosage of orally administered PAL, perhaps in combination with a controlled and moderately low protein diet,*** should effectively control the phenylalanine pool size through its effect on the gastrointestinal tract. **These findings opened a new avenue to the treatment of this classic genetic disorder.** It is hoped that an efficient recombinant approach would be adopted to produce large quantities of PAL enzyme using a construct of the PAL gene from *Rhodosporidium toruloides* and expressing it in a strain of *E. coli* and ***PAL enzyme might become a standard therapeutical tool along with dietary manipulation for the treatment of PKU.***
- ***Liver transplantation*** is not a usual therapy for PKU because of the usually good results achieved with early dietary restriction and because liver disease is not part of the clinical picture of PKU. Still some orthotopic liver transplantation have been successfully tried.
- A low phenylalanine diet is also low in the long-chain polyunsaturated fatty acids (LCPUFA), necessary for cell membrane formation and normal brain and visual development; therefore, ***PCPUFA should also be supplemented in case of PKU.*** The children who receive supplementation show a significant increase in docosahexaenoic acid (DHA) levels of erythrocyte lipids and improved visual function, as measured by a decreased p100 wave latency.
- ***Therapeutic efficacy of tetrahydrobiopterin for the treatment of mild phenylketonuria has also been recommended in PKU,*** particularly for the mild phenylketonuria patients. Phenylalanine oxidation has been shown to be significantly enhanced in 23 out of 31 patients. Conversely, the patients with classic phenylketonuria show no response to tetrahydrobiopterin. Long-term treatment with tetrahydrobiopterin in children increases daily phenylalanine tolerance, allowing them to discontinue their restricted diets. ***Matalon et al. (2004)*** found that 21 out of 36 ***(58.3%) PKU patients responded***

favorably to oral tetrahydrobiopterin (BH4) supplementation. A single dose of 10 mg/kg resulted in a mean decrease of greater than 30% in blood phenylalanine levels. Patients who responded were found to have mutations in the PAH gene within the catalytic, regulatory, oligomerization, and BH4-binding domains.

B. 2 TYROSINEMIAS

Tyrosinemias are a group of inherited disorders ***characterized by levels of amino acid tyrosine and their catabolic intermediates*** in blood and their ***excretion in urine.*** Since the patients might differ in their clinical presentation and the biochemical etiology, tyrosinemias have been classified as follows:

B.2.1 Tyrosinemia, Type I

Alternative titles: Hepatorenal Tyrosinemia, Tyrosinosis, Fumarylacetoacetase Deficiency, Fumarylacetoacetate Hydrolase (FAH) Deficiency.

Among the children of first-cousin parents, **Lelong et al. (1963)** was the first to suggest that ***cirrhosis, Fanconi renotubular syndrome, high plasma tyrosine*** and ***hepatosplenomegaly*** could be due to a defective enzyme involved with tyrosine metabolism.

Tyrosinosis is ***characterized*** by ***accumulation of tyrosine*** and a number of metabolites and derivatives of the intermediates of tyrosine metabolism. ***Biochemical studies show generalized aminoaciduria, marked elevation of methionine*** in the serum in a number of patients, and a disproportionately ***high urinary excretion of methionine.*** The ***hypertrophy of the islets of Langerhans*** is also seen probably ***due to stimulation by methionine*** or one of its metabolites. Hypermethioninemia may be secondary to liver failure.

Biochemical Defect: Any of the enzymes involved in tyrosine metabolism can cuse the features of tyrosinemia but most commonly it is due to the deficiency of fumaryl acetoacetate (EC 3.7.1.2). This ***leads to accumulation of succinylacetone (SA) and succinylacetoacetate (SAC). Porphobilinogen synthase activity*** is always is always ***low*** in these patients as it is also ***inhibited by these substances.*** It has been suggested that the severe liver and kidney damage during tyrosinemia is caused by accumulation of tyrosine metabolites. A puzzling feature of hereditary tyrosinemia has been episodes similar to acute hepatic porphyria, ***with excretion of δ-aminolevulinic acid*** in the urine. The inhibition of porphobilinogen synthase explains this feature.

In Type I tyrosinemia, the defect in FAH, the last enzyme in the tyrosine catabolism pathway, results in accumulation of succinylacetone (SA) that reacts with amino acids and proteins to form stable adducts via Schiff's base formation, lysine being the most reactive amino acid. Patients with this disorder surviving beyond infancy are at considerable ***risk for the development of hepatocellular carcinoma, and a high level of chromosomal breakage is observed n tyrosinemia cells, suggesting a defect in the processing of DNA.*** By *in situ* hybridization, **Berube et al. (1989)** assigned the **FAH gene to 15q23-q25.**

Clinical features: Both acute and the chronic forms of tyrosinemia type 1 are known.

a. **Acute Tyrosinosis:** The infants exhibit diarrhea, vomiting and a ***'cabbage like' odor.*** They do not thrive well and there is usually ***associated liver damage.*** Untreated patients do not survive and death occurs due to liver failure within 6 to 8 months.
b. **Chronic Tyrosinosis:** Clinical features are similar as in acute form but with milder symptoms and course. Children survive and untreated cases lead to death by the age of 10 years.

The disorder usually progresses in ***three stages:***

- Stage I: Infants exhibit hepatic necrosis and hypermethioninemia.
- Stage II: Nodular cirrhosis and chronic hepatic insufficiency without hypermethioninemia are found.

- Stage III: Renal tubular damage ***(Baber syndrome),*** often with hypophosphatemic rickets, appears.

Cardiomyopathy, usually subclinical, is a frequent finding. Neurologic crisis that usually begins at the mean age of 1 year and frequently is the cause of hospitalization. These abrupt episodes of peripheral neuropathy are characterized by severe pain with extensor hypertonia, vomiting or paralytic ileus, muscle weakness and occasionally self-mutilation. The neurologic crisis could be fatal. Low tyrosine diet arrests progression of the disease.

Diagnosis and Biochemical Findings

- ***High levels of Tyrosine can be demonstrated in blood*** (6-10 mg/dl) and urine. The traditional approach to screening for tyrosinemia, was based on the fluorometric determination of tyrosine on the first dried blood spot received by neonatal screening programs.
- ***Loading test with tyrosine and with p-hydroxyphenylpyruvic acid (PHPPA)*** can be used to detect *p*-hydroxyphenylpyruvate oxidase activity, which can be confirmed by enzyme assay in liver biopsy samples.
- ***In the urine, Alpha-keto-gamma-methylbutyric acid is present and may account for the peculiar odor.*** In some patients, PHPPA, *p*-hydroxyphenylacetic acid and *p*-hydroxyphenyllactic acid are excreted in unusually large amounts due to a concomitant lack of liver *p*-hydroxyphenylpyruvate oxidase activity (Tyrosinemia type III). Urinary excretion of δ-aminolevulinic acid, a neurotoxic intermediate of porphyrin biosynthesis, is elevated during crisis as well as during asymptomatic periods.
- ***An enzyme-linked immunosorbent assay (ELISA) to measure the deficient enzyme in dried blood spots has been developed.*** The acute form of hereditary tyrosinemia has absence of FAH enzyme protein, whereas the chronic form has presence of immunoreactive emzyme protein.
- **Prenatal diagnosis** is possible either by the ***detection of succinylacetone in the amniotic fluid or the measurement of fumarylacetoacetate in cultured amniotic cells.*** The enzymatic diagnosis could also be feasible in chorionic villus material. It has been showed that normal red cells have fumarylacetoacetase activity and thus studies of red cells should permit rapid diagnosis and recognition of heterozygotes.
- As an aid to early diagnosis for early institution of drug therapy, **Holme and Lindstedt (1992)** suggested a neonatal screening test based on the measurement of porphobilinogen synthase activity, the activity of this enzyme is almost always lower in patients with tyrosinemia type I.

Treatment

- ***Diet Management:*** Dietary restriction of tyrosine can help the patients to over the acute phase but it has been shown, however, that liver damage is prenatal in onset (as indicated by greatly elevated alpha-fetoprotein in cord blood) and that hypertyrosinemia developed only postnatally. Thus, therapy aimed at reduction of the elevated tyrosine level is unlikely to be of fundamental value.
- ***Liver Transplant: The permanent cure could only be achived by the liver transplant.*** During the pretransplant period, intensive medical support and restriction of dietary tyrosine must be initiated to improve the patient's condition and promote weight gain.
- ***Alternatives to liver transplant:*** Lindstedt et al. (1992) and Holme and Lindstedt (1998) treated type I tyrosinemia patients with a ***potent inhibitor of 4-hydroxyphenylpyruvate dioxygenase*** (EC 1.13.11.27) to prevent the formation of maleylacetoacetate and fumarylacetoacetate and their saturated derivatives. The agent used was ***2-(2-nitro-4-trifluoromethylbenzoyl)-1, 3-cyclohexane-dione (NTBC).***

Signs of improvement included decrease in several metabolites, correction of the almost complete inhibition of porphobilinogen synthase in erythrocytes, decrease in alpha-fetoprotein, improved liver and renotubular functions, and regression of hepatic abnormalities by computed tomography. No side effects were encountered. Inhibition of 4-hydroxyphenylpyruvate dioxygenase may prevent the development of liver cirrhosis and abolish or diminish the risk of liver cancer. Furthermore, normalization of porphyrin synthesis should eliminate the risk of porphyric crisis. Only 10% of the patients had not responded clinically to NTBC treatment.

- Another therapeutic agent, ***Nitisinone, a triketone herbicide that inhibits 4-hydroxyphenylpyruvate dioxygenase*** by rapid, avid and reversible binding has been very successful in the treatment of tyrosinemia type I. *The agent has been approved by the FDA for the treatment of tyrosinemia type I.*

B. 2.2 Tyrosinemia Type II

(Alternative Titles: *Richnar-Hanhart syndrome,* Tyrosine Aminotransferase Deficiency; TAT Deficiency, Keratosis Palmoplantaris With Corneal Dystrophy, Oregon Type Tyrosinemia, Oculocutaneous Type Tyrosinosis)

Richner (1938) and **Hanhart (1947)** described an ***oculocutaneous syndrome characterized*** by herpetiform ***corneal ulcers*** and painful punctuate ***keratoses*** of digits, palms, and soles with severe ***mental and somatic retardation.*** This condition is also known as tyrosinemia with palmar and plantar keratosis and keratitis. Later it was observed that these patients have tyrosinemia and hydroxyphenylpyruvic acid was elevated in the urine and it was labeled as oculocutaneous tyrosinosis. The disorder shows heterogeneity in the clinical presentation and some of the patients might just have the cutaneous features without involvement of the eyes.

The ultrastructural changes show thickening of the granular layer and increased synthesis of tonofibrils and keratohyalin; in the ridged palmar or plantar skin, large numbers of microtubules and unusually tight packing of tonofibrillar masses, which contained tubular channels or inclusions of microtubules. The authors assumed that increased cohesion and tight packing of tonofilaments prevement normal spreading of keratohyalin and result in its globular appearance.

Biochemical Defect: The biochemical basis of tyrosinemia type II is a ***deficiency of soluble tyrosine transaminase*** (EC 2.6.1.5) ***deficiency*** (Fig. 27.14) *p*-hydroxyphenylpyruvic acid oxidase is normal that distinguishes it from tyrosinemia type I. ***Plasma phenylalanine lebels are normal.*** The mitochondrial form of tyrosine amino-transferase (TAT) was present in the liver. The soluble form of TAT was lacking. The patient had markedly elevated tyrosine blood levels aassociated with an increase in urinary *p*-hydroxyphenylacetate and *p*-hydroxyphenyllactate. Levels of *p*-hydroxyphenylpyruvate may be normal. Excessive amounts of intracellular tyrosine enhance crosslinks between aggregated tonofilaments resulting in the skin lesions and the ocular plaque formation.

The tyrosine aminotransferase gene has been assigned to 16q22-q24 by means of a gene clone in somatic cell hybrid analysis. The patients with deletion around this gene could also show the absence of some other genes like hapatoglobin gene which is adjacent to the TAT gene.

The maternal tyrosinemia has an adverse effect on the developing fetus and hence the offsprings, even if with normal TAT, could end up with microcephaly and mental retardation.

Diagnosis: The diagnosis is generally made on the ***basis of skin/eye lesions along*** with ***elevated levels of tyrosine in plasma. The TAT enzyme activity may be measured in the liver*** biopsy samples or skin fibroblasts.

Management: Diet restricted in phenylalanine and tyrosine, particularly if initialized in the early infancy, helps in preventing the mental retardation.

B-2.3 Tyrosinemia, Type III

Alternative titles: 4-α-Hydroxyphenylpyruvic Acid Oxidase Deficienty, 4-α-Hydroxyphenylpyruvate Dioxygenase Deficiency.

Tyrosinemia Type III is an ***autosomal recessive disorder*** caused by a ***deficiency in the activity of p-hydroxyphenylpyruvate dioxygenase (HPPD)*** (Fig. 27.14) and is ***characterized*** by elevated levels of blood tyrosine and massive excretion of its derivatives, *p*-OH-phenylpyruvic and *p*-OH-phenyllactic acid into urine. Patients with this disorder have ***mild mental retardation*** and/or ***convulsions,*** with the ***absence of liver damage.***

The first case was reported by *Giardini et al. (1983)* in a 17-month-old girl who had acute intermittent ataxia and drowsiness. Her psychomotor development was normal. The authors described tyrosinemia without liver dysfunction due apparently to deficiency of 4-hydroxyphenylpyruvate dioxygenase (4HPPD). In liver biopsy tissue there was no detectable activity of 4HPPD, either in the whole homogenate or in the cytosol *fraction.*

Gene Map

The gene for the enzyme 4HPPD has been assigned to ***chromosome 12 at locus*** 12q24-qter and a number of pathogenic mis-sense and nonsense mutations have been reported at the locus.

B. 3 ALBINISM

History

Famous albinos include Noah of flood fame and the Reverend Dr Spooner. Spooner was a brilliant classicist at Oxford whose amusing tendency to errors of speech came to be known as spoonerisms. Although probably elaborated on by students, the aberration appears to have been market. As a classicist, Spooner must have read extensively. The aberration of speech was probably related to his nystagmus which caused a jumbling of information from the printed page. His intelligence was such that his mind comprehended despite the jumbling, but a jumbling of sorts occurred with oral output.

Introduction

Albinism includes a spectrum of clinical syndromes characterized by 'hypomelanosis', arising from ***inherited defects in the pigment cells (melanocytes) of eye and skin.*** Albinism is one of the earliest inherited traits studies.

Biochemical Features

Skin colour of all humans is due to the epidermal pigment, Melanin; the differences in skin colour across the world arise due to the amount of melanin as well as the size and shape of the melanin containing granules. ***Melanin is synthesized from phenylalanine/tyrosine amino acids*** through the intermediates ***3, 4-dihydroxy phenylalanine (DOPA) and DOPA-quinone (see figure 27.14)***

In the albino, the ganglion cell layer does not thin out in the foveolar pit put shows a layer 6 to 8 cells thick where there should be none. There is therefore ample reason for the uncorrectable defective central fixation, and the ocular nystagmus, in this case of the optical variety. The optical coherence tomography (OCT) could be used to document foveal hypoplasia in patients with oculocutaneous albinism.

All types of conditions with oculocutaneous or ocular hypopigmentation in man and animals with nystagmus tested to date have shown either electrophysiologic or anatomic evidence of a decussation defect in the optic tracts.

Using MRI, *Schmitz et al. (2003)* found that the size and configuration of the optic chiasma in humans with albinism are distinctly different from those of normal control subjects.

Amelanic melanocytes are present in the skin of albinos. These contain granules similar to the premelanosomes of normal melanocytes. In the test developed by *King and Witkop (1977)* which determines free (unbound) tyrosine, heterozygotes have shown little or no tyrosinase activity. It was postulated that whatever tyrosinase is

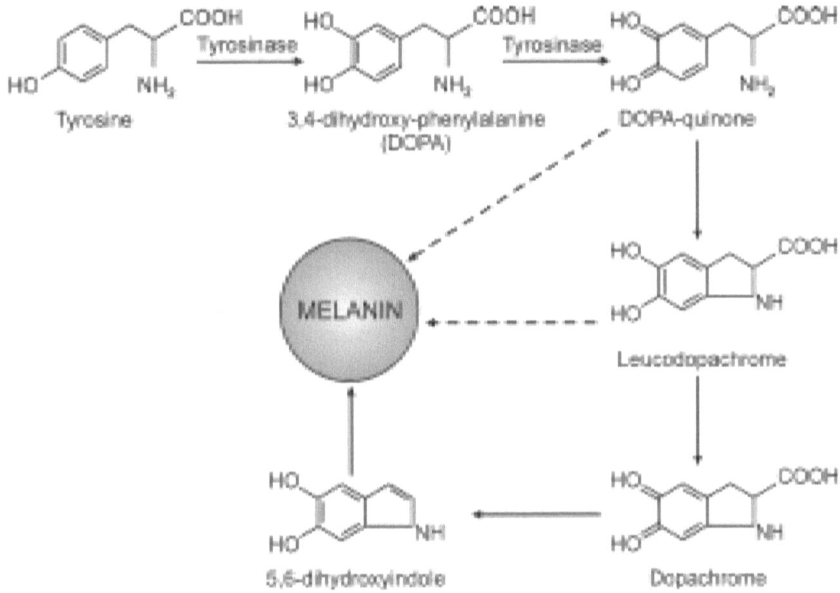

Fig. 27.14: Biosynthesis of Melanin from Tyrosine

synthesized in the heterozygotes is immediately bound to the melanosome matrix.

The yellow form of albinism is clinically similar to the tyrosinase-positive albinism, but that the hair bulbs show organelles similar to the pheomelanosomes of red hair and absence of tyrosinase activity. Unlike OCA1A, the melanosomes in OCAIB contain residual amounts of melanin and may include the more developed stage III premelanosomes and stage IV melanosomes.

MOLECULAR GENETICS

Tyrosinase enzyme gene has been ***mapped to locus 11q14-q21 on chromosome 11.*** In classic tyrosinase-negative OCA, a thr-to-lys substitution that abolished 1 of 6 putative N-linked glycosylation sites was detected. In one of the studies no cases of tyrosinase gene deletions or other rearrangements were found, even in DNAs from patients with both tyrosinase-deficient oculocutaneous albinism and mental retardation. The families studied exhibited several different pigmentation phenotypes suggesting that tyrosinase-deficient OCA results from ***heteroallelism for different small defects of the tyrosinase gene.*** More than 60 independent albinism-producing alleles have been described at the TYR locus.

In patients with yellow OCA, a pro81-to-leu substitution the may interfere with the normal folding of the tyrosinase polypeptide has been reported. In the temperature sensitive phenotype, the R402Q mutation in the tyrosinase gene is responsible for a temperature-sensitive enzyme resulting in peripheral pigmentation.

Types of Albinism

Albinism is divided broadly into **two categories** based on the distribution of the hypopigmented tissues viz. **Oculocutaneous albinism** and **Ocular albinism.** In the first, pigment is absent both in the eyes and in the skin; in ocular albinism, only eye pigment is missing. For both forms of oculocutaneous albinism, affected persons are ***homozygous*** for an ***autosomal recessive gene, wherease ocular albinism is transmitted as an X-linked recessive.*** In addition to these types of albinism, there are several rare forms as well as several other diseases that involve hypopigmentation.

Albinism can be grouped into tyrosinase-positive or tyrosinase-negative:

a. ***Tyrosinase-positive:*** Apparently these albinos have ***normal tyrosinase activity,*** which cannot act on tyrosine *in vivo.* It has been suggested that the ***defect probably lies in the transport of tyrosine into the melanocytes.*** In most cases, they show some degree of pigmentation. Hair colour ranges from white yellow to light tan. Lightly coloured naevi may be present. Hair bulbs from these individuals may be able to convert added tyrosine to pigment "Eumelanin" *in vitro.* ***Melanocytes in these patients contain lightly pigmented melanosomes. Tyrosine-positive albinos may have traces of pigment and acquire more pigment as they age.*** A tyrosinase-positive albino African adult may have darker skin than a normally pigmented blond European.

b. ***Tyrosine-negative:*** These albinos ***completely lack visual pigment.*** The ***melanocytes lack tyrosinase activity,*** and the mutation is thought to be in the structural gene for this enzyme. Tyrosinase-negative albinos are completely without pigment throughout their lives.

B. 3.1 Oculocutaneous Albinism (OCA)

I. Oculocutaneous Albinism Type I (OCAI): Oculocutaneous albinism Type I is an ***autosomal recessive disorder characterized by absence of pigment in hair, skin, and eyes,*** and does not vary with race or age. Severe nystagmus, photophobia and reduced visual acuity are common features. OCAI is devided into the following ***subtypes:***

a. ***Type IA, characterized by complete lack of tyrosinase activity*** due to production of an inactive enzyme.

b. ***Type IB (OCAIB),*** (YELLOW MUTANT TYPE, YELLOW ALBINISM) ***characterized by reduced activity of tyrosinase.*** The homozygote is 'dead white' at birth, with serious ocular abnormalities, but rather rapidly develops normal skin pigmentation and yellow hair. The condition differs from albinism II in the yellow hair and the fact that incubation with L-tyrosine or L-DOPA yields equivocal results.

c. ***Atemperature sensitive phenotype OCA*** has also been reported—the patients have white hair in the warmer areas (scalp and axilla) and progressively darker hair in the cooler areas (extremities) of their bodies. Tyrosinase assay demonstrated a loss of activity above 35-37 °C.

II. Oculocutaneous Albinism Type II (OCA2): In OCA2, some pigment is present at birth but is lost later. Tyrosinase-positive oculocutaneous albinism (OCA, type II) is the most prevalent type of albinism throughout the world; the overall frequency of OCA2 in the United States as approximately 1 per 36,000.

Throughout sub-Saharan Africa, it is responsible for a great deal of morbidity, with skin cancer and gross visual impairment being important sequelae.

The *mutations* causing OCA2 are located on p-locus of the tyrosinase gene.

III. Oculocutaneous Albinism Type III: The phenotype is caused by mutation in tyrosinase-related protein-1 (TYRP1). First detected in Nigeria, the albinos are tyrosinase-positive. Sun sensitivity is less marked and in most cases retinal pigment is present on fundoscopy. Nystagmus and strabismus are present in less than one fifth of the patients. Red reflex on transillumination of the iris and nystagmus are important clues to the diagnosis. In New York City, numerous cases are seen in Puerto Rican families. Albinism in dark-skinned persons such as Puerto Ricans is not always obvious because freckled skin and reddish hair may be present.

Melanocytes from the patients exhibit normal amounts of soluble melanin in the supernatants. However, significant reduction in the amount of insoluble melanin in melanocytes is observed. Ultrastructural studies of cultured melanocytes revealed that the melanocytes of the affected patients contained only early melanosomes.

Absence of Tyrosine-related protein in these patients results in a reduction in tyrosine hydroxylase activity in melanocytes due to the regulatory role of TYRP1 on tyrosine hydroxylase activity of tyrosinase.

Mutation causing OCAIII has been located to Gene map locus 9p23.

IV. Oculocutaneous Albinism Type IV (OCA4): This form of oculocutaneous albinism has been found to be ***caused by mutation in the MATP gene.*** Phenotype is identical to that in OCA2. Owing to the fact that ***several alleles of the mouse 'underwhite' (uw) gene cause generalized hypopigmentation, Newton et al. (2001)*** studied the humen homolog of the mouse underwhite gene, MATP. In a Turkish patient with generalized hypopigmentation and ocular abnormalities 'whithin the phenotypic range commonly associated with OCA2', they identified a homozygous G-to-A transition in the splice acceptor sequence of exon 2. The patient's parents were heterozygous for the mutation. ***OCA4 is one of the most common types of albinism in Japan.***

B-3.2 Ocular Albinism

Ocular albinism Type 1 ***(OCI) (Nettleship-Falls type Ocular Albinism):*** This is ***X-linked ocular type albinism*** with the papillary reflex characteristic of albinism. The fundus is depigmented and the choroidal vessels stand out strikingly. Nystag-mus, head nodding, and impaired vision also occur. ***Pigmentation is normal elsewhere except in the eye.*** In carrier females the fundus. Especially in the periphery, shows a mosaic of pigmentation. Nystagmus is an associated feature. In fact, the ocular albinism has been commented on only obliquely or not at all in some reports of X-linked nystagmus in families that almost certainly had ocular albinism. ***The gene for ocular albinism has been mapped to Gene map locus Xp22.3.***

DIAGNOSIS

The elective abortion of albino fetuses is difficult to defend because of the satisfactory adjustment and even success in some areas of activity of albino individuals. Persistent ocular albinism and nystagmus permit accurate diagnosis in the adult.

Shimizu et al. (1994) made the prenatal diagnosis of tyrosinase-negative OCA by ***an electronmicroscopic DOPA reaction test of fetal skin at 20 weeks' gestation.*** A previous child born with albinism was 9 years old at the time; the pregnancy in which the diagnosis had been made was terminated at 21 weeks.

B.4 ALKAPTONURIA

Alternative titles: AKU, Homogentisic Acid Oxidase Deficiency

Alkaptonuria enjoys the historic distinction of being one of the first conditions in which Mendelian recessive inheritance was proposed (by Garrod, 1902, on the suggestion of Bateson) and of being one of the four conditions in the charter group of inborn errors of metabolism. *Stenn et al. (1977)* provided evidence that the Egyptian mummy Harwa, dating from 1500 BC, had alkaptonuria.

The ***manifestations*** are ***urine that turns dark on standing*** and ***alkalinization, black ochronotic pigmentation of cartilage*** and collagenous tissues, and ***arthritis,*** especially characteristic in the spine. The patients with Alkaptonuria show unusual stress, ochromotic arthropathy and are ***at risk of calcification of coronary artery and aortic valve secondary to ochronosis.*** There are reports of urolithiasis in AKU patients in middle and late adulthood who have already developed the full clinical picture of the disorder, but urolithiasis as early as at two years of age has been reported. Phornphutkul et al (2002) provided a revieew of the natural history of alkaptonuria. They based the review on an evaluation of 58 patients with the disorder ranging in age from 4 to 80 years. They found that joint replacement was performed at a mean age of 55 years and that renal stones developed at 64 years, cardiac-valve involvement at 54 years, and coronary artery calcification at 59 years. Linear regression analysis indicated that the radiographic score for the severity of disease begain increasing after the age of 30 years, with a more rapid increase in men than in women. they reported that kidney stones were documented in 13 male and 3 female patients. Of the 27 men who were 31 to 60 years old, 8 had prostate stones. The development of prostate stones was not associated with the development of kidney stones. Three patients, each over the age of 50 years, had undergone aortic valve replacement.

Biochemical Defect: The ***enzymatic defect*** lies in the ***deficiency of Homogentisic acid oxidase*** involved in the breaking of the phenyl ring to form malleylacetoacetate during the catabolism of phenylalanine and tyrosine. ***Homogentisic acid and its toxic derivative, benzoquinone acetic acid (BQA) bind to the collagenous fibres causing the ochronosis and arthritis.*** Benzoquinone acetic acid is also responsible for the darkening of urine on alkalinization and on standing.

Genetic defect: The gene for homogentisic acid oxidase has been ***mapped on chromosome 3 at the locus 3q21-q23. Co-inheritacne of hypocalcuric hypercalcemia (hyperparathy-roidism) and sucrose-iso-maltase deficiency*** has been observed due to adjacent location of the genes.

Incidence: Alkaptonuria was found to be unusually frequent in the Dominican Republic and in Slovakia. As many as 126 cases had been reported from Czechoslovakia, 108 from Germany and 90 cases of alkaptonuria had been reported from the United States till 1963.

Diagnosis: A. Screening Tests

- ***Benedict's test:*** Homogentisic acid excreted in urine reduce alkaline copper sulphate solution. Thus on boiling with Benedict's Qualitative reagent a *greenish-brown colour* first results givins a ***brownish precipitate*** when allowed to settle
- ***Ferric Chloride test:*** Like Phenylketonuria, a positive ferric chloride test is obtained in alkaptonuric urine.

On adding a few drops of 10% ferric chloride solution to a few ml of urine a ***transient blue or green colour*** is obtained in alkaptonuria.

- ***Ammoniacal silver nitrate test:*** When a few drops of 10% ammonia are added to a mixture of 0.5 ml urine and 5 ml of 3% silver nitrate solution, a *black colour* is produced.

The mixture must not be exposed to direct sunlight.

B. Estimation of Homogentisic Acid

Homogentisic acid can be estimated by using the colour produced with ammonium molybdate and potassium dihydrogen phosphate, using as standard a solution of hydroquinone similarly treafar

Procedure

Take 1 or 2 ml of urine, dilute to 15 ml with water, add 2 ml of 5% ammonium molybdate in 5 N sulphuric acid and 2 ml of 1% of potassium dihydrogen phosphate and dilute to 25 ml. Treat a hydroquinone standard containing 1 mg per ml in the same way. *One mg of hydroquinone equals to 0.79 mg of homogentisic acid.*

Note:

If albumia is present in the urine, it must be removed before the estimation is done.

CLINICAL MANAGEMENT

- The rational and recommended treatment in the management of alkaptonuria is ***long term administration of ascorbic acid (1 g/day). The antioxidant effect of ascorbic acid prevents the oxidation of homogentisic acid to BQA and hence excretion of BQA in the urine is decreased.*** The reduced BQA formation could prevent or slow down the process of deposition of the molecule in connective tissue and hence the development of arthritis and ochronosis. The excretion of BQA in urine is substantially reduced whereas the excretion of homogentisic acid remains almost unaffected.

- The other therapeutic approaches include ***2 (-2-nitro-4-trifluoromethylbenzoyl)-1, 3-cyclohexanedione (NTBC), a potent inhibitor of p-hydroxyphenylpyruvate dioxygenase,*** which catalyzes the formation of homogentisic acid from *p*-hydroxyphenyl-pyruvate acid, and had been used in the treatment of type I tyrosinemia. A dose dependent reduction in the urinary output of homogentisic acid is observed.
- **Phornphutkul et al. (2002)** reported the treatment of a 51-year-old woman with ***nitisinone. Nitisinone is a triketone herbicide that inhibits 4-hydroxyphenylpyruvate dioxygenase by rapid, avid binding that is reversible.*** The agent has been approved by the FDA for the treatment of tyrosinemia type I but can also be useful for the management of AKU. Urinary HGA excretion fell from 2.9 to 0.13 g per day after a 10-day course of nitisinone. Plasma tyrosine levels in the patients rose, with no clinical signs or symptoms. They emphasized that the long-term safety and efficacy of this treatment required further evaluation.

B. 5 HOMOCYSTINURIA

Alternative titles: Cystathionine Beta-Synthase Deficiency, CBS Deficiency.

Homocystinuria was discovered independently by Gerritsen et al. (1962) in Madison, Wisconsin, and by Carson and Neill in Belfast, Northern Ireland. The patients of both groups were studied because of mental retardation and found to be deficient in the enzyme cystathionine synthase.

Homocystinuria is a metabolic disorder ***characterized by increased urinary homocystine and methionine. Major clinical manifestations*** involve ***the eyes*** and the ***central nervous, skeletal,*** and ***vascular systems viz. dislocation of eye lenses, spinal osteoporosis and thromboembolic events (recurrerent strokes).*** Mild to moderate mental retardation is seen in almost two-thirds of the patients and the intelligence quotient (IQ) is lower than normal, with an average of 80.

Based on newborn screening and cases detected clinically, the ***worldwide frequency of homocystinuria*** has been reported to be 1 in 344,000, while that in Ireland is much higher at 1 in 65,000.

Biochemical Defect: The ***autosomal recessive disorder*** is due to the abnormal metabolic block in the metabolism of the sulphur containing amino acid methionin (Fig. 27.15). The ***enzyme cystathionine β-synthase*** (EC 4.2.1.22) ***is deficient or absent*** resulting in the accumulation of homocysteine in plasma and its subsequent excretion in urine.

Heme may be necessary for binding of pyridoxal-phosphate to CBS and for correct CBS foldings, the inability to bind heme may prevent correct folding and subsequent tetramer formation of mutant and, to a lesser extent, normal CBS subunits. It has been postulated that the mutant CBS ***misfolding and aggregation may be the primary defect in a significant proportion of patients with homocystinuria.***

Types

Three types of homocysteinuria have been reported viz.

- With no residual activity
- With reduced activity and normal affinity for pyridoxal-phosphate
- With reduced activity and reduced affinity for the cofactor (pyridoxal-phosphate)

In addition to cystathionine β-synthase deficiency, at least 7 *'causes'* of homocystinuria are know. These are:

- Defect in vitamin B_{12} metabolism
- Deficiency of N (5, 10)-methylenetetrahydrofolate reductase, type 3
- Selective intestinal malabsorption of vitamin B_{12}
- Vitamin B_{12} responsive homocystinuria, cb1 E type
- Methylcobalamin deficiency, cbl G type
- Vitamin B_{12} metabolic defect, type 2
- Transcobalamin II deficiency.

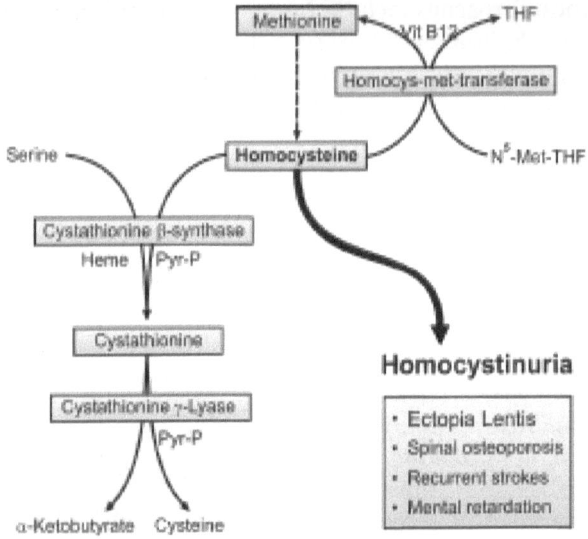

Fig. 27.15: Metabolism of Methionine and Homocysteinuria

The susceptibility of ocular zonule to abnormal formation in diseases of sulphur metabolism has been explained by the fact that the zonular fibres are composed of glycoprotein with a high concentration of cysteine. Excess homocysteine may interfere with the normal synthesis of collagen crosslinks, thus ***accounting for the development of osteoporosis.*** Collagen Type I crosslinks expressed by serum C-terminal telopeptide of collagen Type I in these patients are significantly lower compared to those in healthy individuals.

The ***role of plasma homocysteine in arterial occlusive diseases has been extensively studied*** over the last few years and high plasma homocysteine levels have very strongly emerged as a ***major risk factor for coronary artery disease.***

The ***hypopigmentation in homocysteinuric patients appears to be due to the inhibition of tyrosinase,*** the major pigment enzyme, by DL-homocysteine. ***In vitro, copper sulfate restores homocyst(e)ine-inhibited tyrosinase activity*** when added to the culture cell medium. The results suggested that the probale mechanism of the inhibition is the interaction of homocyst(e)ine with copper at the active site of tyrosinase.

Molecular genetics: The **gene** for the enzyme cystathionine β-synthase has been mapped to chromosome number 21 at the locus 21q22.3. More than 40 CBS mutations in homocystinuria in various ethnic groups have been identified. Most of these were mis-sense mutations; however, 7 deletions have been documented, 2 of which were total deletions of exons 11 and 12. In patients of Celtic origin, a particular mutation i.e. G307S mutation in the CBS gene, is the most common cause of homocystinuria, accounting for about 71% of alleles in Irish homocystinuria.

CLINICAL FEATURES

- ***Mental retardation:*** in children and surviving adults.
- Some affected individuals, are extraordinarily tall, with long extremities, frequently with flat feet with toes out ***(Charlie-Chaplin gait).***
- Liver is enlarged ***(hepatomegaly).***
- ***Skeletal deformities:*** involving spine, (vertebrae), and thorax, resulting to kyphosis, scoliosis, arachnodactyly. May be premature osteoporosis which also accounts to above deformities. X-ray spine: shows ***"cod fish"*** vertebrae.
- ***Ectopia Lentis:*** curious dislocation of lens of the eye. Not seen at birth, may show at the age of 2 to 3 years.

- ***Life threatening arterial/venous thrombosis.***
- Most of the patients show abnormal EEG.

An excellent review of clinical data of 629 patients with homocystinuria collected from all parts of the world by *Mudd et al. (1985)* showed that among patient not discovered by newborn screening, mental capabilities were higher in B6-responsive patients (mean IQ, 79) than in B6-nonresponsive patients (mean IQ, 57). For untreated B6-responsive and B6-nonresponsive patients, these were, respectively: chance of dislocation of eye lenses (ectopia lentis) by age 10, 55% and 82% chance of having clinically detected thromboembolic event by age 15, 12% and 27%; chance of rediologic detection of spinal osteoporosis by age 15, 36% and 64% and chance of not surviving to age 30, 4% and 23%. About one-third of the homocystinuric subjects have normal intelligence. The methionine restriction diet prevents/slows down the appearance of almost all the clinical features. When initiated neonatally, methionine restriction prevents mental retardation, reduces the rate of lens dislocation, and may even reduce the incidence of seizures. Pyridoxine treatment of late-detected B6-responsive patients reduces the rate of occurrence of initial thromboembolic events.

- ***Ectopia lentis is a nearly constant feature*** in patients over the age of 10 years but because of its progressive nature may be absent in younger patients. It may be mentioned here that ectopia lentis along with neurologic defects is also observed in another disorder of sulfur metabolism i.e. sulfocysteinuria.
- ***Skeletal features*** of homocysteinuria patients suggest Marfan's syndrome, but with the limitation of joint mobility and ***generalized osteoporosis.***
- ***Thrombotic lesions of arteries and veins are the features in homocysteinuric patients.*** The risk of thrombolytic events increases when the patients also have the factor V Leiden mutation, which is a common phenomenon in this disorder. The incidence of heart attacks and storke in the parents or grand-parents (heterozygotes) of homocystinuric children is not higher than normal.

Pneumothorax, pseudocysts and reversible hypopigmentation are additional clinical features of homocystinuria.

Diagnosis

- ***Silver-nitroprusside test:*** *Spaeth and Barber (1967)* described a silver-nitroprusside test which is almost completely specific for homocystine.
- The ***enzyme cystathionine synthase activity*** can be measured in ***cultured fibroblasts*** derived from normal skin, as well as in cells of amniotic fluid.
- Homocysteinuric patients also ***show high platelet turnover and enhanced thromboxane biosynthesis.*** High urinary excretion of 11-dehydro-TXB2, a major enzymatic derivative of TXA2, is observed in almost all homocystinuric patients. The elevated thromboxane biosynthesis is thought to reflect, at least in part, the *in vivo* platelet activation.
- The ***abnormal response of total urinary homocysteine after methionine loading was the most sensitive test*** and a satisfactory way for studying mild disturbances in homocysteine metabolism. Testing for heterozygosity, especially in families of homocystinuria patients, may be a very valuable guide to reduced methionine intake and B6 supplementation as preventive measures. Methionine loading has been successfully used to this effect, the heterozygotes show pathologic homocysteinuria about 4 hours after the loading dose. The patients with venous thromboembolism at the age of less than 40 years may be tested for heterozygocity.
- **Screening:** The screening programs to detect neonatal homocysteinuria have been in effect in England for more than four dacades now. A cutoff level for blood methionine of 1 mg/dl in the neonatal screening tests for homocystinuria is successful in identifying the affected infants who have only slightly

elevated concentrations of methionine. Among the 1.1 million infants screened in 8.5 years, 7 with the disorder were identified, giving a frequency of 1 in 157, 000.

CLINICAL MANAGEMENT

- Homocysteine that is not metabolized to cystine is remethylated to methionine in reactions that use either N5-methyltetrahyd-rofolate of betaine (trimethylglycine) as methyl donors. Therefore, ***folic acid in pharmacologic doses is therapeutically valuable*** in the disease, Decrease in urinary excretion of homocystine and increase in methionine has been noted during treatment, whereas additional benefits can be realized from betaine in B_6-responsive patients.
- ***Treatment of B_6 nonresponsive patients*** centers on lowering of homocysteine and its disulfide derivatives by adherence to a ***methionine-restricted diet.*** However, lifelong dietary control is difficult.
- ***Betaine supplementation is used extensively*** in CBS-deficient patients to lower plasma disulfide derivatives. With betaine therapy, methionine levels increase over baseline, but usually remain at levels that are not associated with adverse affects. The methionine levels should be monitored in CBS deficient patients on betaine and betaine should be considered as an adjunct, not an alternative, to dietary control.
- **Pullin et al. (2002)** reported that ***vitamin C ameliorates endothelial dysfunction*** in patients with homocystinuria, independent of changes in homocysteine concentration, and should therefore be considered as an ***additional adjunct to therapy*** to reduce the potential long-term risk of atherothrombotic disease.

B. 6 HISTIDINEMIA

(***Alternative titles:*** Histidine Ammonia-Lyase Deficiency, HAL Deficiency, Histidase Deficiency, HIS Deficiency)

Histidinemia is an ***autosomal recessive metabolic disorder characterized by increased levels of histidine in blood, urine, and cerebrospinal fluid, and decreased levels of the metabolite urocanic acid in blood, urine, and skin cells.*** Although histidinemia was originally associated with mental retardation and speech defects, it is generally considered to be a ***benign disorder.*** However, it is possible that histidinemia may be a risk factor for developmental disorders in certain individuals under specific circumstances, such as perinatal events. The reported ***frequency*** of histidinemia is 1 in 20,000 births.

Biochemical and Clinical Features

The first reported cases and the detection of errors of histidine metabolism came in 1962 when *Ghadimi et al. (1961)* reported 2 patients with histidinemia and suggested that it resulted from a 'familial disturbance of histidine metabolism.' In the same year *Auerbach et al. (1962)* were unable to detect the histidase metabolites urocanic acid or FIGLU (formiminoglutamic acid) in the urine of a patient with histidinemia, whereas loading with urocanic acid produced large amounts of FIGLU, indicating normal urocanase activity. They ***concluded*** that the ***defect was in the histidase enzyme.***

Most of the patients with histidinemia show ***normal speech, weight,*** head circumference, developmental quotient, IQ, and hearing. The CNS symptoms may be observed in less than 1% of individuals with histidinemia. However, histidinemia could be a risk factor for harmful effects under specific circumstances, such as abnormal perinatal events. There was no apparent benefit from a low histidine diet in early childhood. Therefore, histidinemia is a benign metabolic disorder that does not require treatment.

The **HAL gene** has been assigned to **chromosome number 12** and **mutations in the locus** 12q22-q23 have been related to histidinemia.

B.7 MAPLE SYRUP URINE DISEASE

(*Alternative titles*: Branched-Chain Keto-aciduria, Branched-Chain Alpha-Keto Acid Dehydrogenase Deficiency, BCKD Deficiency, Keto Acid Decarboxylase Deficiency, Lipoamide Dehydro-genase Deficiency, Lactic Acidosis Due to LAD Deficiency, Dihydrolipoamide Dehydrogenase Deficiency, DLD Deficiency)

Gene map locus 19q13.1-q13.2, 7q31-q32.

The ***major clinical features*** of maple syrup urine disease are • ***mental and physical retardation,*** feeding problems, and a ***maple syrup odour to the urine.*** The keto acids of the branched-chain amino acids are present in the urine, resulting from a block in oxidative decarboxylation (Fig. 27.16). There are *5 clinical subtypes* of MSUD: • ***the 'classic' neonatal severe form,*** • ***an 'intermediate' form,*** • ***an 'intermittent' form,*** • ***a 'thiamine-responsive' form,*** and • an ***'E3-deficient with lactic acidosis' form.*** All of these subtypes can be caused by mutations in any of the 4 genes viz. BCKDHA, BCKDHB, DBT, and DLD. These genes encode the catalytic components of the branched-chain alpha-keto acid dehydrogenase complex (BCKD), which catalyzes the catabolism of the branched-chain amino acids, leucine, isoleucine, and valine. E3-deficient form of MSUD is caused only by mutation in the E3 gene. ***BCKD enzyme is identical to pyruvate dehydrogenase*** and ***α-ketoglutarate dehydro-genase enzymes*** i.e. has ***three enzyme subunits (E1, E2, and E3) and uses five coenzymes.*** Apart from the three regular enzyme subunits, it also has two extra subunits: BCKD kinase and BCKD phosphorylase.

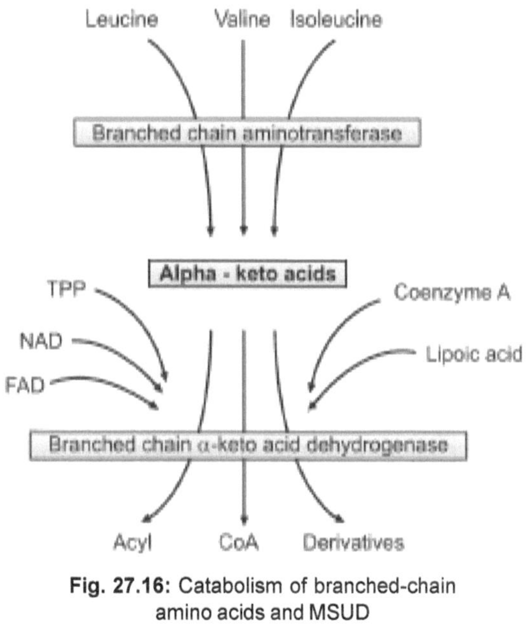

Fig. 27.16: Catabolism of branched-chain amino acids and MSUD

Maple syrup urine disease caused by mutation in the E1-alpha subunit gene is referred to as MSUD type IA; that caused by a mutation in the E1-beta subunit gene as type IB; that caused by defect in the E2 subunit gene as type II; and that caused by defect in the E3 subunit as type III. The BCKD complex also contains 2 regulatory enzymes, a kinase and phosphorylase. Additional forms identified by mutations in the specific kinase and specific phosphatase could be designated as types IV and types V, respectively.

CLINICAL FEATURES OF SUBTYPES

1. **Classic Severe MSUD:** In classic MSUD, which is the most common form of the disorder, ***50% or more of the keto acids are derived from leucine,*** and the activity of the BCKD complex is less than 2% of normal. Affected newborns appear normal at birth, with symptoms developing between 4 and 7 days of age. The infants show lethargy, weight loss, metabolic derangement, and progressive neurologic signs of altering hypotonia and hypertonia, reflecting a severe encephalopathy. Seizures and coma usually occur, followed by death if untreated. Otitis media and the characteristic odour are the tell tale features.
2. **Intermediate MSUD:** The patients with Intermediate form of MSUD have 15 to 25% residual BCKD activity in leucocytes and fibroblasts. The symptoms are accordingly of moderate severity. The physical growth may be normal and most of the symptoms are that of CNS characterized by severe developmental delay. Systemic acidosis may be

present and markedly increased levels of plasma branched-chain amino acids and urinary branched-chain keto acids are observed.

3. **Intermittent MSUD:** Late onset of symptoms and clinical normalcy during the intervening period between attacks differentiates the intermittent form of the disorder from classic MSUD. In addition, the level of leukocyte BCKD complex activity seemed to be higher than in the classic form of the disease and the activity could be normal during the latency period. The episodes present with recurrent acidosis, ataxia, lethargy, semi-coma and elevated urinary branched-chain keto acids following otitis media.
4. **Thiamine-responsive MSUD:** ***Some mutations in E1-alpha as well as E1-beta subunits can reduce the affinity of the enzyme for thiamine pyrophosphate (TPP),*** one of the essential coenzymes. Since the K_m of the enzyme is increased, high concentrations of TPP can restore the enzyme activity. Therefore, a variant of MSUD in which the hyperaminoacidemia can be completely corrected by thiamine hydrochloride (10 mg per day) along with dietary restriction is known as thiamine responsive MSUD. The activity of the BCKDH complex in thiamine-responsive MSUD is about 30 to 40% of the normal rate.
5. **E3-Deficient MSUD with Lactic Acidosis:** E3-deficient MSUD, or MSUD type III, presents a combined deficiency of the branched-chain alpha-keto acid dehydrogenase, pyruvate dehydrogenase, and alpha-keto glutarate dehydrogenase-complexes. This is the result of E3 being a common component of all the three mitochondrial multienzyme complexes *(Chuang and Shih, 2001).*

   The clinical presentation of this form of MSUD, first reported by **Robinson et al. (1977),** includes ***progressive neurologic deterioration and persistent metabolic acidosis.*** The patients have ***elevated blood pyruvate, lactate, alpha-ketoglutarate, and branched-chain amino acids,*** as well as ***occasional hypoglycemia.*** The deficiency of the pyruvate dehydrogenase complex, and specifically of dihydrolipoyldehydrogenase, or E3 can be demonstrated in the biopsy tissues. Thiamine therapy is of no benefit but ***administration of lipoic acid may resolve the abnormal organic aciduria and lactic and pyruvic acidemia,*** with clinical improvement. Intractable metabolic acidosis and multiorgan failure can often be fatal.
6. **MSUD and Fenugreek Tea:** The odor of the urine in MSUD is more reminiscent of fenugreek (*Trigonella foenim* graecum L.) than of maple syrup. Physicians should keep in mind that a fenugreek odor of urine with neurologic distress in newborn infants, without a history of fenugreek ingestion (in the form of 'fenugreek tea' as home remedy for flatulence) should raise a suspicion of MSUD.

A child who presented with neurological symptoms and characteristic odour in urine was found to be a case of 'pseudo-maple syrup urine disease' caused by drinking fenugreek tea. The parents indicated that the child had been given herbal tea (Helba tea) to reduce flatulence and prevent fever. Tea contains seeds of fenugreek. Analysis of the infant's urine revealed the presence of ***sotolone,*** the ***compound responsible for the aroma*** in maple syrup urine disease. Tea prepared from fenugreek seeds was found to contain sotolone. Since herbal teas are popular as home remedies, particularly in Middle Eastern countries, physicians should use caution when they are presented with young infants from such countries, to avoid unnecessary and costly investigations.

Incidence: In a mobile, urban, predominantly white population of New England, a frequency of MSUD of 1 in 290,000 on newborn screening has been documented. The highest reported frequency of MSUD was observed among the Old Order Mennonites of Pennsylvania. In conservative Mennonites of eastern Pennsylvania, classic MSUD has a frequency as high as 1 in 176 births. Further, it has been reported that 33% of the MSUD cases were caused by mutation in the E1-alpha gene, 38% by mutations in the E1-beta gene, and 19% by mutations in the E2 gene. Ten percent of the tested cell lines may show ambiguous results.

B.8 METHYLMALONIC ACIDURIA

Alternative titles: MMA, Methylmalonic Acidemia Due To Methylmalonyl-CoA Mutase Deficiency, MMA Due To MCM Deficiency

Methylmalonic aciduria (MMA) is a genetically heterogeneous disorder of methylmalonate and cobalamin (cbl; vitamin B_{12} metabolism. Isolated methylmalonic aciduria is found in patients with mutations in the MUT gene causing partial, mut(-), or complete, mut (0), deficiency of Methylmalonyl-CoA mutase (MCM) enzyme. The Mut(0) form is unresponsive to B_{12} therapy. Various forms of isolated methylmalonic aciduria also occur in a subset of patients with defects in the synthesis of the MUT coenzyme adenosylcobalamin (AdoCb1) and are classified according to complementation group: cblA, caused by mutation in the MMAA gene on chromosome 4q31, and cb1B, caused by mutation in the MMAB gene on locus 12q24.

Combined methylmalonic aciduria and homocystinuria may be seen in complementation groups cb1C, cb1D, and cb1F.

Biochemical: Enzyme Methylmalonyl-CoA Mutase (MCM) is involved in the conversion of methylmalonic acid to succinic acid that is assimilated in the tricarboxylic acid cycle. The enzyme requires the active vitamin B_{12} (adenosyl cobalamin) as the coenzyme (Fig. 27.17).

Deficiency of the enzyme activity or its coenzyme causes the accumulation of methylmalonic acid in the plasma and its excretion in urine. The cases where MCM expression is normal but coenzyme availability is inadequate respond to the administration of cobalamin.

The mutase enzyme in cells from some MMA patients shows decreased affinity for AdoCbl with abnormally high Km for the coenzyme. These cases are considered to represent a structurally abnormal enzyme and are characteristic of the mut (-) phenotype.

CLINICAL FEATURES

The clinical spectrum of MMA is wide, ranging from a benign condition to fatal neonatal disease.

The **most common presenting symptoms** at the onset are lethargy, failure to thrive, recurrent vomiting, dehydration, respiratory distress and hypotonia. ***Other common features include hepatomegaly,*** developmental delay, and coma. Mut(0) patients present earlier in infancy than the other groups. ***All patients have methylmalonic academia*** and ***normal serum cobalamin,*** and ***most have metabolic acidosis, ketonuria, hyperammonemia, and hyperglycinemia.*** Approximately half of all the patients have pancytopenia.

Although a broad correlation has been found between mutase class and phenotype, survival with good outcome is possible among mut(0) patients and, conversely, significant morbidity occurs among mut(-) patients. Acidosis and metabolic imbalance have been found to be necessary preconditions for significant morbidity.

Renal insufficiency is frequently reported in mutase-deficient methylmalonic acidemia.

Because of improvements in therapy, many patients with MMA reach child-bearing age.

Diagnosis: The primary diagnosis depends upon the ***demonstration of methylmalonic acid*** and ***propionic acid*** in the ***urine*** and ***plasma*** samples on a ***Gas Liquid (GLC) or High Performance Liquid (HPLC) chromatogram.*** It should be kept in mind that the propionic acid peak can be misinterpreted as ethylene glycol (a chemical in anti-freeze) peak and hence a case of ethylene glycol poisoning can be diagnosed as that of MMA and vice versa.

The specific typing can only be done by estimating the enzyme activity in the tissue samples and by cobalamine responsiveness.

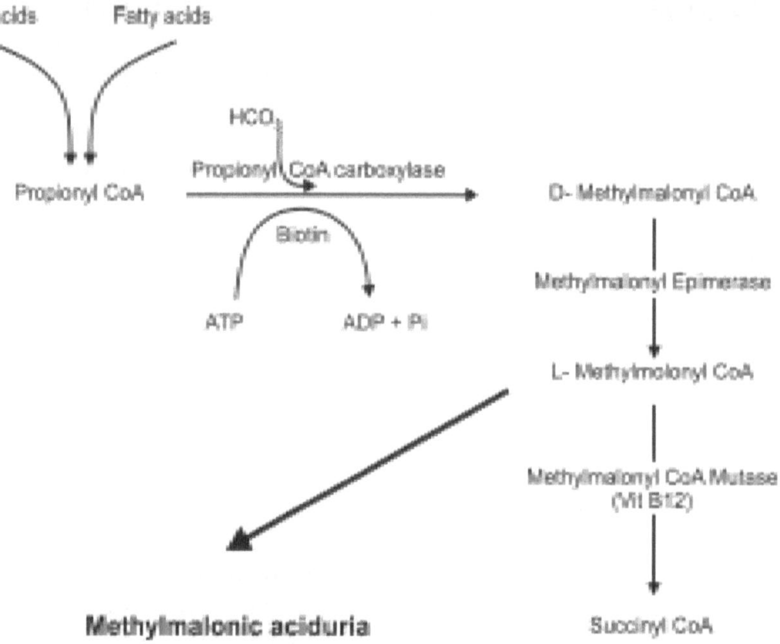

Fig. 27.17: Propionic acid metabolism and methylmalonic aciduria

B.9 GLYCINE DECARBOXYLASE DEFICIENCY

(Alternative titles: Glycine Cleavage System P Protein; GCSP; Glycine Dehydrogenase; Non ketotic glycinemia)

The enzyme system for cleavage of glycine (glycine cleavage system; GCS; EC 2.1.2.10), which is confined to the mitochondria, is composed of 4 protein components:

- P protein (a pyridoxal phosphate-dependent glycine decarboxylase).
- H protein (a lipoic acid-containing protein),
- T protein (a tetrahydrofolate-requiring enzyme), and
- L protein (a lipoamide dehydrogenase).

A ***defect in any one of these enzymes can result in glycinemia*** which may present with ***non-ketotic hyperglycinemia and encephalopathy.*** Minor dysfunctions of the central nervous system may be found in these patients, which may be due to a slightly abnormal degradation of glycine (which has a neurotransmitter role).

Glycine decarboxylase is present in human liver, kidney, brain, and placenta; moderate concentrations are also in brain, small intestine, thyroid gland, and pituitary gland; and small amount may be present in colon, bladder, and lungs.

GENE STRUCTURE AND MOLECULAR GENETICS

Takayanagi et al. (2000) determined the structure of the GLDC gene and its pseudogene. The GLDC gene spans at least 135 kb and contains 25 exons. All donor and acceptor sites adhered to the canonical GT-AG rule, except for the donor site of intron 21, where a variant form GC is used instead of GT. By primer extension analysis, the transcription initiation site was assigned to a residue 163 bp upstream from the translation initiation triplet. The GLDC pseudogene has no introns and shares 97.5% homology with the coding region of functional GLDC, suggesting that it is a processed pseudogene that arose from the GLDC transcript about 4 to 8 million years ago.

A high frequency of glycine encephalopathy has been found in some countries of Finland (von Wendt et al, 1981). It was found that 14 of 20 P protein alleles in heterozygote Finnish patients carried a single nucleotide substitution from G to T in the protein coding region, which resulted in an amino acid alteration from serine-564 to isoleucine.

Using the GCSP cDNA as a probe in Southern blot analysis of genomic DNA from 2 patients with nonketotic hyperglycinema, Tada et al (1990) showed that they had a specific defect in P protein, viz. a partial deletion.

Applegarth and Toone (2001) reviewed the laboratory diagnosis of glycine encephalopathy and confirmed nine mutations in the T protein and eight in the P protein.

GENE MAPPING

The functional GCSP gene has been assigned to chromosome 9 at locus 9p24-p23 and a processed pseudogene to 4q12.

B. 10 HYPERLYSINEMIA

Alternative titles: Lysine: Alpha-Ketoglutarate Reductase Deficiency, Alpha-Aminoadipic Semialdehyde Synthase Deficiency, Lysine Intolerance, L-Lysine: NAD Oxido-Reductase Deficiency.

Clinical Features: The patients with hyperlysinemia may present with ***impaired sexual development, lax ligaments and muscles, convulsions in early life, and perhaps mild anemia. Mild to severe physical and mental retardation*** may be seen with convulsions, muscular and ligamentous asthenia, and normocytic, normochromic anemia which responds to dietary restriction of lysine. ***Subluxation of the lenses develops in some of the patients,*** although it has been suggested to be due to another superimposed disorder. Some patients might present with episodic vomiting, rigidity, and coma; high levels of plasma ammonia may be the causative feature of coma.

Biochemical defect: ***Reduced lysine:alpha-ketoglutarate reductase activity is the primary enzymatic abnormality resulting in hyperlysinemia.*** Lysine is a potent competitive inhibitor of arginase. As a result, urea synthesis and ammonia detoxification are interfered with. High levels of ammonia and arginine may be an additional feature. A defect in L-lysine: NAD-oxido-reductase activity in liver may also cause the accumulation of lysine.

Two successive enzymes viz. lysine ketoglutarate reductase and saccharopine dehydrogenase in the major pathway of lysine degradation have been implicated i.e. the first 2 steps in the mammalian lysine degradation pathway, suggesting the existence of a bifunctional enzyme encoded by a single locus. In hyperlysinemia, both enzymatic functions of Alpha-Aminoadipic Semialdehyde Synthase (AASS) are defective; in saccharopinuria, some of the first enzymatic function is retained.

B.11 CYSTINURIA

Cystinuria is a ***heritable disorder of amino acid transport, transmitted as an autosomal recessive trait.*** It is one of the most common genetic disorders, with an overall prevalence of approximately 1 in 7,000. It is due to ***the defective transport of cystine and dibasic amino acids through the epithelial cells of the renal tubule and intestinal tract.*** Cystine has a low solubility, and its precipitation results in the formation of calculi in the urinary tract, which leads to obstruction, infections, and ultimately renal insufficiency. Causative mutations have been identified in the SLC3A1 gene. SLC3A1 protein is expressed in the brush border plasma membrane of both the proximal straight tubules of the nephron and the small intestine and in considered to be responsible for reabsorption of cystine and dibasic amino acids, most probably by means of a heteroexchange diffusion mechanism of transport with neutral amino acids.

Types

Three types of classic cystinuria have been described:

- ***Cystinuria type I:*** The homozygote patients ***excrete*** relatively large ***amounts of cystine, lysine, arginine and ornithine*** in the urine. Heterozygotes (e.g. parents) have no abnormal amino aciduria. ***Type I is the most frequent*** type and often occurs in compound heterozygotes with type III.
- ***Cystinuria type II:*** The disorder appears to be incompletely recessive because heterozygotes also have a moderate degree of ***amino aciduria,*** mainly cystine and lysine, and may occasionally form ***cystine stones.***
- ***Cystinuria type III:*** In these cases, the intestinal transport of all dibasic amino acids is retained by heterozygotes, and homozygotes excrete cystine in slight excess. Heterozygotes show moderate hyper-excretion of cystine and dibasic amino acids. Homozygotes show a nearly normal increase in cystine plasma levels after oral cystine administration.

The doubly heterozygous persons (I-II, I-III, or II-III) have full-blown cystinuria. The findings are best explained on the basis of allelism of the genes responsible for the 3 types. Actually, 'genetic compound' is a term preferable to 'double heterozygote' when the mutant genes are allelic.

The excretion rates of obligate carriers among the relatives of cystinurics are sufficient to determine the type of cystinuria in the proband. When obligatory heterozygotes show normal amounts of cystine and dibasic amino acids in the urine, they are called type I. When up to twice the normal range is excreted in the urine, they are called type III. When carriers excrete large amounts of cystine and lysine (9-15 times the normal range but less than in most stone-formers), they are called type II.

The International Cystinuria Consortium (1999 and 2001) identified the SLC7A9 gene, which ***encodes a protein,*** termed ***b(0, +) AT,*** that belongs to a family of light subunits of amino acid transporters expressed in kidney, liver, small intestine, and placenta. Co-transfection of b(0,+) AT with rBAT brought the latter to the plasma membrane, and resulted in the uptake of L-arginine in COS cells. They localized the gene to the non-type I cystinuria locus on chromosome 19q. The preliminary results suggested that cystinuria is a digenic disease in some of the mixed type I/non-type I patients and supported the hypothesis of partial genetic complementation. The *consortium* offered 2 hypotheses as to why mutations in the SLC3A1 gene are recessive, whereas mutations in the SLC7A9 gene are incompletely recessive. First, if the active b (0,+) transporter is constituted by more than 1 rBAT and b (0,+) AT subunit, 1 mutated allele of the light subunit might produce a dominant defect, whereas 1 mutated allele of the rBAT heavy subunit would produce a trafficking defect. Second, the light subunit might associate with a protein other than rBAT and express cystine transport activity in a different proximal tubular segment. In situ hybridization and immunolocalization studies showed expression of the light subunit in the epithelial cells of the proximal straight tubule, like the heavy subunit, but higher expression in the proximal convoluted tubule. Most of the renal cystine reabsorption occurs in the proximal convoluted tubule via a low-affinity system not identified at the molecular level. If the SLC7A9 gene also encodes this transport system, a partial defect in this major renal reabsorption mechanism would explain the incompletely recessive phenotype of non-type I cystinuria. The authors presented a genotype-phenotype correlation in non-type I cystinuria, and hypothesized that a mild urinary phenotype in heterozygotes may be associated with mutations permitting significant residual transport activity.

B.12 HARTNUP DISORDER

First described by Baron et al. (1956), this disorder is ***characterized*** by a ***pellagra-like light-sensitive rash, cerebellar ataxia,*** emotional instability, and amino aciduria; and is defined as an inborn error of neutral amino acid transport. ***Two forms*** of Hartnup disease has been discussed: in the classic form the defect is expressed in both intestine and kidney, in a ***variant form*** it is expressed only in kidney. Hartnup disorder has no ill effects on the fetus. Normal ratios of amino acid concentrations between maternal and umbilical veins suggested that placental transport of free amino acids, unlike renal transport, is not reduced. In the United States, cases of the full-blown clinical disorder are not seen, probably because of super-adequate diet.

Incidence

Hartnup disease was found to have about the same frequency in Massachusettes as phenylketonuria, i.e., 1 in 14, 219 births.

BIOCHEMICAL FEATURES

The *defect* in Hartnup disorder ***involves the intestinal and renal transport of certain neutral alpha-amino acids.*** The intestinal transport defect, in some patients might be partially evident only under loading conditions. Methionine and tryptophan transport are affected to larger extent, whereas lysine and glycine transport might be moderately impaired. *Faecal indoles and urinary indican are elevated after oral tryptophan loading.*

Genetic heterogeneity probably exists in Hartnup disease because cases have been described in which only the urinary characteristics of Hartnup disease were present, and there was no evidence of an intestinal transport defect. It has been suggested that Hartnup disorder is multifactorial. Whereas deficient activity of the Hartnup transport system is monogenic, the associated plasma amino acid value is polygenic. By homozygosity mappint, Nozaki et al. (2001) and Seow et al. (2004) assigned the Hartnup disease ***locus to chromosome*** 5p15.33.

B. 13 INHERITED UREA CYCLE DISORDERS

Urea cycle disorders are ***characterized*** by the ***triad*** of ***hyperammonemia, encephalopathy,*** and ***respiratory alkalosis.*** **Five disorders** involving different defects in the biosynthesis of the enzymes of urea cycle have been described:

- ornithine transcarbamoylase deficiency,
- carbamoyl phosphate synthetase deficiency,
- argininosuccinate synthetase efficiency or citrullinemia,
- argininosuccinate lyase deficiency, and
- arginase deficiency.

Since ***generalized seizures are the major clinical complication in almost all the urea cycle disorders,*** the patients many times require ***antiepileptic treatment. Sodium valproate should never be administered to these patients.*** Valproate inhibits ureagenesis and can be toxic to mitochondria, therefore, sodium valproate may precipitate acute liver failure in males with urea cycle defects. The vulnerability of toxic effects of valproate extends to heterozygotes as well.

Frequency

In Japan, the total frequency of the urea cycle enzymopathies, carbamoyl phosphate synthetase deficiency, ornothine transcarbamoylase deficiency, argininosuccinate synthetase deficiency, argininosuccinate lyase deficiency and arginase deficiency has been reported to be 1 in 46,000.

1. CARBAMOYL PHOSPHATE SYNTHETASE I DEFICIENCY

Carbamoyl phosphate synthetase I (CPS-I) deficiency is an ***autosomal recessive*** inborn error of metabolism of the urea cycle which causes hyperammonemia. The gene for carbamoyl phosphate synthetase has been mapped to locus **2q35** on ***chromosome number 2*** and mis-sense mutation (s) in the gene has been linked with the disorder.

Incidence

The estimated *incidence* of CPS I deficiency in Japan has been reported as 1 in 800, 000.

CLINICAL FEATURES

Two forms of carbamoyl phosphate synthetase (CPS) deficiency are recognized: a lethal neonatal type and a less severe, delayed-onset type.

- ***Early-onset form*:** This disorder is characterized by moderate to severe ***cerebral damage*** and ***hyperammonemic coma in neonates.*** Histopathologic examination of the liver shows diffuse microvesicular steatosis, distinct focal hepatocellular and Kupffer cell glycogenosis. The ***CPS enzyme is totally absent.*** The disorder is fatal within a few postnatal days of life.
- ***Delayed-Onset Form:*** This form of the disorder is due to the *partial deficiency of CPS enzyme.* The patients present in early childhood or even in adulthood with *hyperammonemic coma* simulating Reye syndrome. *Intermittent seizures* may be present with episodes of vomiting, mild abdominal pain, and muscle weakness. The psychomotor development is slow.

  The patients who progress to adulthood have intermittent seizures and might complain of spells of confusion and disorientation. They are always at risk of hyperammonemic coma. Valproate administration to control generalized seizures should be avoided as valproic acid-induced coma has been reported. 'Valproate sensitivity' has been observed also with ornithine transcarbamoylase deficiency and citrullinemia, the other two causes of hyperammonemia.

DIAGNOSIS

Prenatal Diagnosis: By chorionic villus sampling, Finckh et al. (1998) diagnosed a 12-week-old fetus with CPS I deficiency. Pathologic examination of the fetal liver showed hepatocellular changes consistent with the disorder.

CLINICAL MANAGEMENT

The treatment of the patients with inborn errors of urea synthesis is targeted at activation of alternative pathways of waste nitrogen synthesis and excretion. ***Intravenous administration of sodium benzoate, sodium phenylacetate and arginine diverts the ammonia destined for urea synthesis to the formation of hippuric acid*** and is successful in keeping the ammonia levels in check. When other measures fail, dialysis should be considered.

2. ORNITHINE TRANSCARBAMOYLASE DEFICIENCY

Ornithine transcarbamoylase (OTC) deficiency is an ***X-linked inborn error of metabolism*** of the urea cycle which causes ***hyperammonemia, encephalopathy and respiratory alkalosis.***

Frequency

OTC deficiency has a frequency of 1 in 80,000 births in Japan.

CLINICAL FEATURES

Chronic ammonia intoxication and mental retardation are the major features. The clinical picture of OTC deficiency during acute exacerbations with microvesicular fat accumulation in the liver may suggest Reye syndrome.

Both milder and severe form of the disorder are known depending upon the activity of enzyme OTC in the liver. The age of presentation ranges from 2 months to 44 years.

In the ***milder form*** activity of the enzyme might be up to 25% of that in healthy individuals, whereas in *severe form total absence* or minimal (5-7%) OTC acitivity is found. The patients with milder form would have raised plasma ammonia levels and generalized aversion to proteins. During childhood, they might be called as 'very difficult, introverted with volcanic tempers'. Some patients may be normal initially but gradually develop severe spasticity due to cerebral atrophy.

The ***neuropathologic findings*** in cases of OTC deficiency may include ***astrocyte transformation to Alzheimer type II glia,*** a feature of any form of hyperammonemia. Gliosis confined to the brainstem or widespread and ulegyria of the cerebral xortex, as well as atrophy in the internal granular layer of the cerebellum could be found in some of the cases.

Skin lesions like acrodermatitis enteropathica-like dermatosis may be found in a number of urea cycle disorders. Since arginine represents such a lerge proportion of the amino acid composition of epidermal keratins, arginine deficiency associated with urea cycle defects may contribute to compromised epidermal barrier function and skin lesions in affected infants.

High orotic acid levels following high protein diet are associated with hyperammonemia.

Valproate sensitivity: Valproate inhibits ureagenesis and can be toxic to mitochondria. Therefore, sodium valproate may precipitate acute liver failure in males with OTC deficiency. The vulnerability of toxic effects of valproate extends to heterozygotes as well.

INHERITANCE

The ***gene for OTC enzyme*** has been mapped to the ***X-chromosome at locus X2.21.*** Ornithine transcarbamoylase deficiency is an X-linked disorder, but the inheritance seems to be dominant in nature. The ***evidence of X-linked dominant inheritance is based*** on (1) the severe nature of the disorder in males with almost complete absence of enzyme in most cases; (2) wide variation in clinical severity and in enzyme level in heterozygous women; and (3) demonstration of the cellular mosaicism in liver (two type of cells i.e. one with and the other without OTC enzyme activity).

DIAGNOSIS

- Family history, dietary history, episodic nonspecific symptoms, response to withdrawal of protein, and other characteristics should permit early diagnosis. OTC is expressed in the liver and in the mucosa of the small intestine.
- Hamano et al. (1988) described the identification of a carrier of OTC deficiency ***by means of immuno-cytochemical examination of a biopsy specimen from the duodenal mucosa.*** OTC-negative cells were distributed around I side of some villi, whereas OTC-positive cells were located on the othe side.
- Hauser et al. (1990) *described a test* that can be substituted for nitrogen loading for identification of heterozygous females.
- In the nitrogen loading test, there is intramitochondrial accumulation of carbamoyl phosphate. The excess carbamoyl phosphate is diffused into the cytosol where it functions as a substrate to *enhance the biosynthesis of pyrimidine, resulting in the accumulation and excretion of orotic acid.*
- *A single oral dose of allopurinol substitutes for the nitrogen load.* The effectiveness of the method depends on the inhibitory effect of oxypurinol ribonucleotide (a metabolite of allopuril) on orotidine monophosphate decarboxylase, which leads to the accumulation of orotidine monophosphate and its precursor orotic acid, and ultimately to orotic aciduria and orotidinuria.
- Application of RFLP-based diagnosis is limited in this disorder due to genetic heterogeneity of the mutations but the use of DNA polymorphisms in the prenatal diagnosis of OTC deficiency may show some promise.
- Yudkoff et al. (1996) developed a new technique that uses mass spectrometry to measure conversion of $^{15}NH_4Cl$ to ^{15}N-urea and 5-^{15}N-glutamine following an oral load of $^{15}NH_4Cl$.

CLINICAL MANAGEMENT

The disorder is treatable with ***supplemental dietary arginine and low protein diet.***

Administration of sodium benzoate diverts ammonium nitrogen from the defective urea pathway to hippurate synthesis by way of the glycine cleavage complex in ornithine transcarbamylase deficiency just like in other urea cycle disorders.

3. N-ACETYLGLUTAMATE SYNTHASE DEFICIENCY

The formation of N-acetylglutamate, a known activator of carbamoylphosphate synthetase, is catalyzed in the liver by mitochondrial N-acetylglutamate synthetase (NAGS).

Clinical Features: The presentation of the disorder is similar to the other urea cycle disorders characterized by ***high plasma concentrations of ammonia and glutamine.*** The ***neurologic presentation*** ranges from recurrent episodes of vomiting, psychotic behaviorand confusion to features like uncontrollable movements, developmental delay, visual impairment, failure to thrive etc. The hyperammonemia is precipitated by the introduction of high-protein diet or febrile illness. Orotic acid as well as orotidine levels are not raised. ***A deficiency of N-acetylglutamate synthetase should be considered in cases of hyperammonemia without increased excretion of orotic acid.***

Gene Map

Very few cases of NAGS deficiency have been reported till date. The gene for NAGS has been mapped to chromosome # 17 at the locus **17q21.31** A number of mutations in the gene have been assigned to NAG deficiency and are inherited as autosomal recessive.

Treatment: with carbamoylglutamate if initiated early stabilize the clinical feature.

4. ARGININOSUCCINIC ACIDURIA

Alternative titles: Argininosuccinase Deficiency, Argininosuccinate Lyase Deficiency

Argininosuccinic aciduria is an ***autosomal recessive disorder*** of the urea cycle. The gene for the enzyme argininosuccinate lyase is located on ***chromosome # 7 at locus 7cen-q11.2.***

The enzyme argininosuccinate lyase cleaves the argininosuccinate molecule into Arginine and fumarate. Therefore deficiency of the enzyme would be ***characterized by low arginine as well as hyperammonemia*** due to block in the normal functioning of urea cycle.

Onset of symptoms of argininosuccinic aciduria occurs in the first few weeks of life. ***Features include mental and physical retardation, convulsions, episodic unconsciousness, liver enlargement, skin lesions*** and dry and brittle hair showing trichorrhexis nodosa microscopically and fluorescing red. Astrocyte transformation to Alzheimer type II glia may be a consistent feature of any form of hyperammonemia.

Types

Two forms of argininosuccinic aciduria have been recognized: an early-onset, or malignant type and a late-onset type.

- Early onset type is fatal in almost all the cases whereas
- Late onset type patients might survive into adulthood. The surviving individuals have to be maintained on antiepileptic medication. In case of any surgical requirement, general anaesthesia, including enflurane, should be avoided in patients with argininosuccinic aciduria.

  There are some patients of argininosuccinate lyase deficiency, who are characterized by residual activity of argininosuccinate lyase and who present with a less severe clinical course.

DIAGNOSIS

- Prenatal diagnosis of argininosuccinate lyase deficiency has been made by ***trans-abdominal chorionic villi sampling*** at about 10 weeks of gestation.

CLINICAL MANAGEMENT

The patients of argininosuccinase deficiency may be treated to a reasonable success with low protein and arginine supplemented diet. The treatment favours the formation of argininosuccinic acid (ASA); since ASA contains the 2 waste nitrogen atoms later excreted in urea in healthy persons, and since it has a renal clearance similar to urea, hyperammonemia might be relieved by arginine therapy, provided stoichiometric amounts of ornithine are available.

Early treatment, particularly in partial argininosuccinate lyase deficiency, results in normal intellectual and psychomotor development.

5. CITRULLINEMIA

Alternative titles: Citrullinemia, Citrullinuria, Argininosuccinate Synthetase (ASS) Deficiency

The classic citrullinemia is caused by mutations in the gene encoding argininosuccinate synthetase (ASS) ***located on chromosome # 9 at locus 9q34.*** The synthetase enzyme **(EC 6.3.4.5),** ligates the citrulline with aspartate and thus introduces the second nitrogen that is finally excreted as urea. Deficient activity of the enzyme results in accumulation of the substrate citrulline and block in the normal functioning of urea cycle.

CLINICAL FEATURES

Severe vomiting spells beginning at the age of 9 months and ***mental retardation*** were features of the first reported case. Most cases of citrullinemia have pursued a severe course with symptoms from birth and death in the neonatal period. In more than half of cased, ***Orotic aciduria*** as well as hyperammonemia are present.

Types

- The **classical, Type I,** citrullinemia has been found to be due to the changes in the kinetic properties of the enzyme rather than the quantitative levels.
- A distinct, **late-onset form** of citrullinemia has been reported from Japan classified as **citrullinemia type II.** Symptoms included enuresis, delayed menarche, insomnia, sleep reversal, nocturnal sweats and terrors, recurrent vomiting (especially at night), diarrhoea, tremors, episodes of confusion after meals, lethargy, convulsions, delusions and hallucinations, and brief episodes of coma. Delayed mental and physical development was shown by some patients.

Most had a *peculiar fondness for beans, peas, and peanuts from early childhood and a dislike for rice, other vegetables, and sweets.* Since the preferred foods are high in arginine, the dietary predilection of these patients may reflect an *arginine deficiency.* As the patients get older, episodic disturbances become more frequent and bizarre behavior, including maniac episodes, echolalia, and frank psychosis, appears. Citrulline concentrations in the plasma are increased and ASS activity is deficient. Most adult citrullinemic patients in Japan have a quantitative type of abnormality of ASS (Type II), Only one patient of citrullinemia Type II has been reported from USA.

BIOCHEMICAL FEATURES

Type I citrullinemia shows kinetically abnormal ASS in the liver, kidney and cultured fibroblasts. ***In Type II, low ASS is found in the liver but not in kidney*** or cultured skin fibroblasts. Residual enzyme in the liver has normal kinetic properties. In Type II citrullinemia, the decrease in the enzyme protein is due either to increased degradation of the enzyme or to decreased or inhibited translation in the liver.

Another type of citrullinemia, which was classified as ***Type III has been reported*** and is characterized by ***no detectable enzyme activity for ASS*** and no translation activity for ASS mRNA.

CLINICAL MANAGEMENT

With the expansion of newborn screening programs to include citrullinemia, numerous asymptomatic infants and children have been indentified. With improvements in neonatal intensive care and the ***early use of sodium benzoate and phenyl acetate*** to remove nitrogen by alternative pathways, the outcome for newborns with hyperammonemia may not always be as poor as previously thought.

6. ARGININEMIA

Alternative titles: Arginase Deficiency, Hyperargininemia

Arginase deficiency is an ***autosomal recessive*** inborn error of metabolism caused by a defect in the final step in the urea cycle, the hydrolysis of arginine to urea and ornithine. ***The failure to cleave arginine in the patients leads to hyperargininemia and hyperammonemia.***

Biochemical and Clinical Features

The patients present with • ***psychomotor retardation,*** • ***epileptic seizures and*** • ***spastic paraplegia.*** The children may have episodes of vomiting, hypotonia, irritability, and ataxia. ***'Valproate sensitivity' has also been observed*** in the patients with argininemia and any valproate therapy to control seizures might push the patients into stupor with marked hyperammonemia. In general, arginase deficiency does not commonly have the severe hyperammonemia seen with other urea cycle disorders.

The activity of argininase I is very low or absent in the tissues but that of argininase II in kidney might be enhanced multi-fold by exposure to elevated arginine levels. The presumably is the mechanism for the high level of the enzyme in the patients and explains the fact that there is persistent ureagenesis in this disorder.

CLINICAL MANAGEMENT

Therapy with sodium benzoate and dietary restriction of arginine causes an impressive improvement.

7. ORNITHINE AMINOTRANSFERASE DEFICIENCY

Alternative titles: OAT Deficiency, Ornithine Keto Acid Aminotransferase Deficiency, OKT Deficiency, Ornithine-Delta-Aminotransferase Deficiency, Hyperornithinemia with Gyrate Atrophy of Choroid and Retina; HOGA

Ornithine-delta-aminotransferase (EC 2.6.1.13) catalyzes the major catalytic reaction for ornithine. Ornithinemia presumably due to deficiency of ornithine ketoacid aminotransferase (OAT) was reported in 9 patients with ***gyrate atrophy of the choroid and retina by Simell and Takki (1973).***

Early degenerative and atrophic brain changes and abnormal EEG are features of gyrate atrophy, in addition to the well-characterized eye and muscle manifestations. The clinical history of gyrate atrophy is usually ***night blindness*** that begins in late childhood, ***accompanied by sharply demarcated circular areas of chorioretinal atrophy.*** During the second and third decades the areas of atrophy enlarge. Ornithine levels are 10 to 20 times higher than normal in plasma, urine, spinal fluid and aqueous humor. Generally, no consistent clinical abnormality other than the ocular one is found. ***Hyperammonemia is absent in the fasting state or after meals or even on stress testing.***

Despite the selected atrophy of Type 2 fibres with tubular aggregates, gyrate atrophy patients usually have no muscle symptoms, although they may show impaired performance when speed or acute strength is required.

It has been suggested that changes in skeletal muscle, as well as the ocular changes, may be mediated by hyperornithinemia-induced deficiency of high-energy creatine phosphate.

Some cases of OKT deficiency are pyridoxine (B_6)-responsive. Both the B_6 responsive and nonresponsive forms contain intermediate levels of OKT activity. The variants could be distinguished, however, by the *in vitro* responsiveness of OKT activity to pyridoxal phosphate (PLP) stimulation. The apparent Km for PLP is lower in non-responsive patients than in patients responsive to pyridoxine.

CLINICAL MANAGEMENT

The main source of ornithine is arginine in dietary protein, and ***restriction of arginine in the diet appears to have therapeutic value.*** If started at an early age, long-term substantial reduction of plasma ornithine levels might appreciably slow the progression of the chorioretinal lesions and, to a lesser extent, the progressive loss of retinal function in patients with gyrate atrophy.

8. HYPERORNITHINEMIA-HYPERAMMONEMIA-HOMOCITRULLINURIA SYNDROME

Alternative titles: HHH syndrome; Ornithine Translocase Deficiency

The ***hyperornithinemia-hyperammonemia-homocitrullinuria (HHH) syndrome*** is an autosomal recessive disorder characterized by hyperammonemia and increased excretion of ***homocitrulline.*** The ***clinical symptoms*** are related to hyperammonemia and resemble those of other urea cycle disorders e.g. episodes of vomiting, tonic-clonic convulsive seizure, Pyramidal signs, decreased vibration sense, buccofaciolingual dyspraxia and learning difficulties or subnormal intelligence. No visual problems or fundus changes like those in ornithinemia with gyrate atrophy have been observed.

Plasma ornithine concentrations in HHH patients ***range from 380 to 630 μ M/l*** on a self-restricted protein diet and are usually slightly lower than in gyrate atrophy. The pathophysiology of the disease may involve diminished ornithine transport into mitochondria, resulting in ornithine accumulation in the cytoplasm and reduced ability to clear carbamoyl phosphate and ammonia loads. ***Two ornithine transporter proteins*** are implicated **ORNT1** and **ORNT2;** the defect in one or both result in clinical diversity of the syndrome. Ornithine-delta-aminotransferase, the enzyme deficient in ornithinemia, is normal. Homocitrulline is thought to originate from transcarbamoylation of lysine.

Gene Map

The ***genetic cause*** of the HHH syndrome is assigned to the ***mutation(s)*** in the ***SLC25A15 gene.***

CLINICAL MANAGEMENT

A ***low protein diet*** initiated early in life permitted normal development. Ornithine supplementation and restricted protein intake appeared to be useful in treatment.

9. THE ORGANIC ACIDEMIAS

The term "organic acidemia" or "organic aciduria" (OA) applies to a ***diverse group of disorders characterized by the excretion of non-amino organic acids in urine.*** The organic acidemias share many clinical similarities. The majority of the classic organic acid disorders result from abnormal amino acid catabolism of branched chain amino acids or lysine. They include maple syrup urine disease (MSUD), propionic acidemia, methylmalonic acidemia (MMA), isovaleric acidemia, biotin-unresponsive 3-methylcrotonyl-CoA carboxylase deficiency, 3-hydroxy-3-methylglutaryl-CoA (HMG-CoA) lyase deficiency, ketothiolase deficiency, and glutaric acidemia Type I (GA I).

Clinical Presentation: A neonate affected with an OA is ***usually well at birth*** and for the first few days of life. The usual clinical presentation is that of ***a toxic encephalopathy*** and includes vomiting, poor feeding, neurologic symptoms such as seizures and abnormal tone, and lethargy progressing to ***coma.*** In the older child or adolescent, variant forms of the OAs can present as loss of intellectual function, ataxia or other focal neurologic signs, Reye syndrome, recurrent ketoacidosis, or psychiatric symptoms. A variety of MRI abnormalities have been described in the OAs, including ***distinctive basal***

ganglia lesions in GA I, white matter changes in MSUD, and abnormalities of the globus pallidus in methylmalonic acidemia.

Despite appropriate management, individuals with organic acidemias have a ***greater risk of infection*** and ***a higher incidence of pancreatitis,*** which can be fatal. Methylmalonic acidemia is associated with an increased frequency of renal failure and the cblC variant of methylmalonic acidemia is associated with pigmentary retinopathy.

Diagnosis/testing:

- The probability of a positive outcome is enhanced by diagnosis in the first ten days of life. Clinical laboratory findings that should suggest an organic acidemia include ***acidosis, ketosis, hyperammonemia, abnormal liver function tests, hypoglycemia and neutropenia*** Propionic acidemia may present with isolated hyperammonemia early in its course.
- ***First-line diagnosis*** in the organic acidemias is ***urine organic acid analysis using gas chromatography with mass spectrometry (GC/MS),*** utilizing a capillary column. The organic acids found in the urine provide a high degree of suspicion for the specific pathway involved. The urinary organic acid profile is nearly always abnormal in the face of acute illness with decompensation.
- Depending on the specific disorder, ***plasma amino acid analysis*** can also be helpful. Plasma amino acid analysis requires a quantitative method such as ***column chromatography, high-performance liquid chromatography (HPLC),*** or ***GC/MS.*** Once the detection of specific analytes narrows the diagnostic possibilities, the ***activity of the deficient enzyme is measured in lymphocytes or cultured fibroblasts as a confirmatory test.***
- Because many laboratories have difficulty performing and/or interpreting urine organic acids analyzed by GC/MS, it is important that the ***biochemical genetic testing*** be performed in an experienced laboratory and interpreted by an individual trained in biochemical genetics.

Organic aciduria. Several disorders, not classified as primary disorders of organic acid metabolism, have a characteristic urinary organic acid profile that suggests the appropriate diagnosis (Table 27.7).

- ***Mevalonic aciduria,*** a disorder of cholesterol biosynthesis, shows mevalonic acid in the urine.
- ***Glutaric acidemia II (GA II, EMA-adipic aciduria),*** a disorder of fatty acid oxidation, ***characterized by multiple organic acids in abnormal concentration in urine. These organic acids include ethylmalonic acid, glutaric acid, dicarboxylic acids and glycine conjugates*** of medium chain dicarboxylic acids.
- The fatty acylCoA-glycine conjugates that signal incomplete fatty acid oxidation may be identified during GC/MS analysis of urine and serve as signals to the diagnosis of MCAD deficiency and other disorders of fatty acid oxidation and transport.
- Biotinidase deficiency, a disorder of biotin recycling, results in the urinary excretion of several unusual organic acids, including 3-hydroxy-isovaleric, 3-methylcrotonic, 3-hydroxypropionic, methylcitric, 3-hydroxybutyric acids and acetoacetate. Propionyl glycine and tiglylglycine may also be seen.
- Mitochondrial diseases with disordered oxidative phosphorylation often demonstrate the presence of abnormal organic acids in the urine, ***including lactate and 3-methylglutaconic, 2 hydroxybutyric, 3 hydroxybutyric, 2-methyl-3-hydroxybutyric, and ethylmalonic acids.***

Pathogenesis

The pathophysiology results from accumulation of precursors and deficiency of products of the affected pathway. The accumulated precursors are themselves toxic or are metabolized to produce toxic compounds. The ***pathophysiology of these disorders is the result of toxicity of small molecules to brain, liver, kidney, pancreas, retina, and other organs. Some of these molecules, such as the glutaric acid metabolites, are thought to be excitotoxic to neurons and may affect NMDA***

Table 27.7: Metabolic Findings in Organic Acidemias

Disorder	*Amino Acid Pathway(s) Affected*	*Enzyme Defect*	*Organic acid/ amino acid in Urine*
Maple syrup urine disease (MSUD)	Leucine, isoleucine, valine	Branched chain ketoacid dehydrogenase	Branched chain ketoacids and hydroxyacids in urine; alloisoleucine in plasma
Propionic acidemia	Isoleucine, valine, methionine, threonine	Propionyl CoA carboxylase	Propionic acid, 3-OH propionic acid, methyl citric acid, propionyl glycine in urine; propionyl carnitine, increased glycine in blood
Methylmalonic acidemia (MMA)	Isoleucine valine, methionine, threonine	Methylmalonyl CoA mutase	Methylmalonic acid in blood and urine; propionic acid, 3-OH propionic acid, methyl citrate in urine; acyl carnitines, increased glycine in blood
Isovaleric acidemia	Leucine	Isovaleryl CoA dehydrogenase	3-OH isovaleric acid, isovalerylglycine in urine
Biotin-unresponsive 3-methylcrotonyl-CoA carboxylase deficiency	Leucine	3-methylcrotonyl-CoA carboxylase	3-hydroxy-isovaleric acid, 3-methylcrotonyl glycine in urine
3-hydroxy-3-methylglutaryl-CoA(HMG-CoA) lyase deficiency	Leucine	HMG-CoA lyase	3-OH-3-methyl glutaric acid, 3-methylglutaconate, 3 OH-isovalerate, 3-methylglutarate in urine
Ketothiolase deficiency	Isoleucine	Mitochondrial acetoacetyl-CoA thiolase	2-methyl-3-hydroxybutyric acid,2-methylacetoacetic acid,tiglylglycine in urine
Glutaric acidemia Type I (GA I)	Lysine, hydroxylysine	Glutaryl CoA dehydrogenase	Glutaric acid 3-OH-glutaric acid in urine

receptors. Evidence suggests that ***methylmalonic acid is excitotoxic to neurons.*** In maple syrup urine disease (MSUD), ***leucine is believed to be toxic to neurons.*** In addition, because catabolism of amino acids provides energy for other cellular processes, energy deficiency during metabolic crisis may contribute to the clinical syndrome.

Several rare OAs present with neurologic signs without concomitant biochemical manifestions. They include 4-hydroxybutyric aciduria, D-2-hydroxyglutaric aciduria, 3-methylglutaconic aciduria caused by 3-methylglutaconic acid dehydratase deficiency, and malonic aciduria. Methylmalonic aciduria, cblC variant, may present with developmental delay, minor dysmorphology, and hypotonia without acidosis. Late-onset 3-methylcrotonyl carboxylase deficiency may present as developmental delay without Reye-like syndrome, in contrast to the early-onset form.

C. Disorders of Lipid Metabolism

C1 DEFECTS IN FATTY ACID OXIDATION METABOLISM

Mitochondrial oxidation of fatty acids provides the chief source of energy during prolonged fasting as well as for skeletal muscle during exercise and for cardiac muscle. ***Ten genetic defects*** in this pathway have been recognized in infants and children, including:

a. Long Chain Acyl CoA Dehydrogenase (LCAD) deficiency,
b. Medium Chain Acyl CoA Dehydrogenase (MCAD) deficiency,
c. Short Chain Acyl CoA Dehydrogenase (SCAD) deficiency,
d. Deficiency of the plasma-membrane carnitine transporter,
e. Carnitie palmitoyltransferase I (CPT I) deficiency,
f. Carnitine palmitoyltransferase II (CPT II) deficiency.

Patients with these defects ***present with coma after a period of starvation and have hypoketosis,*** i.e., their serum ketone concentrations are low. They may also have ***cardiomyopathy*** and ***muscle weakness.*** Urinary excretion of products of fatty acid oxidation through alternate pathway (e.g. omega-oxidation) is specific for each kind of disorder and urinary analysis looking for these acids makes a major tool in the diagnosis. Myoglobinuria may also be accompanied with the muscular features particularly in the acute phase of the disease.

(A) ACYL-COA DEHYDROGENASE DEFICIENCY

β-oxidation of fatty acids takes place inside the mitochondria for which the activated fatty acids (acyl CoAs) are transported across the mitochondrial membranes with the help of carnitine. Inborn errors of mitochondrial fatty acid β-oxidation include the deficiency of β-oxidation enzymes, particularly the first enzyme of the pathway i.e. Acyl CoA dehydrogenase (ACD). Different chain length fatty acyl CoAs are acted upon by different enzymes because the fatty acyl CoA can only accept a limited range of carbon atoms in the fatty acids. Therefore, the deficiency of different enzymes leads to slightly varying signs and symptoms; the enzymes with known inherited deficiency are: • short-chain acyl-CoA dehydrogenase deficiency, • medium-chain acyl-CoA dehydrogenase deficiency, • long-chain acyl-CoA dehydrogenase deficiency and • very long-chain acyl-CoA dehydrogenase deficiency.

In a prospective tandem ***mass spectrometry screening*** of 9,30,078 blood spots from neonates in the US population, ***a frequency of MCAD deficiency*** of 1 in 15,001 was documented.

1. Very Long Chain ACD Deficiency (VLCAD)

VLCAD deficiency can be classified clinically into 3 ***forms:***

a. ***Severe early-onset form:*** Presents within 4 months of birth with ***high incidence of cardiomyopathy*** and high mortality. All patients would have liver dysfunction.
b. ***Intermediate childhood onset form:*** Usually presents with ***hypoketotic hypoglycemia.*** This is the form with more favorable outcome.
c. ***The adult-onset myopathic form:*** Presents with isolated skeletal muscle involvement, ***rhabdomyolysis,*** and ***myoglobinuria*** after exercise or fasting (Andresen et al., 1999). Elevated serum creatine kinase could also be found.

Depending upon the severity of the disease, hepatocellular injury and marked lipid accumulation in many tissues is observed.

Laboratory findings might include hyperammonemia and increased urinary levels of adipate and sebacate.

2. Long Chain ACD Deficiency (LCAD)

- ***Nonketotic hypoglycemia*** and ***episodes of cardiorespiratory arrest associated with fasting are characteristic.*** Other features included ***hepatomegaly, cardiomegaly, and hypotonia.*** Total plasma carnitine concentration is low.
- ***Specific assay*** show that the ***activity of long-chain acyl-CoA dehydrogenase is very low (<20%)*** compared to control values in ***fibroblasts, leukocytes and liver.***

Treatment with frequent low-fat high-carbohydrate feedings, riboflavin and carnitine reduced the frequency and intensity of crises.

(B) MEDIUM CHAIN ACD DEFICIENCY (MCAD)

Reported mostly from children and young adolescents with unexplained episodes of lethargy and unconsciousness and C_6-C_{10} dicarboxylic aciduria. Inherited deficiency of medium-chain acyl-CoA dehydrogenase is ***characterized by intolerance to prolonged fasting,*** recurrent episodes of hypoglycemic coma with medium-chain dicarboxylic aciduria, ***impaired ketogenesis,*** and ***low plasma and tissue carnitine levels.*** The disorder may be severe, and even fatal, in young patients.

As in long chain ACD deficiency, dicarboxylic acids and 3-hydroxydicarboxylic (3OHDC) acids can be demonstrated in the urine arising from the alternate (omega) oxidation of fatty acids and their intermediates. ***Adipic and monounsaturated sebacic, seburic and ozeleic acids are among those elevated in urine and serum.***

(C) SHORT CHAIN ACD DEFICIENCY (SCAD)

Two distinct clinical phenotypes of hereditary short-chain acyl-CoA dehydrogenase deficiency have been identified:

- One type has been observed in infants with acute acidosis and muscle weakness;
- The other has been observed in middle-aged patients with chronic myopathy. SCAD deficiency is generalized in the former type and localized to skeletal muscles in the latter.

Cases with neonatal onset have a variable phenotype that includes metabolic acidosis, failure to thrive, developmental delay, and seizures, as well as myopathy. There are no episodes of non-ketotic hypoglycemia, which are characteristic of mediun-chain and long-chain acyl dehydrogenase deficiencies. ***All patients with SCAD have neurologic deficits:*** hypotonia/hypertonia, hyperactivity, and/or developmental delay.

Ethylmalonic aciduria, is commonly found in short chain ACD deficiency, but the disorder cannot be taken as conformatory to short chain ACD deficiency. It appears to be a complex multifactorial/polygenic condition where a number ofother genetic and environmental factors are involved.

BIOCHEMICAL FEATURES AND DIAGNOSIS

- **Rinaldo et al (1988)** found that ***measurement of urinary hexanoylglycine and phenylpropionylglycine by a method of stable-isotope dilution*** is a fast and reliable method for diagnosis of Medium Chain ACD deficiency. It can be applied to random urine specimens without pretreatment such as fasting.
- The diagnosis of MCAD deficiency, including presymptomatic neonatal recog-nition, can be made reliably through the ***analysis of acylcarnitines in blood. Tandem mass spectrometry*** is a convenient method for fast accurate determination.
- **Clayton et al (1998)** reported their experience in diagnosing MCAD deficiency using the ***technique of electrospray ionization tandem mass spectrometry (ESI-MS/MS) analysis*** of butylated carnitine species from dried blood spots. The authors concluded that if neonatal screening was undertaken at 7 to 10 days of age, this technique was both sensitive and specific and would therefore be suitable for a national neonatal screening program.
- **Onkenhout et al. (2001)** ***determined the fatty acid composition of liver, skeletal muscle, and heart obtained from postmortem patients***

with deficiency of 1 of the 3 types of acyl-CoA dehydrogenase: medium-chain, very long-chain, and multiple. ***Increased amounts of multiple unsaturated fatty acids were found exclusively in the triglyceride fraction.*** They could not be detected in the free fatty acid or phospholipids fractions. They concluded that intermediates of unsaturated fatty acid oxidation that accumulate in these disorders are transported to the endoplasmic reticulum for esterification into neutral glycerolipids. ***The pattern of accumulation was characteristic for each disease, making fatty acid analysis of total lipid of postmortem tissues a useful tool in the detection of mitochondrial fatty acid oxidation defects*** in patients who have died unexpectedly.

- **Ohashi et al (2004)** demonstrated that the ***immuno-histochemical technique was an effective diagnostic tool for ACD deficiency.*** They identified 13 patients with the myopathic form of VLCAD deficiency using immuno-histochemistry to ***analyze the VLCAD protein in skeletal muscle biopsies.*** Biochemical analysis confirmed that all 13 patients had low enzymatic activity and reduced amounts of VLCAD protein. Genetic analysis confirmed that they all had mutations in the ACADVL gene.
- The definitive diagnostic test for SCAD deficiency is ***an ETF-linked enzyme assay with butyry1-CoA as a substrate,*** performed after immunoactivation of MCAD, which has similar activity.

CLINICAL MANAGEMENT

ACD deficiency is one of the few ***directly treatable causes of cardiomyopathy in children.*** After initial treatment with intravenous glucose and carnitine, the patient thrives on a low-fat diet supplemented with medium-chain triglyceride oil and carnitine accompanied with avoidance of fasting. Multiple meals (at least five meals a day) are recommended and raw corn-starch after the last meal has been found to be helpful.

Some of the authors have cautioned against the administration of carnitine in Medium Chain ACD deficiency saying this is either of no consequence or harmful for the patient.

Avoidance of fasting and prompt institution of glucose supplementation in situations when oral intake is interrupted remain the mainstays of therapy.

5. Jamaican vomiting Sickness: The disease is caused by ***eating the unripe fruits of 'Akee' tree*** found on the Caribbean islands. The fruit contains a ***toxin, hypoglycin*** that inactivates the medium chain and short chain fatty acyl CoA dehydrogenase enzyme. The resultant inhibition of the oxidation of medium and short chain fatty acids causes ***hypoglycemia*** with ***excretion of medium and short chain mono-or*** di-carboxylic acids. Some of the other features of the ACD deficiency discussed above may also be present.

(D) CARNITINE-ACYLCARNITINE TRANSLOCASE DEFICIENCY

Carnitine-acylcarnitine translocase (CACT) is 1 of 10 closely related ***mitochondrial-membrane carrier proteins*** that shuttle substrates between cytosol and the intramitochondrial matrix space. CACT transfers fatty acylcarnitines into mitochondria in exchange for free carnitine. The ***CACT gene shows differential expression in different tissues.*** High level are found in heart, skeletal muscle and liver, and much lower levels in brain, placenta, kidney, pancreas, and especially in the lungs (Fig. 27.18).

Gene Mapping

By fluorescence *in situ* hybridization, Viggiano et al. in 1997 ***mapped the CACT gene to 3p21.31 and its pseudogene, CACTP, to 6p12.***

Clinical/Laboratory Features: The ***newborn infants present with seizures, apneic periods and bradycardia.*** The attack is mostly provoked by fasting. The patients might have recurrent premature ventricular contractions, ventricular tachycardia, hypotension and ***episodes of***

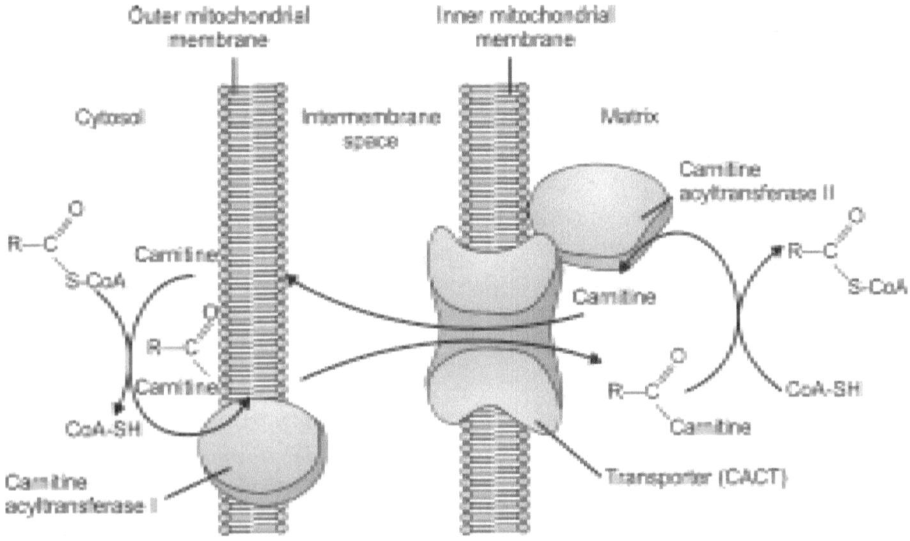

Fig 27.18: Transport of fatty acyl CoA across the mitochondrial membranes

hypoglycemic coma. Hyperammonemia is persent in some patients.

The disorder is fatal in a number of cases terminating with increasing weakness, hepatomegaly, and reduced liver function; cardiorespiratory arrest is another cause of sudden death.

Urine analysis: Urine organic acid analysis shows ***elevated lactate, dicarboxylic, and hydroxydicarboxylic acids with no ketones.***

Management: The prognosis of the patients with CACT deficiency is very poor, but attempts have been made to stabilize the condition and prevent the sudden death.

Treatment includes peritoneal dialysis with a permanent Tenckof catheter *in situ*, enteral feeding with high calories, low protein, long-chain fatty acids, medium-chain triglyceride oil, and frequent feedings.

In a child with CACT deficiency who was the product of a consanguineous marriage, lacobazzi et al in 2004, therapy with a formula which ***provided most of the fat in the form of medium chain triglycerides*** as well as ***carnitine supplementation reduced*** the concentration of long chain acylcarnitines and reversed cardiac symptoms and hypoglycemia.

(E) CARNITINE PALMITOYLTRANSFERASE DEFICIENCY

The carnitine palmitoyltransferase (CPT; EC2.3.1.21) enzyme system, in conjunction with acyl-CoA synthetase and carnitite/acylcarnitine translocase, provides the mechanisam whereby ***long-chain fatty acids are transferred from the cytosol to the mitochondrial matrix to undergo beta-oxidation for energy production.***

The CPT I isozymes (CPT1A and CPT1B) are located in the mitochondrial outer membrane and are detergent-labile, whereas CPT II is located in the inner mitochondrial membrane and is detergent-stable. Disorders due to the deficiency of either of the two transferases (CPT I and CPT II) have been reported.

Gene Mapping

By fluorescence *in situ* hybridization, *Britton et al. (1997)* ***mapped the CPT1A gene to chromosome 11q13.1-q13.5.***

Major control over fatty acid oxidation process is exerted at the level of CPT I by virtue of the unique inhibitability of this enzyme by malonyl-CoA. This fuel 'cross talk' was first recognized in the context of hepatic ketogenesis and its regulation thereafter emerged as a central component of metabolism in a variety of tissues.

For many years, it was unclear whether of not there were 2 distinct CPT proteins associated with mitochondrial beta-oxidation because CPT I and CPT II have similar physical characteristics, including molecular mass and kinetic properties, and that antibodies raised against each enzyme crossreacted with the other. During the last decade only, it has been shown that the respective causative mutations of CPT I and CPT II deficiencies reside in distinct genes.

Liver and fibroblasts express the same isoform of mitochondrial CPT1, therefore, ***fibroblast assays may be used in the differential diagnosis of the 'muscle' and 'hepatic' forms of CPT deficiency.***

To investigate the mechanism by which central metabolism of lipids can modulate energy balance, *Obici et al. (2003)* selectively reduced lipid oxidation in the hypothalamus. Either genetic or biochemical inhibition of hypothalamic CPT1 activity is sufficient to diminish food intake and endogenous glucose production substantially. They concluded that ***changes in the rate of lipid oxidation in selective hypothalamic neurons signalled nutrient availability to the hypothalamus, which in turn modulated the exogenous and endogenous inputs of nutrients into the circulation.***

Clinical Features: ***Episodic periods of hypoglycemia*** owing to reduced gluconeogenesis due to impaired fatty acid oxidation. ***Recurrent muscle weakness and myoglobinuria.***

C2 REFSUM'S DISEASE

Alternate Title: Phytanate α-oxidase deficiency

Refsum's disease is a rare ***autosomal recessive*** disorder characterized by neurological mani-festations like ***chronic polyneuropathy, distal muscular atrophy and night blindness.***

Biochemical Defect: The ***enzyme deficient is phytanate α-oxidase, which is involved in the conversion of phytanic acid*** (product of a number of plant phytols) ***to pristanic acid. Phytanic acid accumulation in the blood as well as tissues is responsible for most of the clinical manifestations.***

Clinical Presentation: Manifestations are principally ***neurological*** e.g. early chronic polyneuropathy with distal muscular atrophy and progressive paresis of the distal extremities. Sensory disturbances my include paresthesiae, occasional severe pain especially in the knees. ***Cerebellar involvement*** causes ataxia and nystagmus.

- ***Ocular involvement*** can manifest as ***pigmentary retinitis, night blindness and concentric narrowing of the visual fields.***
- ***Mental development*** is usually normal.

Diagnosis: ***Demonstration of phytanic acid in plasma or in tissue lipids is pathognomonic.***

Management: Management is primarily ***dietary. Restriction of dietary phytols can help in showing down the disease progress.***

C3 ZELLWEGER'S SYNDROME

Zellweger's syndrome (Hepato-renal syndrome): Rare inherited disorder. There is inherited absence of peroxi-somes in all tissues. Due to the absence of peroxisomes and its enzymes, fail to oxidize long-chain FA in Peroxisomes. As a result there is accumulation of FA C_{26}-C_{38} chain-length in brain tissue and other tissues like liver/ kidney.

C4 NORUM'S DISEASE

A genetic deficiency of LCAT produces Norum's Disease due to the failure of esterification of cholesterol at the cost of lecithin. The disease is characterized by:

- Rise in free cholesterol ↑
- Rise in lecithin in plasma ↑ and
- Fall in cholesterol ester, ↓ lysolecithin ↓ and α-lipoproteins ↓ in plasma.

C5 NIEMANN-PICK DISEASE

Large accumulations of sphingomyelins may occur in brains, liver and spleen of some persons suffering from Niemann-Pick disease.

It is an inherited disorder of sphingomyelin metabolism in which sphingomyelin is not degraded, as a result sphingomyelin accumulates. It is a lipid-storage disease (Lipidoses).
Inheritence: Autosomal recessive.
Enzyme defect: Deficiency of the enzyme *sphingomyelinase*, a lysosomal enzyme.
Clinical Features: Affects children, arises at birth or infancy. The child presents with gradual enlargement of abdomen, enlargement of liver ***(hepatomegaly)***, enlargement of spleen ***(splenomegaly)***, and manifests progressive mental deterioration (due to accumulation of sphingomyelins in brain). Other lipids and cholesterol are usually normal or may be slightly elevated.
Prognosis: Usually fatal, progressive downhill course. Over 80% of infants die within 2 years.

C6 GAUCHER'S DISEASE

An inherited disorder of cerebrosides metabolism (lipidosis).

- ***Inheritance:*** It is autosomal recessive.
- ***Enzyme defect:*** Deficiency of the enzyme ***β-Glucocerebrosidase,*** a lysosomal enzyme. Normally this enzyme hydrolyzes glucocerebrosides to form ceramide and glucose. In absence of the enzyme, the cerebrosides cannot be degraded in the body, as a result large amounts of glucocerebrosides, usually ***'kerasin'*** accumulate in RE cells viz., liver, spleen, bone marrow and also brain. Complex lipids appear to collect within mitochondria of the RE cells.

Biochemically, there is characteristically elevation in serum acid phosphatase level.

Clinical features: Adults as well as infants are affected.

(a) In infancy and childhood: Fairly acute onset, with rapid course and death in several years. The infant loses weight, fails to grow, progressive mental retardation. Initially there is spasticity, later on followed by flaccidity.

(b) In adult: Progressive enlargement of spleen ***(splenomegaly)*** which may reach to umbilicus or below. Characteristic **"bone pain"** due to marrow cells replaced by histiocytes loaded with the lipids. As a result leads to ***progressive anemia, leucopenia and thrombocytopenia,*** tendency to get secondary infections and bleeding tendency.

C7 TAY-SACH'S DISEASE (GM_2 GANGLIOSIDOSIS)

Accumulation of gangliosides in brain and nervous tissues takes place. The affected ganglioside is GM_2. ***The Enzyme deficiency is hexosaminidase A***.
Inheritance: autosomal recessive.

Normal degradation of GM_2 requires the action of a specific hydrolyzing enzyme ***hexosaminidase A,*** which removes the terminal Gal-NAc. Subsequently the other components are hydrolyzed by other specific enzymes. In absence of the enzyme *Hexosaminidase A*, GM_2 cannot be degraded and accumulates.

This rare inherited disorder is associated with:

- Progressive development of ***idiocy and blindness in infants*** soon after birth. This is due to widespread injury to ganglion cells in brain (Cerebral cortex) and retina.
- ***A cherry-red spot about the macula, seen ophthalmoscopically is pathognomonic*** and is caused by destruction of retinal ganglion cells, exposing the underlying vasculature.
- There may be seizures and association of macrocephaly.

Prognosis is bad, usually death follows.

GM_1 Gangliosidosis: It is due to a deficiency of the enzyme **β-galactosidase,** leading to accumulation of GM_1 gangliosides, glycoproteins and the mucopolysaccharide Karatan sulphate.

The inheritance pattern and symptoms are similar to Tay-Sach's disease.

C8 METACHROMATIC LEUKODYSTROPHY (MLD)

It is an inherited disorder in which sulfatide accumulates in various tissues. Sulfatide is formed from "galactocerebroside" through esterification of OH group on C_3 of galactose with H_2SO_4 (SO_4 at C_3 of Gal). ***Ratio of cerebroside: to sulfatide in brain normally is 3:1. In this disorder, it is altered to 1:4.***

Enzyme deficiency: Deficiency of enzyme *sulfatase* called as ***Aryl sulfatase A.***

Sulfatides	Sulfatase H_2O	Galactocerebroside H_2SO_4

Types: Two clinical types are seen.

(a) Late infantile type: Usually manifests before 3 years, gross involvement of CNS:

- Defects in locomotion, weakness, ataxia, hypotonus, and paralysis
- Difficulties in speech
- There may be optic atrophy.

(b) Adult type: Initially associated with psychiatric manifestations but subsequently progressive dementia.

C9 FABRY'S DISEASE

Fabry's Disease: An inherited disorder, a lipid storage disease (lipidosis).

- ***Inheritance:*** X-linked dominant, full symptoms only in males.
- ***Enzyme deficiency: α-galactosidase.*** The enzyme is found normally in liver, spleen, kidney, brain, and small intestine.
- ***Nature of lipid*** that accumulates: ***ceramide trihexoside*** (globotriosyl ceramide)
- ***Clinical manifestations:***
- ***Skin rash*** (reddish purple)
  - Pain in lower extremities *(painful neuropathy),*
  - Lipid accumulates in the endothelial lining of blood vessels, may produce *vascular thrombosis.*
  - Progressive ***renal failure:*** due to extensive deposition of lipids in glomeruli. Occasionally manifestations of cardiac enlargement.
  - ***Eye involvement:*** corneal opacities, cataracts, vascular dilatation.

C10 KRABBE'S DISEASE

- An inherited disorder of lipid metabolism, a lipid storage disease (lipidosis)
- ***Enzyme deficiency: galactocerebrosidase* (*β-galactosidase*).** The enzyme normally catalyzes the hydrolysis of galactocerebrosides and it splits the linkage between ceramide and galactose

Galactocerebrosides
α-galactocerebrosidase ↓ H_2O
Ceramide + Galactose

- ***Nature of lipid*** accumulating: ***Galactosyl ceramide***
- ***Clinical manifestations:***
  - Severe mental retardation in infants
  - Total absence of myelin in central nervous system
  - Globoid bodies found in white matter of brain.

Note: Galactocerebroside is an important component of myelin

- ***Diagnosis:*** Depends on the determination of galactocerebrosidase activity in leucocytes and cultured skin fibroblasts.
- ***Prognosis:*** fatal.

C11 Primary Hyperlipoproteinaemias

Already dealt in this book. Please refer to Chapter 13.

D. Inborn Errors of Defective DNA Repair and Purines/Pyrimidine Metabolism

INTRODUCTION

Eukaryotic cells have one or two sets of DNA. The DNA being the genetic material, has to be preserved in its entirety to maintain the functionality and progression of the cells/ organisms. Cellular DNA is subjected to an onslaught of damaging insults which threaten cellular control and replication. ***DNA damage can result from exposure to exogenous agents,*** such as radiation and chemicals in the environment, ***as well as from endogenous DNA-damaging agents that arise as by-products of cellular metabolism.*** Damage can also occur during DNA replication, and from such spontaneous events as depurination and de-amination of nucleotides. The range of lesions arising in DNA is large, but they can be subdivided into **four distinct classes:**

- ***strand breaks,***
- ***damage or modification to a single base,***
- ***dimmer formation or cross-links between adj-acent or apposing bases, and***
- ***damage to the phospho-diester backbone.***

It is, therefore, not suprising that a plethora of ***damage response mechanisms operate to maintain genomic stability.*** These include processes that • recognize and repair the damage, • cell cycle checkpoints that prevent cell cycle progression in the presence of damage, and • mechanisms, such as ***apoptosis, that remove damaged cells.*** The DNA repair mechanisms are dependent upon a complex molecular interaction between the various component proteins. It is very much expected that the transcription and translation of these repair proteins can also be defective or the genes for these proteins could also be damaged and mutated. Such a situation would result in a compromised repair mechanism, making the cellular DNA susceptible to the damage by external assault.

Individuals with defective DNA repair mechanisms have pleiotropic phenotypes including a predisposition to cancer, neuro-degeneration and developmental abnormalities. Increasingly, immunodeficiency is recognized as a feature of some of these syndrome. Further evidence for the overlap between DNA repair and immune development is the finding that some individuals with poorly understood immunodeficiencies exhibit cellular ionizing radiation sensitivity, probably as a consequence of defective repair of radiation-induced DNA damage. This review discusses the common molecular defects identified in DNA repair-defective syndromes associated with immuno-deficiency, as well as detailing the clinical features seen in affected individuals.

Classification

A ***classification*** of the repair mechanisms that operate to deal with these lesions together with details of human syndromes known to be defec-tive in these processes is given in Table 27.8.

1. XERODERMA PIGMENTOSUM

Xeroderma pigmentosum (XP) is a ***rare autosomal recessive disease*** associated with sun sensitivity and a high risk of cutaneous malignancy in sun-exposed areas. It is due to ***defective repair of nucleotide excision repair caused by mutation of at least 7 genes called XPA to XPG.*** Patients are highly sensitive to sunlight or UV light and their skin is damaged and is liable for multiple cancer, scarred and atrophied eyelid, ulcerated cornea, may lead to death in a few decades, about 2/3rd of the patients die before adulthood.

Table 27.8: Genes involved in common DNA repair pathways and identified hereditary disorders with identified defects in these pathways

Repairs pathway	*Genes involved*	*Hereditary disorders*
Base excision repair	Glycosylases; HAPI; DNA pol; XRCCI, DNA ligase III, PARP	None yet identified
Nucleotide excision repair	XPA-G, DNA pol; PCNA, RFC; RPA, transcription complex. CSA, CSB	*Xeroderma pigmentosum*
Mismatch repair	HMsh2, 3 and 6; M1h1; hPms2	*Hereditary colon cancer*
Homologous recombination	HRad 51; hRad52, hRad 54; XRCC2 and XRCC3	None yet identified*
Non homologous end joining	DNA-PK (Ku70, Ku80 and DNA-PKcs); XRCC4, DNA Ligase IV	Possibly rare cases of severe combined immunodeficiency

*BRCA1 and BRCA2 may also operate in homologous recombination (HR), but this has not yet been definitively proven.

Phenotype and Clinical Characteristics

- ***Severe sun photosensitivity (poikilodermia):*** induced precocious cutaneous lesions concomitant to first sun exposures on the exposed areas (hands, arms, face); dry skin, senile-like, cutaneous retraction (premature aging of the skin) (Fig. 27.19).
- ***Photophobia,*** often the first sign, before cutaneous lesion; followed by bilateral cataract; increased risk of benign and malignant ocular tumors.
- ***Neurological signs*** (14 to 40% of patients): mental retardation, pyramidal syndrome, peripheral neuropathy; more severe central nervous system (CNS) disorders are observed when mutations occur in XPA DNA binding site.
- ***Clinical heterogeneity:*** related to genetic heterogeneity of the disease (7 known complementation groups A, B, C, D, E, F, G and 7 characterized genes). Intensity and precocity of signs are dependent on the gene involved; groups A, C, D and G are associated with a more severe disease.

Note

The ***same genes are implicated in two related diseases:*** Cockayne syndrome (groups B, D and G) and trichothiodystrophy (groups B and D).

Mutability

The cell cultures/skin fibroblasts show hypermutability after UV irradiation. The spontaneous chromosome abnormalities in lymphocytes fibroblasts are not increased; however, after UV-exposure an increased number of sister chromatid exchanges (SCE) and chromosomal aberrations are observed (mainly chromatid-type abnormalities); fibroblasts express an increased sensitivity to chemical mutagens.

Genes and Proteins Involved

All XP genes are implicated in various steps of the NER (nucleotide excision repair system, except the XP variant that is mutated in a mutagenic DNA polymerase (Pol H) able to by pass the UV-induced DNA lesions; various alterations of the same gene may involve various phenotypes *Cockayne syndrome, trichothiodystrophy.*

- The clinical and cytologic XP heterogeneity is the consequence of the genetic heterogeneity: 7 complementation groups (XPA to G) plus an additional variant form, evidenced by somatic cell fusion experiments.
- **The genes involved are:**
  a. XPA, located in 9q22,
  b. XPB, also called ERCC3* located in 2q21,
  c. XPC, located in 3p25,
  d. XPD, also called ERCC2, located in 19q13,
  e. XPE, located on chromosome 11,
  f. XPF, also called ERCC4, located in 19q13,
  g. XPG, also called ERCC5, located in 13q32, and
  h. XPV, also called Pol eta, and located in 6p12-21.

*ERCC: Excision-Repair Cross Complementing rodent repair deficiency.

Defects in any of seven gene products, designated XPA to XPG, can confer an XP phenotype. These proteins jointly operate in nucleotide excision repair (NER), a repair mechanism that handles the damage induced by UV exposure. Consistent with this, XP cells are highly sensitive to UV irradiation. Immunodeficiency has been reported in some but not all XP patients. ***Impaired natural killer cell cytotoxicity in particular*** has been described, and whilst defective interferon production has been suggested as the mechanism, the basis is currently unknown. UV damage is known to suppress the immune response in normal cells and the presence of elevated unrepaired DNA damage in XP patients is likely to enhance this immunosuppression. Thus it appears that at least some of the immunosuppression in XP develops as a consequence of the repair defect rather than as a direct result of the abnormal XP proteins impairing immune development. In support of this, defective post-UV immunity has been observed in XP-A mice.

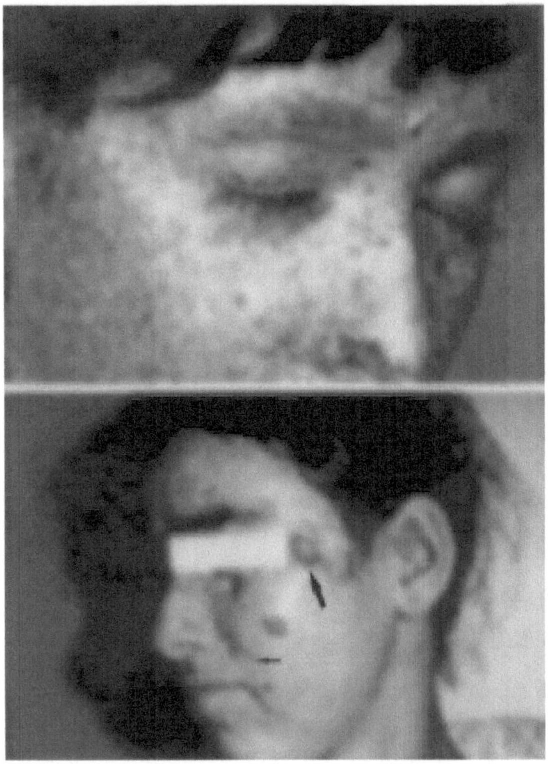

Fig. 27.19: Above: Characteristic aspect of evolved lesions of the face in an XP patient. To be noted multiple scars of carcinomas and an aged aspect of the skin with poikilodermia. Below: Multiple basocellular carcinomas on the face of an XP patient. Thick arrow points to a recent lesion, and thin arrow to a scar of an old lesion

2. ATAXIA TELANGIECTASIA

Alternate Title: Louis-Bar Syndrome, AT, Cerebello-Oculocutaneous Telangiectasia

Clinical Presentation

Ataxia telangiectasia (AT) is a ***complex genetic neurodegenerative disorder*** that may become apparent during infancy or early childhood. The ***disorder is characterized*** by progressively • impaired coordination of voluntary movements (ataxia); the • development of reddish lesions of the skin and mucous membranes due to permanent widening of groups of blood vessels (telangiectasia), and • impaired functioning of the immune system (i.e., cellular and humoral immunodeficiency), resulting in ***increased susceptibility to upper and lower respiratory infections (sinopulmonary infections).*** Individuals with AT also have ***an increased risk of developing certain malignancies,*** particularly of the lymphatic system ***(lymphomas),*** the blood-forming organs (e.g., ***leukemia***), and the ***brain.***

Telangiectasias typically develop between 3 and 5 years of age. The earlier ataxia can be misdiagnosed as ataxic cerebral palsy before the appearance of oculocutaneous telangiectases.

In those with AT, progressive ataxia typically develops during infancy and may initially be characterized by abnormal swaying of the head and trunk. As the disease progresses, the condition ***leads to an inability to walk*** by late childhood or adolescence. Ataxia is often accompanied by ***difficulty in speaking (dysarthria);*** drooling; and ***an impaired ability to coordinate certain eye movements (oculomotor apraxia),*** including the occurrence of involuntary, rapid, rhythmic motions (oscillations) of the eyes while attemp-ting to focus upon certain objects ***(fixation nystagmus).*** Affected children may also develop an unusually stooped posture and irregular, rapid, jerky movements that may occur in association with relatively slow, writhing motions (choreoathetosis). In addition, telangiectasias may develop by mid-childhood, often appearing on sun-exposed areas of the skin, such as the bridge of the nose, the ears, and certain regions of the extremities, as well as the conjunctiva.

Biochemical Basis

AT is inherited as ***an autosomal recessive trait.*** The disorder is ***caused by changes (mutations) of a gene known as ATM*** (for "AT mutated") that has been mapped to the ***long arm (q) of chromosome 11 (11q22.3). The ATM gene controls (encodes for) the production of an enzyme that plays a role in regulating cell division following DNA damage.***

Some of the clinical heterogeneity may be explained by the nature of the ATM mutation. Whilst the majority of 'classical' A-T patients have frameshift mutations that are likely to inactivate gene function and express no (or undetectable quantities of) protein, a subset of milder 'AT variants' have mis-sense mutations which allow the production of some normal

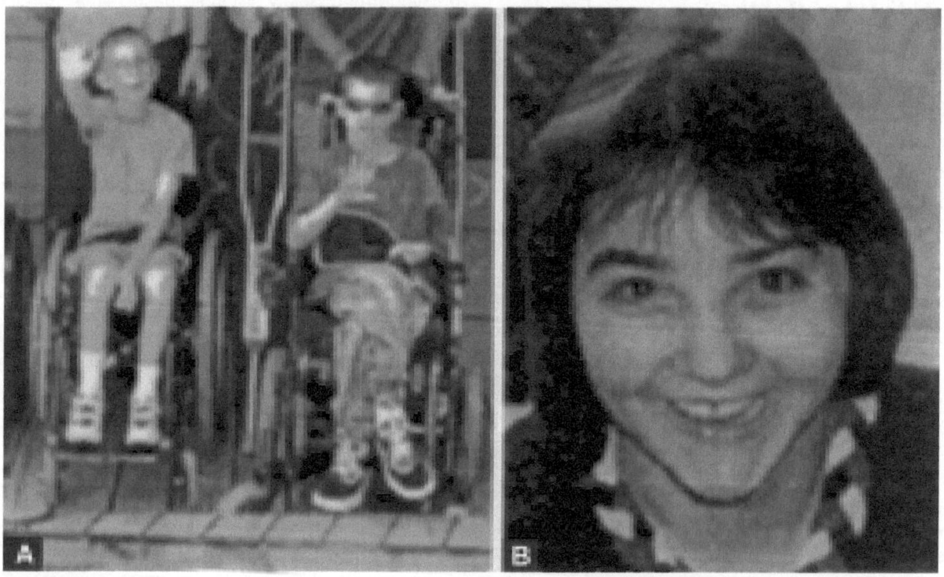

Figs 27.20 A and B: Photographs of AT patients (A) Jeremy and Alex (B) Siam Watkins

protein. At least 4 of these (A, C, D, and E) map to chromosome 11q23 and are associated with mutations in the ATM gene.

The defective protein in A-T cells is a member of the phosphoinositol 3-kinase (PI 3-K) family of kinases, has serin threonine protein kinase activity and is implicated in the phosphorylation of a range of proteins involved in damage response mechanisms, including p53 and Chk1. Taken together, these and additional findings suggest that this protein acts as an early sensor of DNA damage, and activates by phosphorylation, a number of damage response mechanisms including a ***p53-dependent pathway that controls apoptosis and G1/S arrest.*** The ATM gene is central in location for the phase arrest of the cell cycle as well as for the Nijmegen breakage syndrome (NBS) and Fanconi's anemia and Breast cancer (BRCA1 & BRCA2) proteins (Fig. 27.21) since the phosphorylation of all of these proteins is carried out by the ATM protein.

The wide range of clinical characteristics of A-T is coupled with a pleitropic phenotype at the cellular level. A-T cell lines display radiation sensitivity, defects in cell cycle checkpoint control including an inability to arrest at the G1/S and S phase checkpoints and, for cells in G2 at the time of irradiation, an impaired G2/M

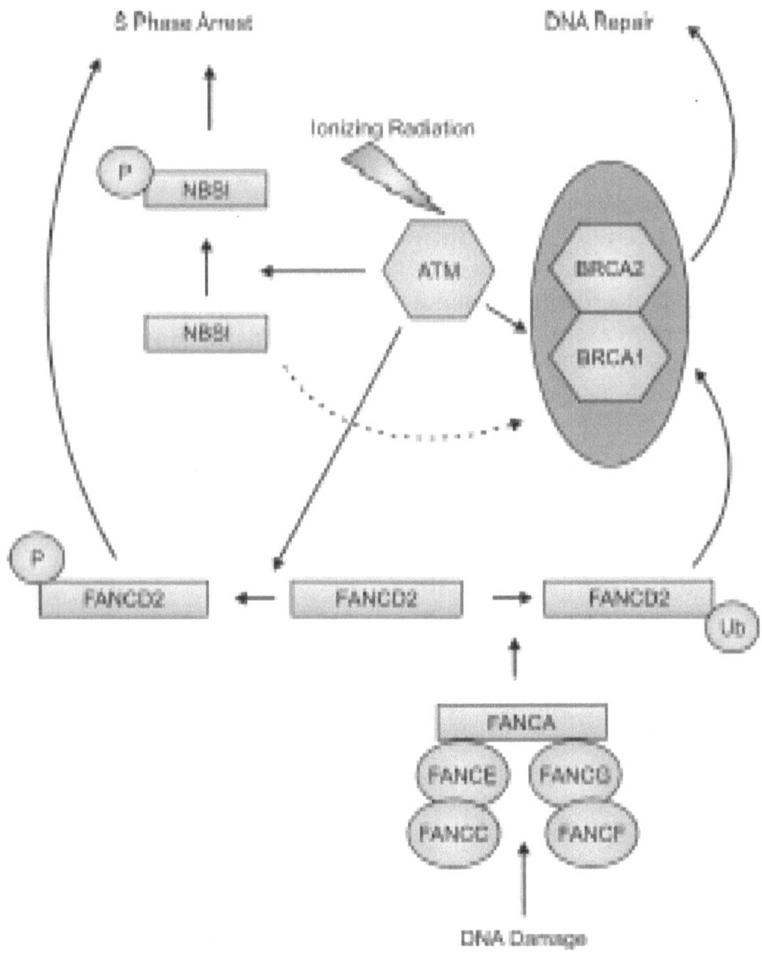

Fig. 27.21: ATM protein and its relation with Fanconi's anemia and Nijmegen breakage syndrome

arrest. Furthermore, p53, a key protein involved in signal transduction and required for G1/S arrest, fails to be stabilized following radiation exposure. However, *the radio-sensitivity of A-T cells appears to be distinct from the checkpoint defects and there is circumstantial evidence that A-T cells also have a DNA repair defect.*

Immunodeficiency

The *immunodeficiency is characterized by both cellular and humoral impairment,* but clinical manifestations are extremely variable, ranging from normal to profoundly reduced responses to bacterial antigens. • *Recurrent sinopulmonary infection is common, occasionally leading to finger clubbing and bronchiectasis, and is associated with hypogammaglobulinemia.* • *Low or absent IgA, IgE or IgG, particularly IgG2 subclass,are frequently found and are due to a defect in B cell maturation,* rather than B cell lymphopenia. • *Autoantibodies have also been documented in some A-T pateints.* • Cellular immunodeficiency is characterized by defective thymic development, with macroscopic absence of the thymus at postmortem examination. A-T patients are proficient in V (D) J recombination but significantly, translocations involving the immunoglobulin and TCR loci are found at elevated frequency in A-T lymphocytes.

Diagnosis

- The *presence of early-onset ataxia with oculocutaneous telangiectases permits diagnosis of AT.* The clinial diagnosis of AT can be problematic before the appearance of telangiectases. *Oculomotor apraxia is a useful aid to early clinical diagnosis.* Early-onset cerebellar ataxia and oculomotor apraxia are also typical of X-linked Pelizaeus-Merzbacher disease and can be seen in Joubert syndrome. These disorders can be distinguished by leukoencephalopathy in the former, and by profound cerebellar hypoplasia in the latter.
- *Elevated levels of alpha-fetoprotein and carcinoembryonic antigen* are the most useful readily available markers for confirmation of the diagnosis of AT.
- Dysgammaglobulinemia, decreased cellular immune responses, and peripheral lymphopenia are supportive findings but are not invariable.
- Henderson et al in 1985 devised a *rapid diagnostic method based on the hypersensitivity of AT lymphocytes to killing by gamma irradiation.* Similar studies in fibroblasts require skin biopsy and a prolonged culture time.

  Chorionic villus sampling, gamma radiation is a reliable way of discriminating between unaffected fetueses and those with AT.
- **Rosin and Ochs in 1986** applied the *exfoliated cell micronucleus test* to the question of in vivo chromosomal instability in AT. This test is performed on exfoliated cells from the oral cavity collected by swabbing the mucosa with a moistened tongue depressor and also on urinary bladder cells obtained by centrifugation of freshly voided urine specimens. Micronuclei in these cells result from fragmentation of chromo-somes in dividing cells from the epithelium, resulting in acentric fragments, which are excluded from the main nucleus when the cell divides. These fragments from their own membrane and can be identified as extra-nuclear Feulgen-positive bodies in daughter cells which migrate up through the epithelium to be exfoliated. They found that *AT Homozygotes had a 5-to 14-fold increase in the frequency of exfoliated cell micronuclei.* Heterozygotes can be reliably identified by this method.

Clinical Management

Patients with AT and their cultured cells are unusually sensitive to X-rays just as patients and cells with xeroderma pigmentosum are sensitive to ultraviolet rays. Treatment of malignancy with conventional dosages of radiation can be fetal to AT paitents.

3. FANCONI'S ANEMIA

Alternate Titles: Fanconi's Anemia, Type I (FAI), Fanconi Pancytopenia, Fanconi's Anemia: Estren-Dameshek Variant, Aplastic anemia with Congenital anomalies, Congenital Pancytopenia, Constitutional Aplastic Anemia, Fanconi Panmyelopathy.

Fanconi's Anemia is a rare genetic disorder that may be apparent at birth or during childhood. The disorder is ***characterized by deficiency of all bone marrow elements including red blood cells, white blood cells and platelets (pancytopenia).*** Fanconi's anemia may also be associated with heart (cardiac), kidney (renal), and/or skeletal abnormalities as well as patchy, brown discolorations (pigmentation changes) of the skin. There are several different subtypes (complementation groups) of Fanconi's anemia, each of which is thought to result from abnormal changes (mutations) of differnt disease genes. Each subtype appears to share the same characteristic symptoms and findings (phenotype). It is ***associated with increased susceptibility to malignant neoplasms and chromosomal instability. It is due to failure of correction of cross-linkage damage.***

Clinical Presentation

The following set of physical abnormalities occur in 80% of the cases:

- Skin pigment change--darkened areas of the skin , cafe-au-lait spots, vitiligo
- Short stature
- Upper limb anomalies --missing, extra or misshapen thumbs; underdeveloped or absent radius bone in the forearm; anomalies of the hands; abnormalities of the ulna.
- Small testicles, genital changes
- Other skeletal anomalies--congenital hip abnormality, scoliosis, spinal or rib malformations small head
- Eye/eyelid anomalies
- Kidney malformations
- Ear anomalies/deafness
- Hip, leg, and toe abnormalities
- Gatrointestinal/cardiopulmonary malformations

Other associated symptoms inlcude: mental retardation, learning disability, low birth weight, failure to thrive.

Biochemical Basis

Fanconi anemia has 8 identified complementation groups (A, B, C, D1, D2, E, F, and G) and genes for at least 7 of these groups have been identified. ***Fanconi anemia genes, FancB and FancD1, have been identified as the Early onset breast cancer gene BRCA2*** (Fig. 27.21). Five of the Fanconi Anemia genes (FancA, FancC, FancE, FancF, and FancG) form a complex which interacts with DNA and leads to the monoubiquitination of the FancD2protein. Through an association with BRCA1 and BRCA2 in nuclear loci, this leads to activation of the processes that lead to DNA repair. The ATM kinase can be activated by ionizing radiation, which in turn activates many targets. One of these, the FancD2 protein,is phosphorylated by ATM, which then leads to S phase arrest. An additional link in this pathway includes the phosphorylation by ATM of the protein encoded by the gene of the Nijmegen Breakage Syndrome (NBSI) and BRCA1. The NBSI protein is part of a complex which, in turn, also leads to phosphorylation of FancD2 by ATM. NBS1 appears to have two independent functions, one is inducing S-phase arrest where FancD2 is not required and the second in interacting with FancD2 in promoting DNA repair. Thus, ***FancD2 is at the cross roads of two pathways • one leading to S: phase arrest which functions from ATM through NBS 1 and associated proteins and the • other in response to DNA damage acting through the Fanconi complex.***

Diagnosis

The laboratory tests performed in evaluating Fanconi's anemia include:

- ***Complete blood count initially demonstrates low platelets (thrombocytopenia), then low neutrophils (Neutropenia), and finally low hemoglobin*** (anemia), which develops over months to years.
- ***Bone marrow biopsy.***
- ***Clastogenic stress-induced chromosomal breakage analysis on blood cells*** of patients and their siblings to diagnose the disease. In this test, drugs are added to a blood sample to check for abnormal damage to chromosomes.
- Hand X-ray, and other imaging studies (X-ray, CT scan, MRI) to evaluate any anomalies.
- Hearing tests
- Developmental tests
- Ultrasound of the kidneys.
- Amniocentesis or chorionic villus sampling has been used for prenatal diagnosis.

Management

- If the hematological changes are mild to moderate and the patient does not require transfusions, a period of observation is currently recommended with frequent blood count checks and yearly bone marrow examinations. Observations for the development of secondary malignancies are also performed. In the short term, growth factors (such as erythropoietin, G-CSF, and GM-CSF) can be used to improve blood counts. Other growth factors for platelet stimulation are currently under investigation.
- ***Bone marrow transplantation*** can cure the blood count problems associated with Fanconi's anemia. An HLA matched sibling is the best donor source, although umbilical cord blood cells and unrelated bone marrow can also be used. This therapy is very effective, and although there are associated toxicities, there has been improvement in the care of Fanconi patients during the transplant. There is approximately a 70% success rate for those patients fortunate enough to have a donor.
- Prior to bone marrow transplantation, ***androgen therapy*** (oxymetholone, nandrolone decanoate) ***combined with low doses of steroids*** (hydrocortisone, prednisone) was the standard treatment, and this approach is currently used if the patient does not have an appropriate bone marrow donor. Typically, 50-70% of patients initially respond to androgen therapy, however, all patients will rapidly relapse when the drug is stopped. In most cases, these drugs eventually become ineffective.
- Symptoms due to low blood counts, such as bleeding, infections, or symptomatic anemia (fatigue, shortness of breath, chest pain, dizziness), are treated with transfusions or antibiotics as needed. Patients with low neuterophil counts, who develop a fever, are usually treated with intravenous antibiotics.

Prognosis

The reported survival of patiens with Fanconi's anemia is highly varied, ranging from 2 to 25 years. The prognosis is especially poor if blood counts are low. Survival has likely been improved by the development and refinement of therapies, such as bone marrow transplantation.

Although bone marrow transplantation can restore blood counts, patients with Fanconi's anemia remain predisposed to a variety of cancers (leukemia, myelodysplastic syndrome, liver cancer,and others).

Women with Fanconi's anemia who become pregnant should be watched carefully as they often require transfusions throughout pregnancy. Men with Fanconi's anemia have decreased fertility, although a small number have fathered children. It is an autosomal recessive anemia.

4. HEREDITARY NONPOLYPOSIS COLORECTAL CANCER (HPCC)

Alternaitve title: Lynch Syndrome

Lynch syndrome is a rare disorder also known as ***hereditary nonpolyposis colorectal cancer (HNPCC) syndrome.*** Though not a cancer in its own right, Lynch syndrome strongly predisposes people who have this inherited defect to develop colorectal cancer as well as several other types of cancer. The condition is named after Henry Lynch, a doctor and authority on inherited cancers.

Hereditary nonpolyposis colorectal cancer (HNPCC), also referred to as Lynch syndrome I and II, is one of several hereditary colorectal cancer syndrome.

- ***Lynch syndrome I is an autosomal, dominantly inherited predisposition to colorectal cancer*** with right-sided predominance (70% proximal to the splenic flexure) and an excess of multiple primary colorectal cancer (45% 10 years after incomplete colonic resection as opposed to subtotal colectomy).
- ***Lynch syndrome II*** not only shows all of the features of Lynch syndrome I, but also involves an enormous array of extracolonic colorectal cancers, particularly ***endometrial carcinoma, followed by carcinoma of the ovary, small bowel, stomach and pancreas, and transitional cell carcinoma of the ureter and renal pelvis.***

Germ-line mutations in the mismatch-repair genes MLH1, MSH2, MSH6, and PMS2 lead to the development of the Lynch syndrome (hereditary nonpolyposis colorectal cancer), conferring a strong susceptibility to cancer. People with Lynch syndrome have more than 80 percent chance of developing colorectal cancer during their lifetime. Colorectal cancer is relatively common, but only about 3 to 4 percent of all colon cancer cases are attributable to Lynch syndrome.

Clinical Presentation

Although the term "nonpolyposis"appears in the name "hereditary nonpolyposis colorectal cancer", people with Lynch syndrome actually do have ***polyps in the lining of the colon or rectum.*** However, these polyps tend to be fewer in number compared with the number present in other forms of inherited colorectal cancers such as familial adenomatous polyposis (FAP).

When cancer does occur in people with Lynch syndrome, most cases arise in the right side of the colon. ***Colorectal cancer associated with Lynch syndrome tends to occur in people at a younger age than for people*** with the more common non-hereditary forms of colorectal cancer. Lynch syndrome is an ***autosomal dominant inherited disorder.*** Lynch syndrome subjects are not only more susceptible to colorectal cancer, but also at increased risk of other types of cancer. For example, women with Lynch syndrome have a ***greater likelihood of developing cancer of their ovaries or the endometrium.*** More than one in three women with Lynch syndrome will develop ***endometrial cancer*** in her lifetime. ***Cancers of the stomach, small intestine, urinary tract, liver, prostate, pancreas, brain and skin are also more common in people with Lynch syndrome.***

Frequency of HNPCC

The lowest known estimate of HNPCC occurrence is 1% which translates into 1500 new cases of HNPCC annually in the United States. Estimates of HNPCC incidence range as high as 5%, or 7500 new occurrences of HNPCC in the United States each year. Either estimate indicates that HNPCC poses a major public health problem, since each new case would signify a family prone not only to colorectal cancer, but also to a variety of extracolonic cancers.

Molecular Genetics and HNPCC

Molecular genetic studies have identified germline mutations in an increasingly large numbe of hereditary cancer syndromes. The genetic basis for HNPCC has been proven by-genetic linkage between cancer occurrences and chromosome 2p in some families and 3p in others.

Localisation of a DNA mismatch repair gene in the critical region of chromosome 2p was documented with the ***discovery of hMSH2 mutations in this gene in several HNPCC families.*** Subsequently, a second mismatch repair gene was found in the critical region of 3p, and ***mutations of that gene (hMLH1)*** were found in the HNPCC families previously linked to chromosome 3p. ***Mutations in these genes appear to account for 90% of all known HNPCC families; hPMS1 and hPMS2 also are mismatch repair genes in HNPCC.***

Defective DNA mismatch repair results in a steady accumulation of mutations. The mutation load can be detected as errors in long tandem repeat sequences, which are errors that produce microsatellite instability. ***A tumour with microsatellite instability is defined as showing replication error (RER) phenotype.***

While the reasons for the accelerated progression of polyps to colorectal cancer in HNPCC remain enigmatic, it is hypothesised that ***loss of the wild-type gene in HNPCC usually is necessary to bring about the DNA repair defect, a concept in accordance with the belief that HNPCC genes are tumour suppressor genes.*** Random loss of the wild-type allele would be expected to occur quite frequently (analogous to loss of the wild-type antigen-presenting cells [APC] gene in polyposis), yet few neoplasms are seen. It is possible that loss of DNA repair proficiency has little or no effect on the stage of initiation but has impact on subsequent progression.

Molecular Diagnosis

Routine molecular screening for Lynch syndrome or hereditary nonpolyposis colorectal cancer is useful in patients with colorectal adenocarcinoma. The screening involves genotying of the tumour for microsatellite instability as the primary screening method. In patients with positive screening results for microsatellite instability, germ-line mutations in the MLH1, MLH2, MLH6, and PMS2 genes should be observed, using immunohistochemical staining for mismatch-repair proteins, genomic sequencing, and deletion studies.

5. FRAGILE X SYNDROME

It is due to microsatellite unstability. Fragile X syndrome is the most common inherited form of mental retardation currently known. Fragile X syndrome is ***a defect in the X chromosome*** and its effects are seen more frequently, and with greater severity, in males than females. In normal individuals, the FMR1 gene is transmitted stably from parent to child. However, in fragile X individuals, there is a mutation in one end of the gene (the 5′-untranslated region), consisting of an amplification of a CGG repeat. Patients with fragile X syndrome have 200 or more copies of the CGG motif. The huge expansion of this repeat means that the FMRI gene is not expressed, so no FMR1 protein is made. Although exact function of FMR1 protein in the cell is unclear, it is known that it binds RNA.

6. NIJMEGEN BREAKAGE SYNDROME

Nijmegen breakage syndrome (NBS) is another ***rare autosomal recessive disorder*** also associated with diverse clinical features overlapping with, but distinct from those of A-T. In common with A-T, ***NBS patients manifest humoral and cellular immune dysfunction, clinical radiosensitivity, chromosome instability and a predisposition to cancer. In contrast to A-T, they display a • characteristic 'bird-like' facial appearance, • microcephaly and growth retardation.*** Whilst the clinical phenotype is variable, most affected children have • ***recurrent bacterial sinopulmonary infections*** which may lead to ***bronchiestasis. Hypogammaglobulinaemia is common, particularly IgA and IgG subclass deficiency,*** and impaired antibody responses to antigens are reported. ***Mild to moderate lymphopenia*** is present with impaired *in vitro* lymphocyte proliferative responses to mitogens. • ***Autoimmune phenomena have occasionally been reported.*** At the cellular level, A-T and NBS cells also show overlapping but distinct phenotypes. In addition to radiosensitivity, NBS cells also display some cell cycle checkpoint defects. ***The protein defective in NBS, NBS1, nibrin or p95, has been identified*** and shows functional homology but only limited sequence homology to Xrs2, a protein that participates in the DNA repair response mechanism in yeast, ***p95 interacts with HMre11 and Hrad 50,*** homologues of two proteins with which Xrs 2 interacts in yeast. Yeast mutants defective in any of these components are impaired in NHEJ as well as HR. However, NBS1 cells are proficient in DSB repair and thus do not appear to be defective in the NHEJ process in higher organisms. NBS1 appears to be recruited to the site of DNA DSBS and thus may function together with ATM to sense DNA DSBs. A number of NBS variant patients have also been described. Significantly, at least a subset of these do not have mutations in NBS1, showing that defects in a second protein can confer NBS-like characteristics.

G. Bloom's Syndrome

Bloom's syndrome (BS) is another ***rare autosomal recesive disorder associated*** with • ***immunodeficiency,* • *genomic instability and a* • *predisposition to cancer.*** Additional ***characteristics include* • *growth deficiency,* • *sun-sensitive erythema of the face, and* • *impaired fertility.*** The clinical phenotype is variable, with respiratory infection leading to chronic lung disease being the most common manifestation of immunodeficiency. ***Prolonged low levels of IgM have been reported*** and sinopulmonary infection is associated with hypogammaglobulinemia. ***Cells from BS patients characteristically show an increased frequency of chromatid gaps, breaks and rearrangements,*** most particularly quadriradials, and increased sister chromatid exchanges (SCEs). The latter two features are indicative of aberrant HR events. ***Recently, the protein defective in BS has been identified*** and belongs to the RecQ helicase family, named after a homologous *Escherichia coli* protein. Homologues in yeast have also been identified and additional related proteins in human cells include RECQC and WRN, the protein defective in the aging disorder Werner's syndrome. Current evidence, including the presence of abnormal replication intermediates and retarded replication fork progress in BS cells, suggests that the Bloom's protein may function either during replication or in a post-replication recombination process that resolves aberrant structures generated during replication. However, BS cells do not display any appreciable sensitivity to either UV or IR.

Disorders of Purine and Pyrimidine Metabolism

1. **Primary metabolic gout:** It is due to inherited metabolic defect in purine metabolism leading to excessive rate of conversion of glycine to uric acid. X-linked recessive defects enhancing the *de novo* synthesis of purines and their catabolism can also lead to hyperuricemia. For example, such defects of PRPP synthetase may make it feedback resistant. X-linked recessive defects of hypoxanthine guanine phosphoribosyl transferase may reduce utilization of PRPP in the salvage pathway. Increased intracellular PRPP enhances *de novo* purine synthesis.
2. **Lesch-Nyhan Syndrome:** Only males are affected by this. It is X-linked recessive defect of *hypoxanthine-guanine phosphoribosyltransferase.* The enzyme is almost absent and leads to increased purine salvage pathway from PRPP. This can result in severe gout, renal failure, poor growth, spasticity and ***tendency for selfmutilation.***
3. **Xanthinuria:** An autosomal recessive deficiency of *xanthine oxidase,* blocks the oxidation of hypoxanthine and xanthine to uric acid. It can cause xanthine lithiasis and **hypouricemia.**
4. **Adenosine Deaminase Deficiency:** An autosomal recessive deficiency of *adenosine deaminase.* It is associated with severe immunodeficiency and both **T cells** and **B cells**

(lymphocytes) are deficient. There occurs an accumulation of deoxyribonucleotides which inhibit further production of precursors of DNA synthesis especially d CTP. **Hypouricemia** occurs which is due to defective breakdown of purine nucleotides. Recently **Gene replacement therapy** has been used successfully in a few cases.

5. **Nucleoside Phosphorylase Deficiency:** An autosomal recessive deficiency of *purine nucleoside phosphorylase,* causes the urinary excretion of guanine and hypoxanthine nucleosides. There is reduced production of uric acid. There is severe deficiency of cell-mediated and humoral immunity.
6. **Orotic Aciduria:** It is of 2 types:
   - ***Type I orotic aciduria:*** It is an autosomal recessive genetic disorder of a protein acting as both *orotate phosphoribosyl-transferase* and *OMP decarboxylase.* Orotate fails to be converted to uridylate. This results in accumulation of orotate in blood elevating its level, growth retardation and **megaloblastic anemia.**
   - ***Type II orotic aciduria:*** It is autosomal recessive, affecting *OMP decarboxylase* and is characterized by megaloblastic anaemia and the urinary excretion of asididine in higher concentrations than orotate.

References

1. Alberti KGMN (Ed): *Recent Advances in Clinical Biochemistry*, Churchill Livingstone, 1978.
2. Annino JS: *Clinical Chemistry, Principles and Procedures* (3rd edn), J & A Churchill Ltd., London, 1964
3. Baron DN: *A Short Textbook of Chemical Pathology* (4th edn), 1982.
4. Burtis CA, Ashwood ER: *Tietz Textbook of Clinical Chemistry* (2nd edn), WB Saunders Company, Philadelphia, 1994.
5. Cheyne GA: *Techniques in Chemical Pathology* (1st edn), Blackwell Scientific Publication, Blackwell, Oxford, 1964.
6. Coodley EL: *Diagnostic Enzymology*, Lea and Febiger, Philadelphia, 1970.
7. Dacie JV, Lewis SM: *Practical Haematology* (6th edn), Churchill Livingstone, Edinburgh, 1984.
8. Dixon M, Webb EC: *Enzymes* (2nd edn), Academic Press Inc., New York, 1964.
9. Firkin F, Chesterman C, Penington D *et al: de Gruchy's Clinical Haematology in Medical Practice* (5th Indian edn), Oxford University Press, Delhi/Mumbai, 1990.
10. Harrison A: *Chemical Methods in Clinical Medicine* (4th edn), J and A Churchill Ltd., 1957.
11. *Hawk's Physiological Chemistry* (14th edn), (Ed-Osler, BL): Blakiston Division, McGraw-Hill Book Co., New York, 1965.
12. Hoffman WS: *The Biochemistry of Clinical Medicine* (4th edn), Yearbook of Medical Publishers Inc., Chicago, 1970.
13. Hyde TA, Draisey TF: *Principles of Chemical Pathology* Butterworths and Co. Ltd., London, 1974.
14. King J: *Practical Clinical Enzymology*, D Van Nostrand Co., London, 1965.
15. Latner AL: *Cantanow and Trumper's Clinical Biochemistry* (7th edn), Saunders, Philadelphia, 1975.
16. Mollison PL, Engelfriet CP Contreras M: *Blood Transfusion in Clinical Medicine* (9th edn), Blackwell Scientific Publication, Oxford, 1993.
17. Smith LC: Plasma Lipoproteins: Structure and Metabolism, *Ann. Rev. Biochem* 1978.
18. Thompson RHS, King EJ: *Biochemical Disorders in Human Diseases* (3rd edn), J and A Churchill Ltd., London, 1970.
19. Thompson RHS, Wootton IDP: *Biochemical Disorders in Human Diseases* (3rd edn), J and A Churchill Ltd., London, 1970.
20. Varley H: *Practical Clinical Biochemistry*, ELBS edn), William Heinemann Medical Books Ltd., London, 1969.
21. Varley H, Bowenlock AH, Bell M: *Practical Clinical Biochemistry* (5th edn), William Heinemann Medical Books Ltd., London, 1980.
22. Wilson JD: *Harrison's Principles of Internal Medicine* McGrow Hill Inc., 1991.
23. Wintrobe MM, Lee GR, Boggs DR *et al: Clinical Haematology* (7th edn), Lea and Febiger, Philadelphia, 1975.
24. Wootton IDP: *Microanalysis in Medical Biochemistry* (6th edn), J and A Churchill Ltd., London, 1982.
25. Zilva JF, Pannall PR, Mayne PD: *Clinical Chemistry in Diagnosis and Treatment* (5th edn) ELBS, Clays Ltd., St. Ives Ple., 1987.

Index

D

E

F

G

H

J

K

L

M

N

Q

R

S

T

U

V

W

X

Z